Also by Charles W. Kane

Medicinal Plants of the Western Mountain States (2017)

Wild Edible Plants of Texas: A Pocket Guide to the Identification, Collection, Preparation, and Use of 60 Wild Plants of the Lone Star State (2016)

Southern California Food Plants: Wild Edibles of the Valleys, Foothills, Coast, and Beyond (2013)

Sonoran Desert Food Plants: Edible Uses for the Desert's Wild Bounty (2011 and 2017)

Herbal Medicine: Trends and Traditions (A Comprehensive Sourcebook on the Preparation and Use of Medicinal Plants) (2009)

Medicinal
PLANTS
of the American
SOUTHWEST

Charles W. Kane

Lincoln Town Press

Medicinal Plants of the American Southwest
Lincoln Town Press

First edition (revised), Fifth printing

This text first appeared as Herbal Medicine of the American Southwest ©
2006, 2007 (reprint), and 2009 (second edition) by Charles W. Kane.

Library of Congress Control Number: 2011906043
ISBN 10: 0977133370
ISBN 13: 9780977133376

Medicinal Plants of the American Southwest is intended solely for educa-
tional purposes. The publisher and author disclaim any liability arising
from the use of any plant listed in this book.

Printed and bound in the United States of America

Contents

Photographs

1. Acacia (Acacia greggii).
2. Aloe (Aloe vera).
3. Antelope horns (Asclepias asperula).
4. Baccharis (Baccharis salicifolia).
5. Beargrass (Nolina microcarpa).
6. Beebrush (Aloysia wrightii).
7. Bird of paradise (Caesalpinia gilliesii).
8. Bouvardia (Bouvardia ternifolia).
9. Bricklebush (Brickellia californica).
10. Brittlebush (Encelia farinosa).
11. Buttonbush (Cephalanthus occidentalis).
12. California poppy (Eschscholzia californica subsp. mexicana).
13. Caltrop (Kallstroemia grandiflora).
14. Camphorweed (Heterotheca subaxillaris).
15. Canadian fleabane (Conyza canadensis).
16. Canyon bursage (Ambrosia ambrosioides).
17. Canyon bursage (Ambrosia ambrosioides).
18. Canyon walnut (Juglans major).
19. Chaste tree (Vitex castus–angus).
20. Chinchweed (Pectis papposa).
21. Clematis (Clematis ligusticifolia).
22. Cocklebur (Xanthium strumarium).
23. Copperleaf (Acalypha neomexicana).
24. Cottonwood (Populus fremontii).
25. Creosote bush (Larrea tridentata).
26. Crownbeard (Verbesina encelioides).
27. Crucifixion thorn (Castela emoryi).
28. Cudweed (Pseudognaphalium leucocephalum).
29. Cypress (Cupressus arizonica).
30. Cypress (Cupressus arizonica).
31. Datura (Datura wrightii).
32. Desert anemone (Anemone tuberosa).
33. Desert barberry (Berberis fremontii).
34. Desert barberry (Berberis trifoliolata).
35. Desert cotton (Gossypium thurberi).
36. Desert lavender (Hyptis emoryi).

37. Desert milkweed (Asclepias subulata).
38. Desert willow (Chilopsis linearis).
39. Dogweed (Dyssodia acerosa).
40. Elder (Sambucus nigra subsp. cerulea).
41. Elephant tree (Bursera microphylla).
42. Filaree (Erodium cicutarium).
43. Flat–top–buckwheat (Eriogonum fasciculatum).
44. Globemallow (Sphaeralcea coulteri).
45. Golden smoke (Corydalis aurea).
46. Greenthread (Thelesperma megapotamicum).
47. Hopbush (Dodonaea viscosa).
48. Jojoba (Simmondsia chinensis).
49. Jumping cholla (Cylindropuntia fulgida).
50. Juniper (Juniperus scopulorum).
51. Kidneywood (Eysenhardtia orthocarpa).
52. Leadwort (Plumbago zeylanica).
53. Limberbush (Jatropha cardiophylla).
54. Mallow (Malva parviflora).
55. Manzanita (Arctostaphylos pungens).
56. Mesquite (Prosopis velutina).
57. Mimosa (Mimosa dysocarpa).
58. Mormon tea (Ephedra aspera).
59. Mountain marigold (Tagetes lemmonii).
60. Night blooming cereus (Peniocereus greggii).
61. Ocotillo (Fouquieria splendens).
62. Passionflower (Passiflora mexicana).
63. Penstemon (Penstemon parryi).
64. Periwinkle (Vinca major).
65. Pipevine (Aristolochia watsonii).
66. Poliomintha (Poliomintha incana).
67. Poreleaf (Porophyllum gracile).
68. Poreleaf (Porophyllum ruderale subsp. macrocephalum).
69. Prickly pear (Opuntia engelmannii).
70. Prickly poppy (Argemone pleiacantha).
71. Puncturevine (Tribulus terrestris).
72. Purple gromwell (Lithospermum multiflorum).
73. Ratany (Krameria erecta).
74. Rayweed (Parthenium incanum).

75. Red betony (Stachys coccinea).

76. Sage (Salvia apiana).

77. Sagebrush (Artemisia tridentata).

78. Scouring rush (Equisetum hyemale).

79. Senna (Senna covesii).

80. Snakeweed (Gutierrezia microcephala).

81. Soapberry (Sapindus saponaria var. drummondii).

82. Spanish needles (Bidens pilosa).

83. Sumac (Rhus ovata).

84. Syrian rue (Peganum harmala).

85. Tamarisk (Tamarix chinensis).

86. Tarbush (Flourensia cernua).

87. Texas ranger (Leucophyllum frutescens).

88. Tobacco (Nicotiana obtusifolia).

89. Tree of heaven (Ailanthus altissima).

90. Trixis (Trixis californica).

91. Trumpet flower (Tecoma stans).

92. Turpentine bush (Ericameria laricifolia).

93. Velvet ash (Fraxinus velutina).

94. Verbena (Glandularia gooddingii).

95. Western black willow (Salix gooddingii).

96. Western black willow (Salix gooddingii).

97. Western mugwort (Artemisia ludoviciana).

98. Western peony (Paeonia californica).

99. Western peony (Paeonia californica).

100. Wild lettuce (Lactuca serriola).

101. Wild licorice (Glycyrrhiza lepidota).

102. Wild licorice (Glycyrrhiza lepidota).

103. Wild oats (Avena fatua).

104. Wild rhubarb (Rumex hymenosepalus).

105. Wolfberry (Lycium pallidum).

106. Wolfberry (Lycium pallidum).

107. Yerba mansa (Anemopsis californica).

108. Yerba mansa (Anemopsis californica).

109. Yerba santa (Eriodictyon angustifolium).

110. Yerba santa (Eriodictyon trichocalyx var. lanatum).

111. Yucca (Yucca baccata).

112. Yucca (Yucca elata).

Acknowledgments

As a community user I am grateful to have access to the University of Arizona's health and science library's journal collection. The information derived through numerous studies was (and continues to be) invaluable in rounding out the historical/empirical precepts presented in this book. The Missouri Botanical Garden's on–line database has been indispensable in listing updated plant names – in today's shifting world of classification things have come a long way since Kearney and Pebbles.

Mac 'pitcher' Macbride, Edward Hacskaylo, Jim Verrier, Adam Seller, Howie Brounstein, Martha Burgess, Joe Billings, Douglas Dunn, Michael and Lynie Stone, Petey Mesquitey, Frank Rose, Donna Chesner, Pamela Hyde–Nakai, Phyllis Hogan, Peter Bigfoot, Becki Garza, Allen and Joan Spencer, Donna and John Albertsen, and the Kane family all deserve thanks for their support of this project. Southwestern plant medicine man, Michael Moore, whose teachings touched an 'abundant stand', deserves a big node. R.I.P. old bear.

Introduction

The history of American southwestern medicinal plant use is similar to that of other regional plant groups within the Americas. A progression of utilizers and related methodologies, each characterized by time and culture, has marked (and continues to) this profound, yet often misunderstood subject. Past waves of primitive, transitional, ethnic, and even religious thought systems continue to infuse the currently accepted scientific model with a calliope of accents, often making today's medicinal plant utilization a conflicted weave of the rational and ideological.

I consider myself (and therefore this book) a follower of scientific thought and western definition. Within the following pages, I have attempted to overlay a modern perspective on subject matter that is very primitive, or at least thought of as primitive. A blending of ethnobotanical accounts with scientific research and personal observation is this information's creative foundation. Through writing this material, my aim is to present a guide or reference on how to best utilize this region's plant life, not only in an understandable way, but in a way that best directs what plant medicines have to offer.

In order to effectively apply any plant medicine, there first and foremost needs to be an accurate understanding of what effectively applied plant medicine actually is *and is not*. The importance of grasping this simple premise can not be stressed more. For the beginner, this understanding does not come easily, mainly due to distracting elements that are considered sacrosanct to many plant medicine enthusiasts, teachers, and relayers of related information. Besides utilizing this book and other well–informed sources in the learning process, stay focused and keep your 'eye on the ball' of *rational* medicinal plant learning. The minefield of herbal counter-culture with it focus on green spiritualism and nouveau–bohemianism can be a massive distraction to the sincere and open–minded student.

The first thing to understand about effectively applied plant medicine: medicinal plants act as therapeutic agents because of our body's response to the chemical elements they contain. More specifically, when medicinal plants are ingested, they stimulate, suppress, or alter a specific area, not by some anthropomorphic activity, but due to our body's attempt to eliminate what is deemed foreign. Expectorant, diaphoretic, diuretic, and other activities are determined by how our bodies process and expel the offending plant material. If we dose these low–level irritants intelligently they will trigger appropriate physiological changes. At this level of activity themes are duplicated: chemically or botanically related plants will reliably produce associated and repeatable outcomes.

Beyond the 'low–level irritant' backdrop, some plant medicines have very specialized qualities or activities – mostly due to a particular set of compounds that do not occur elsewhere – even in related species. These plants are unique in that they trigger very specific physiological changes, which if channeled intelligently will therapeutically impact a particular complaint, problem, or tendency.

As long as the information ahead is properly understood and is applied with a conservative mind–set (skip using herbs alone for cancer or serious organic disease) it will have an enormous impact on health and illness. Though the majority of these plants hail from the American Southwest, the therapeutic framework set forth in this book can be applied to any other group of plants. Due to their botanical and chemical affiliations, even exotic Chinese and Indian medicinal plants have similar if not identical activities to these listed here. The key to making sense of what appears like a vast number of independent specimens with seemingly unrelated uses, be them regional or global, is to start seeing corollaries or similarities in the information or observation. Get the overview, then flesh–out the specifics.

Does this information count? Is using plants for medicine still relevant today even when life expectancy continues to increase due to advances in modern medicine? Both yes and no. Medicinal plant application is still relevant due to modern medicine's shortcomings. I do believe the time approaches when tomorrow's medical science fiction will become today's medical science fact. When that day arrives, and it will, when our understanding of the body and corresponding technologies results in the eradication of illness as we know it, then herbal medicine as a viable chronic disease treatment should be allowed to rest.

In the meantime, choose standard medical treatment, not as fearful robotic followers, but as the (rationally) informed. Choose plants as medicine when too the situation fits (and not as radical 'health' or 'green lifestyle' zealots). The best mental approach in applying this book's information is sensibility. Simply view this material as a tool in the shed: when a power–tool (conventional medicine) is too coarse or overwhelming, when the job needs the finesse of a hand–tool (plant medicine), you will be well prepared.

Format Explanation

Plant Names

Each profile is headed by the main common name, followed by a current scientific name in italics, the accepted author in regular text, and synonyms. Secondary common names follow. The main common name assigned to each plant is generally accepted as the most common and longest in current usage.

It is important to note that most common names as well as many scientific names for any given plant change from generation to generation. No name is set in stone. Botanical classifiers can be fickle in applying and reapplying nomenclature depending on the classifying systems/politics of the day. When you know the plant, you know the plant, names be damned.

Description and Distribution

Look to these sections for the plant's botanical description, growth tendencies, and geographical range. When pertinent, state–to–state location, elevation ranges, topographies, and micro–climates are also covered.

Chemistry

In this section each plant's known chemical composition is listed. Readers will note that some profiles have a smaller chemistry listing than others. This is not due to a lack of compounds, but of available research.

Medicinal Uses

The plant's effect on organ systems, tissue groups, and medical symptoms are described in this section. Application to organic disease syndromes has been keep to a minimum but occasionally it is pertinent – how the plant affects stress patterns and its mechanism of action are preferred.

Plants are multi–directional. Rarely do they affect just one area of the body. They influence physicality by how an organ or tissue group eliminates or detoxifies the compounds they contain. In other words, it is not the plant that is the remedy for the ailment or discomfort, but it is what the plant does to the body, organ system, or group of tissues that then affects the manifested problem. For example, an aromatic–bitter herb stimulates secretion and dilates stomach lining vasculature thereby quieting indigestion. Technically speaking, there is no such thing as an herb for a 'stomach-ache' or for 'arthritis'...but there are numerous herbs that influence these symptoms by their effects on related physiological process.

Indications

Under this listing readers can find the truncated medicinal use (or what symptoms indicate each plant's use) for each plant. If '(external)' is not by the indication then that application is designed for internal use.

Collection

Depending on the plant, virtually any part can be medicinally potent. Mostly though, roots, bark, leaves, flowers, seeds, and sap or exudate provide the strongest medicines. Stems, branches, and core wood are less likely to give benefit. The former parts are functional, having an array of chemical processes taking place within them. The latter parts are structural, serving mainly as a skeletal support for the functional parts – much like our bodies.

When preparing to collect medicinal plants, beyond having the obvious implements (shovel, knife, pruners, etc.), it is sensible to first have a mental understanding of the process and to at least intellectually grasp what the activity entails. The reason why there exists today such a booming herbal market is because collecting plants is hard (roots and bark) and tedious (flowers, leaves, and seeds) work. The average consumer just does not have the time for the activity...and you may not either. If this is the case, then purchase the herb instead. With today's abundance of home–grown 'microbrew' herbal product lines, I guarantee some herbalist has even the most obscure medicinal plant in this book for sale.

Of course plant collecting is not like ditch–digging (well...it occasionally can be), but still, there needs to be a degree of 'stick–with–it–ness' in order to successfully complete the process. A basic understanding of natural environments and a degree of ecological sensitivity are also of equal importance (most herbal medicine enthusiasts are low on 'stick–with–it–ness' but off the chart on ecological sensitivity). The following list of guidelines/ questions will help in determining when, where, and how to properly collect plant medicines.

» First and foremost, be sure that the plant of interest has been accurately identified.
» Is the plant threatened, endangered, on 'at–watch' lists, or just locally scarce? If so it may be better to find an alternative herbal medicine or make a trip to more abundant picking grounds.
» What are the local/state/federal policies in your area regarding plant

collection? Will a ticket be issued if discovered by authorities or do 'personal collection' laws exist?

» If harvesting on private land have arrangements with the owner been made? You'll likely find a majority of land owners interested in the subject and if they are respectfully approached you may have a reliable gathering area for years to come.

» Are seasonal conditions proper?

» Are the plants of the stand healthy and without insect and/or microbial damage?

» Are sources of contamination close by? It is best to collect away from roadsides, city and town areas, industrial sites, agricultural areas, and heavily traveled foot trails.

» Is the plant being collected properly? Take your time and enjoy the experience. The goal should not be quantity, but quality and thoroughness.

» Clean up before leaving – fill in holes, and if preparing medicines in the field, spread around core wood and other unusable plant materials in order to lessen the visual impact of collection.

» Not collecting the plant due to other–than–optimal circumstances is always an option.

Drying Plants

» Dry plant materials out of direct sunlight. Herbage can be placed loosely in paper bags or laid well–spaced on cardboard flats. Small bundles of leafing tops, with the topmost portions of the plant hanging down are secured from ceiling rafters until dry.

» Once dry, garble the leaves and flowers from the stems; discard the stems (unless otherwise directed).

» Chop roots into ¼"–½" pieces or longer longitudinal strips. Both these and bark strips dry adequately if well–spaced.

» For quicker drying or to ensure no mold growth occurs if in a humid environment a dehydrator can be used.

Preparations

Readers will find this section either joined with the dosage heading or listed independently if there are important details that need to be relayed separately from the plant's dosage. See the main Preparations section for complete instructions on how to prepare a DPT (dry plant tincture), FPT (fresh plant tincture), infusion, decoction, etc.

Dosage

The dosage listings in this section are meant as starting points for an average–weighted adult. Depending on weight and sensitivity, in order to achieve the desired result, dosage may need to be decreased or increased.

For children and infants reduce the dose according to weight. For example, if a dose for a 150lb. adult is 30–60 drops 3 times daily, then for a 50lb. child, 10–20 drops 3 times daily is the correct reduction. All percentages for DPT and fluidextract listings apply to alcohol and glycerin contents.

It is important to note that like herbal medicine in general, dosing crude herbal medicines is not a precise science. The variables that come into play when attempting to achieve an effective dose for most herbs are myriad. Most herbs have a wide safe range (unless otherwise noted) and can be increased (within reason) until their therapeutic effects become apparent.

Cautions

If the following precepts are adhered to when using medicinal plants there will be little to fear from potential adverse reactions.

» Quantity: a little will help, a lot may harm. Any plant properly dosed can be medicinal. The same plant may be toxic in larger amounts.

» As a society, we are over medicated. If taking pharmaceuticals or OTC medicines for a particular problem, throwing an herb or two into the mix to affect the same organ or tissue group may be OK...or not. Do some interaction research before playing herbal doctor, or consult with a professional versed in such matters.

» Herbal medicines during pre– and post–operation times may conflict with existing medical programs/physician recommendations. Be extremely cautious when considering herbs that influence clotting time or that are strongly sedating or stimulating.

» Children, the elderly, and those with sensitive constitutions tend to be more prone to adverse effects with larger herbal doses.

» If any herb causes sickness, headaches, diarrhea, nausea, dizziness, or other unwanted sensations, then lessen the dose or discontinue the herb. In my experience most 'cleansing reactions' are actually toxic reactions from taking too much of or the wrong herbal medicine. Most herbal 'mega–doses' are only going to sicken the recipient. So much more can be achieved with moderation and consistency.

» If an herb affects the mother to be, then it is affecting the fetus. The herb's activity is usually delivered to the baby through breast milk as well. While pregnant or nursing limit herbs that have strong physio-logic activities. In these times think of food as medicine.

» Aside from the fundamental social and moral wrong of abortion, and the medical procedure's link to breast cancer, a number of herbs dis-cussed in this book have abortifacient potential. As a rule, they are un-reliable and if used in sufficient quantity are apt to cause harm to the 'mother' as well.

A Note on Formulas

This book is lacking formulas for a reason: one size does not fit all. If you think the situation calls for a formula then keep it simple. A formula com-prised of over five or six herbs is likely to cause more physiologic chatter than therapeutic direction and stems from Man's well known ability to complicate. A well–formulated mixture should be direct, elegant, and un-fettered. Keep in consideration the multi–systemic nature of herbs; they usually affect more than one organ system. When it comes to designing formulas: don't elaborate. Edit.

Excessive polypharmacy is rampant in the natural supplement indus-try. Read the label of most herbal supplement combinations; if the ingre-dient list is filled with numerous herbs then that formula has absolutely no direction, and only can help someone through placebo or by creating a little physiological 'noise' in the body by its elimination through various pathways.

Preparations

Introduction

Medicinal plant preparation can be summed up in one simple premise: how an herb is prepared is of equal importance to what herb is dispensed. Superior plant medicines are made that way by a delivery method that suites each particular plant being utilized. When a plant medicine has been potentiated through proper preparation its activity becomes more distinct and less will be needed for an effective dose.

In determining which methods are optimal for delivery, each plant should be taken on a case by case basis. That said, groupings or corollaries that help in preparation specifics become more evident when focus is placed on a particular plant's family or related constituent groups. Chances are Marshmallow, Mallow, and Globemallow, all Mallow family plants, will be best prepared through water–based preparations. Not only are they closely related botanically but their chemistries are similar; therefore preparations will be similar, if not identical. Torchwood family plants (Myrrh, Frankincense, Guggul, and Elephant tree), due to their resins and non–polar compounds, should be tinctured with a higher percentage of alcohol. In essence: botanically related plants are often chemically related and consequently preparations (and uses) are related.

It is often forgotten that up to the mid–20th century, half of what doctors prescribed (and pharmacists filled), were plants or derivatives thereof. Prior to WWII, the national formulary and US dispensary (both standard references for doctors/pharmacists) had more print related to whole plants, their derivatives, and related preparations, than synthetically created drugs.

It is a misconception that the area of herbal preparation (herbal medicine for that matter) is uncertain and untried. For over a span of two centuries, preparation (and use) was developed, expanded upon, and peaked (then withered due to its replacement with modern medicines). Just as there is no need to reinvent the wheel, there is no need to alter traditional (and often simple) plant preparation technique in the name of the latest exclusive, propriety, or specialized preparation process that usually was developed as a marketing point anyway.

What follows are the main preparations standard in past and present–day herbal medicine. They are simple and time–tested methods designed to achieve the most from each plant.

Bath

1. Draw a hot bath.
2. Add 1 gallon of tea to the bath water.
3. Soak until the water has cooled, or otherwise directed.

Capsule

Capsules come in various sizes with 'o' (250 mg.), 'oo' (500 mg.), and 'ooo' (1000 mg.) being the most common. To fill simply immerse the two halves in an herbal powder, then fit the capsule together. Encapsulation machines speed up the process. They are available in various designs by different makers.

Cough Syrup

Method 1: Honey Steep

1. Take 5½ ounces of finely chopped, fresh plant material; pack into a pint mason jar and fill to the top with honey.
2. Secure the lid and set aside for several weeks. Squeeze or press the honey from the herb and bottle the infused honey.
»   *Ratio: 1 part herb (weight) to 2 parts of honey (volume).*

Method 2: Tincture in Honey/Glycerin Base

1. Mix together 8 ounces of the appropriate tincture(s) with 4 ounces of honey and 4 ounces of glycerin.
2. Bottle.
»   *Ratio: 2 parts tincture (volume) to 1 part honey (volume) to 1 part glycerin (volume).*

Method 3: Tincture with Simple Syrup

1. Mix together 8 ounces of tincture(s) and 8 ounces of simple syrup.
2. Bottle.
»   *Ratio: 1 part tincture (volume) to 1 part simple syrup (volume).*

Considerations

These preparations do not need to be refrigerated. Method 2 and 3 are basically diluted tinctures and are stronger than the honey steep. 1–2 teaspoons is an average adult dose, verses 1 tablespoon for the honey steep.

Douche

1. Make a half–strength tea.
2. Cool until warm.
3. Add ½ teaspoon of table salt per pint of tea in order to increase the solution's salinity.
4. Use as directed.

Considerations

Like any water–based preparation, be sure to make this herbal solution fresh daily. No need to potentially add bacterial or fungal elements to sensitive tissues by using old tea.

Eyewash

Method 1

1. Make 1 pint of tea with distilled or filtered water through the properly designated method (infusion, decoction, etc.)
2. Strain well through a paper towel or cloth.
3. Add ½ teaspoon of table salt.
4. Stir until dissolved.
5. Apply as needed.

Method 2

1. Add 10 drops of appropriate tincture to 2 ounces of isotonic water (¼ teaspoon of table salt to 1 cup of distilled or filtered water).
2. Apply as needed.

Considerations

It is important to make any non–preserved eyewash solution fresh daily.

Fluidextract

First introduced into the U.S.P. of 1850, the fluidextract is an official pharmaceutical preparation. More concentrated than a tincture it is 1:1 in strength, meaning each milliliter of extract contains a representation of 1 gram of dried herb (i.e. 1 ounce of fluidextract will be derived from and have the potency of 1 ounce of dried herb).

Not all plants lend themselves well to fluidextracts, but the ones that are suited for this preparation are mentioned in each plant profile. To make a fluidextract a basic tincture needs to be made through percolation. It is then concentrated to a 1:1. Essentially fluidextracts enable a lower dose, and are convenient if making formulas. See *Herbal Medicine: Trends and Traditions* for step–by–step instructions.

Fomentation

1. Soak a cloth or towel in a warm herb tea.
2. Squeeze the excess tea from the cloth.
3. Apply the cloth to the affected area.
4. Re–soak and apply as needed.

Hydrosol

Also called floral water, a hydrosol is created through essential oil distillation. Actually considered a by–product of the distillation process, it is composed of the condensed steam (water) that was initially in contact with the plant material. Filled with hydroscopic volatile compounds and traces of colloid–formed essential oil, hydrosols share some therapeutic characteristics with essential oils; the main exception being potency. Dilute and mild, hydrosols can even be used as replacements for standard teas. Often they are used as facial sprays or washes. Additionally they make a fine replacement for the water portion when making ointments.

Liniment

A liniment is essentially an externally applied tincture. Isopropyl alcohol can be used instead of ethyl alcohol for this preparation (do not use isopropyl alcohol internally). Due to alcohol's dermal penetrating ability it is common for liniment combinations to contain one or more analgesic/anti-inflammatory oriented herb.

Oil, Essential

Typically prepared through steam distillation, an essential oil represents the volatile or aromatic fraction of a particular plant. Non–polar terpenes make up the bulk of any essential oil constituent list.

It is important to note that essential oils differ greatly from herbal oils. Two very different processes are employed to reach two very different finished products. The two are not interchangeable.

Pure essential oils can be used both externally and internally. Because they represent a potentiated fraction of a plant care should be taken when they are used, especially when ingested. Undiluted they represent some of the strongest topical medicines we employ. As antiinflammatories, analgesics, and antimicrobials/antivirals they excel. Applied undiluted to sensitize tissue/mucus membranes they may cause some irritation; diluting 100–200% with a carrier oil (olive, almond, etc.) usually is sufficient in reducing this tendency. They can be added to an herbal oil in a wide range of ratios – just enough to impart a fragrance, or enough to be the main topical agent.

Ingested, essential oils should be approached with prudence as toxicity due to overdose is a pertinent issue. Unlike tinctures, where 30–60 drops (for many plants) is a normal therapeutic dose, 2–3 drops for an essential oil is roughly equal in potency. For this preparation several drops are placed in a gelatin capsule and then swallowed. See Spirit for another internal preparation utilizing essential oils.

Most plants with a distinctive smell can be used as essential oils: many plants in the Mint, Sunflower, Cypress, and Pine families are well utilized. Although this preparation excludes many other constituents (vitamins/minerals, glycosides, and most alkaloids) due to their nonvolatile nature, if used properly the right plant can be better directed and potentiated.

Essential oils are easily added to tinctures. They are particularly useful, like fluidextracts, when keeping volume low is important.

When purchasing essential oils the label will typically state 'not for internal use'. This has more to do with the potential of toxicity from a high dose rather than any innate poisonous quality. Check that they are not preserved or diluted with synthetics (some 'natural' perfumes).

For those inclined to personally render essential oils, there are many decent distillers on the market today. Most fall into two camps – the 'lab equipment' type and the old–school copper type. Both work; if nothing else the decision to purchase one or the other is often based on size and visual appeal. *See Hydrosol for a useful distillation by–product.*

Oil, Herbal

Herbal oils are usually applied to unbroken skin for their interaction with the epidemic/keratin (surface) layers. They soften the skin, retain the active medicine, and provide a limited protective coating, enabling skin conditions to better respond to the herbal medicine within the oil. Herbal oils are the base for both ointments and salves. Ointments are better at penetrating; salves at protecting.

Vegetable oils can be broken into several classes depending on viscosity or thickness and to what degree they dry or thicken when exposed to air. Olive, almond, and peanut oils are thicker than most, and create less of a film when exposed to air. Mustard seed, canola, sesame, sunflower, pumpkin, soy, and corn oils thicken to a moderate degree, but are less viscous. Hemp, linseed (flax), safflower, sunflower, and walnut oils are the least viscous, and upon air contract, produce a gummy film.

Rancidity is a factor with all fats. If an herbal oil is being stored for over several months use olive as the base oil. It is greatly resistant to oxidation and rancidity. Even compared to grapeseed, known for its high antioxidant activity, olive oil will be found more stable.

Once made store the oil in an air–tight, darkened glass container. Refrigeration is not necessary, but nonetheless should be kept at cool temperatures.

Method 1: Alcohol Intermediate

Best for herbs that are high in volatiles, resins, and other non–polar constituents, this method stands out as one of the better herbal oil techniques, demonstrated by the vibrant color imparted to the oil.

1. Mix 1 ounce of dried, coarsely powered herb with ½–1 ounce of 190 proof ethyl alcohol.
2. Cover and let stand for an hour.
3. Pour 7 ounces of olive oil into a blender.
4. Add the alcohol–saturated herb.
5. Blend on high for 15 minutes or until blender container is very warm to hot.
6. Strain the oil/herb through a piece of cloth.
7. Discard the herb and bottle the oil.
» *Ratio: 1 part herb (weight) to ½–1 part 190 proof ethyl alcohol (volume) to 7 parts olive oil (volume).*

Method 2: Wilted Herb

This method works best for herbs that become less potent upon fully drying. Here we are taking advantage of the herb's fresh state but need to reduce the water content to lessen possible microbial fermentation.

1. Wilt the plant to half of its original weight; this often takes 8–12 hours.
2. Chop or dice the herb. Be careful not to make a puree, as this will release too much water into the oil, encouraging fermentation.
3. In a jar combine 1 ounce of chopped herb in 7 ounces of olive oil.

4. Mix thoroughly.
5. Seal and let stand in a warm (90–100 degrees) place, out of direct sunlight, for 14 days. Covered, exposed to the sun or next to a stove or heat duct are some good places.
6. Strain, but do not press the oil from the herb.
7. Let stand until any residual water and the oil completely separate. Pour off the oil, or with a basting syringe collect the oil apart from any water layer.
8. Bottle the oil. Discard the water.
» *Ratio: 1 part herb (weight) to 7 parts olive oil (volume).*

Method 3: Old Standard

1. Combine 1 ounce of dried, powdered herb with 7 ounces of olive oil.
2. Using a blender thoroughly mix the combination.
3. Pour into a sealable jar.
4. Seal and let stand in a warm (90–100 degrees) place, out of direct sunlight, for 14 days. Covered while exposed to the sun or next to a stove or heat duct are some good places.
5. Agitate the mixture several times a day.
6. After 14 days, blend (electric blender) until the container is very warm–hot.
7. Strain the oil from the powdered herb through a piece of cloth.
8. Discard the herb and bottle the oil.
» *Ratio: 1 part herb (weight) to 7 parts olive oil (volume).*

Method 4: Heat

This method is particularly useful when the alcohol intermediate technique is not preferred. Use this method with plants high in stable oleoresins, such as Cayenne pepper, Ginger, or Myrrh.

1. Combine 1 ounce of dried, powdered herb with 7 ounces of olive oil.
2. Mix thoroughly and place the mixture in a sealable jar. Secure the lid.
3. Submerged in a heated pot of water, heat to 140–160 degrees for 4–5 hours.
4. Remove from heat and let stand for an additional 4 hours.
5. Strain and bottle.
» *Ratio: 1 part herb (weight) to 7 parts olive oil (volume).*

Ointment

Ointments are best used when there is call for a penetrating topical medicine. They affect a deeper array of tissues (compared to salves) but need to be applied more often.

1. Combine 7 parts base oil (almond/olive/pre–made herbal oil) with 1 part beeswax.
2. Slowly heat until the beeswax is dissolved in the oil.
3. Let the oil–beeswax mixture cool until it starts to faintly harden on the sides of the container. At this point you should be able to put your finger into the oil without it being too hot.
4. In a blender pour 12 parts of distilled water/herb tea/hydrosol (it is bet to have this mixture ready to go in a blender before the oil–beeswax begins to cool).
5. Blend on low.
6. Slowly pour the oil/beeswax mixture into the blender.
7. Blend for only 10–15 seconds (the mixture should have a creamy consistency).
8. Blot any extra liquid from the top of the ointment.
9. Mix in any additional essential oils at this point (1 ml. per 5–7 ounces or so).
10. Scoop into containers and refrigerate.
» *Ratio: 7 parts herbal oil (volume) to 1 part beeswax (weight) to 12 parts water/tea/hydrosol (volume).*

Considerations

Depending on what tea/hydrosol or essential oil is added, the refrigerated ointment will last without spoilage for several months – some longer.

Poultice

Method 1: Basic

1. Moisten with warm water and knead a pre–determined amount of dried and powdered herb with warm water until a porridge–like consistence is reached.
2. Apply directly to the affected area, or cover the area first with muslin cloth, then apply.
3. Secure poultice with a covering and/or bandage.
4. Change 2–3 times daily, or when cool.

Method 2: Field Poultice
1. Bruise and/or puree the fresh plant.
2. Apply to affected area and secure.
3. Change 2–3 times daily.
4. A 'spit poultice' can be quickly made by chewing the intended herb (make sure it is internally non–toxic) and applying it to the affected area.

Powder

Depending on the part of the plant some dried materials are harder than others to powder. Roots, bark, and stems are more difficult than leaves, flowers, and lightweight parts. For lighter materials an average blender with a metal or glass container is adequate; for tougher materials a vita–mix works well, or an industrial grinder/mill. Once the plant is powdered it can then be used as a dust, or as a starting point for DPTs, poultices, etc.

Salve

1. While slowly heating 7 ounces of an herbal oil add 1 ounce of beeswax.
2. Let the beeswax slowly dissolve.
3. While still hot, pour the mixture into containers.
4. As the salve cools, it will solidify.
» *Ratio: 7 parts herbal oil (volume) to 1 part beeswax (weight).*

Considerations
Salves will be best applied when there is need of a protective skin coating.

Sitz Bath

Best used for skin, trauma (post–delivery for example), and bacterial/fungal conditions of the genital, anal, and related pelvic tissues, a traditional sitz bath uses a small 'sitting tub'. The updated version of the traditional sitz bath is more superficial in design. It is a small tub of sorts that fits over a toilet bowl. Accompanying this is a gravity–fed solution bag and tubing for specific area application. For simple washes this modern version of the sitz bath is fine. But for more effective treatments longer soaking times will necessitate the traditional design.

1. Prepare a half–strength or full strength tea.
2. Apply/soak until tea is cool.

Spirit

A spirit is simply an essential oil diluted with a specific amount of alcohol. This preparation is mainly designed to make essential oils more palatable for internal use. It also makes essential oils more suitable as formula ingredients.

1.   Take 1 part essential oil and dilute with 9 parts 190 proof ethyl alcohol.
2.   Mix; bottle; store.
»   *Ratio: 9 parts alcohol (volume) to 1 part essential oil (volume).*

Suppository

Suppositories are preparations made for either vaginal or rectal insertion (less commonly for the urethra). Two types of suppositories are covered here. The first has a glycerin/gelatin base and works well with tinctures and fluidextracts as the added medicinal agent. The second type is Cocoa butter based and is better suited for added herbal oils and essential oils.

Method 1: Glycerin/Gelatin

1.   Mix together 6.5 parts glycerin with 2.1 parts of tincture or fluidextract.
2.   Heat for several minutes using low temperatures.
3.   Add 1.4 parts of powdered gelatin.
4.   Mix thoroughly and remove from heat.
5.   Pour into suppository molds and let cool.
»   *Ratio: 6.5 parts glycerin to 2.1 parts tincture/fluidextract to 1.4 parts gelatin (all totaling 10 parts).*

Method 2: Cocoa Butter

1.   Using low heat melt 1 part Cocoa butter.
2.   Add ½ part herbal oil and mix together.
3.   Add any essential oil at this time (1 ml. per 5–7 ounces of oil is a good starting point).
4.   Pour into suppository molds and let cool.
»   *Ratio: 1 part Cocoa butter to ½ part herbal oil.*

Considerations

»   The ratios presented here are meant as guides and can be altered if the suppository's consistency needs to be changed.
»   Placing the suppositories in a refrigerator or freezer for a short period

of time can help in their solidification.

» Suppositories are best used before bed when the body is in a horizontal position.

» If at any time the suppository causes irritation, discontinue or change the recipe.

» Pharmaceutical grade gelatin, suppository molds (both the disposable plastic type and the aluminum/metal block type) are available through pharmacy suppliers. Check on–line or with compounding pharmacies.

Syrup, Simple

Simple syrup is called for in some respiratory formulations and in any other formula where a preparation's sweetness and soothing qualities are called for.

1. In a pot combine 32 ounces of refined white sugar and 16 ounces of water.

2. Slowly heat and stir until the sugar is fully dissolved. Occasionally 1 or 2 additional ounces of water will be needed to fully dissolve the sugar.

3. Let cool and bottle. The syrup does not need to be refrigerated.

» *Ratio: 2 parts sugar (weight) to 1 part (volume) water.*

Considerations

» Any tea can be converted into a syrup by simply adding sugar in the proper ratio. Senna, Marshmallow, Wild cherry, Rhubarb, and Ginger are a number of classics. Tinctures/fluidextracts can also be added to simple syrups, usually in a 1 part to 1 part ratio.

» Other sweeteners will ferment and spoil if used without added alcohol.

Tea

Tea preparations are best applied to plants that have a large array of water–soluble compounds. Plants that are being used for tannins, starches, minerals, and other polar compounds are best taken as teas. All plants are dried first and then infused or decocted.

Making tea with a fresh plant is a waste. Intact, living plant cells are adept at holding on to their vital cellular compounds, not giving them up to water. Through drying this force is disrupted – cell walls are broken making the plant's various constituents permeable to water. Make tea or any water–based preparation fresh daily.

Infusion

1. Bring 1 quart of water to a boil.
2. Turn off heat.
3. Stir in 1 ounce of dry, fragile plant materials – leaves, flowers, thin stems, etc.
4. Cover and steep for at least 15 minutes.
5. Uncover and strain.

» *Ratio: 1 part herb (weight) to 32 parts water (volume).*

Decoction

1. Bring 1 quart of water to a slow simmer.
2. Stir in 1 ounce of thicker, dried plant materials – bark, roots, stems, pods, etc.
3. Cover and simmer for at least 15 minutes.
4. Turn heat off.
5. Steep for 15 minutes.
6. Uncover and strain.

» *Ratio: 1 part herb (weight) to 32 parts water (volume).*

Cold Infusion

1. In a mesh tea bag or colander suspend 1 ounce of dried plant materials in 1 quart of water.
2. Steep over night at room temperature. Strain.
3. Make fresh daily.

» *Ratio: 1 part herb (weight) to 32 parts water (volume).*

Tincture, Overview

» Plants that are high in volatile oils, complex starches, and other non–polar constituents are best prepared through tincturing.

» A 1:2 FPT (fresh plant tincture) means that in each fluid ounce of tincture produced there is contained the therapeutic constituents of ½ ounce of fresh herb. The herb/menstruum ratio generally corresponds to this as well: 1 part of fresh herb to 2 parts of menstruum. A 1:5 DPT (dry plant tincture) means 1 part of dried herb to 5 parts of menstruum or in each fluid ounce of tincture produced there is contained the therapeutic constituents of ⅕ ounce of dried herb.

» A 1:2 FPT is equal in strength to a 1:5 DPT. Since the dried plant lacks water it is being added back into the menstruum to properly extract the plant's constituents.

» The alcohol percentage of the FPT is high. What is being relied upon in this tincture preparation is the hydroscopic (hygroscopic) activity of alcohol. The alcohol literally dehydrates the fresh plant. It pulls all of the plant's constituents/cytoplasm out into the surrounding alcohol. The result is a highly potent, intact representation of the fresh plant. FPTs with lower alcohol contents are inferior; water limits the pulling activity of alcohol.

» 1:2 for a FPT and 1:5 for a DPT are standard ratios originated by chemists in western medicine's past when plants were the main medicines.

» Depending on the plant, lower tincture and extract ratios (1:1 or 2:1, etc.) are not necessarily better or stronger. One characteristic of a good quality tincture is its lack of particulate matter, or sediment. Often many plants respond poorly to a 1:1 or more concentrated preparations because their constituents are not able to remain in suspension and 'salt out' through being too concentrated. This limits the body's ability to properly absorb the preparation.

» All tinctures are made with 190 proof ethyl alcohol (with the exception of several herbs that are extracted well with vinegar – see Acetum Tincture), commonly called Everclear. Look to liquor stores or the liquor section of grocery stores. Availability varies from state to state.

» Glycerin and vinegar (with several exceptions – see Acetum Tincture) are incredibly poor solvents. Even store–bought liquid glycerin 'extracts' begin as alcoholic extracts. The alcohol is then removed and the condensed extract is added to a glycerin medium and sold as a 'glycerite', 'glycerin tincture', etc. The best use for glycerin, associated with tinctures that is, is its addition to an alcoholic menstruum. Its job here is not as a solvent, but to inhibit the formation of unwanted complexes. That is, it keeps a high tannin–content tincture from forming into a curd–like gelatinous mass. Compared to glycerin and vinegar, even water (tea) is a far superior extractive medium.

Tincture, Dry Plant

Method 1: Maceration

1. Place 2 ounces of dried and powered plant material in a glass jar.
2. Add 10 ounces of alcohol/water mixture – see each plant's preparation/

dosage for the correct alcohol/water percentage. (If a plant calls for 60% alcohol then add 6 ounces of grain alcohol and 4 ounces (40%) of water).

3. Combine together with the powdered herb in a glass jar. Secure lid and then shake well for several minutes.

4. Let stand for 2 weeks – shaking every day for 5 minutes.

5. Press the tincture from the marc. Or squeeze by hand using a large piece of flannel or cheese cloth.

6. Discard the marc.

7. Bottle the tincture.

» *Ratio: 1 part dried herb (weight) to 5 parts menstruum (volume).*

Considerations

» When using this tincture method with high tannin–content plants the menstruum should consist of 10% glycerin. This inhibits the tannins from binding together and with other constituents.

Method 2: Percolation

Percolation is a tincturing technique regarded as superior to maceration. Fresh menstruum with full extractive potential is always in contact with the powdered herb; by the time it drains from the cone to be caught below it is 'full' with compounds. The concept is the same when percolating coffee.

Powdered and moistened herb is packed into a glass cone or funnel. This is suspended over, via a stand, or inserted into, a suitable receiving container. Menstruum is added topside into the large opening of the cone. As it descends, the menstruum's flow rate is controlled by a cap or valve. The menstruum that is caught in the receiving vessel is now the percolate (or tincture). *See Herbal Medicine: Trends and Traditions for step–by–step instructions.*

Method 3: Vinegar (Acetum Tincture)

Using either the maceration or percolation technique, vinegar (apple cider vinegar is fine) is used as a solvent. Only useful for several herbs such as Artemisia and Lobelia, its main drawback is a short storage time.

Tincture, Fresh Plant
Method 1: Old standard

1. Place 2 ounces of fresh, chopped plant material in a glass jar.
2. Add 4 ounces of alcohol.
3. Secure the lid. There is no need to shake the mixture. After 14 days, press or squeeze the tincture from the herb.
4. Discard the marc (spent herb).
5. Bottle the tincture.
» *Ratio: 1 part fresh herb (weight) to 2 parts 190 proof ethyl alcohol (volume).*

A Simplified Method
1. Place 5½ ounces of fresh, chopped plant material in a pint mason jar.
2. Fill to the top with alcohol.
3. Secure the lid and follow the instructions mentioned previously.
» *Ratio: 1 part fresh herb (weight) to 2 parts 190 proof ethyl alcohol (volume).*

Considerations
» Filling the jar to the top with alcohol will not amount to exactly 11 ounces (or 2 parts), but it will be close enough.
» After the jar is sealed and several days have passed often the alcohol fully settles to where the level is below the jar's lip. Remove the jar's lid and top–off with alcohol. Secure the lid. Press after the initial 14 days.

Wash

A wash is simple a topically applied herb tea. Using a spray bottle for this preparation in cases of sunburn or skin inflammation for example is a handy way of applying an herbal wash.

Wash, Nasal

The principal use of this preparation is as wash for the sinuses. It is a somewhat bizarre experience that goes against instinct (inhaling water in through the nose, instead of blowing it out). But the result is worth the strangeness, particularly if there is a sinus infection.
1. Make an isotonic solution by adding ½ teaspoon of table salt to 1 pint of warm water or an appropriate tea.
2. Pour the solution into a bowl. It should be shallow enough so liquid is close to the bowl's lip.
3. While plugging one nostril, submerge the open nostril into the solution.
4. *Slowly* inhale through the submerged nostril.

5. The solution will be drawn in through the nostril and collect in the mouth.

6. Spit out the solution.

7. Change nostrils and repeat.

Considerations

»   In acute conditions this wash can be repeated every hour or so.

»   A special container called a 'neti pot' is made for this application. It is basically a miniature watering can. It holds no significant advantage over simply using a bowl.

»   Be sure to use distilled or at least 'purified' water. Although rare, upper respiratory tract infections due to water–borne microorganisms have been reported with contaminated water sources.

Materia Medica

Acacia
Fabaceae/Pea Family

Acacia constricta Benth. *(Acaciopsis constricta, Vachellia constricta)*
White thorn acacia

Acacia angustissima (Mill.) Kuntze *(Acaciella angustissima, Mimosa angustissima, Senegalia angustissima)*
Fern acacia, Prairie acacia

Acacia greggii A. Gray *(Acacia durandiana, Senegalia greggii)*
Catclaw acacia

Description
Out of the three plants profiled here, Acacia angustissima tends to be the most herbaceous. The plant is rarely woody and typically is no more than 4' tall by 4' wide. The branch stems are deeply grooved and woolly. Each large–bipinnate leaf has 2–14 sets of primary leaflets and 9–33 sets of secondary leaflets. The white, ball–like flower clusters are arranged in racemes originating from leaf axils. The brown seedpods are 1½"–3" long and up to ½" wide. The seeds are small and dark brown.

At maturity, Acacia constricta is a large shrub, reaching heights of 6'–8' and often nearly as wide. At branch nodes there are 2 large white thorns; these diminish in size and eventually disappear as the branch or trunk ages and increases in girth. The leaves are composed of 1–7 sets of primary leaflets and 6–16 pairs of secondary leaflets. The small yellow flowers form into ball–like clusters that are between ½"–1" in width; they are very fragrant and sweet smelling. The seedpods that develop in June are light reddish–brown, smooth, and 1½"–4" long. The small black and gray seeds are mottled and between ½"–¼" long.

Acacia greggii is a large shrub or multi–trunked small tree occasioning 15'–20' in height. Like many Acacias, A. greggii has a bipinnate leaf pattern; each leaf has 2–4 sets of leaflets comprised of 4–6 pairs of secondary leaflets or pinnae. The thorns are recurved, solitary, and alternately spaced along the branches. The small flowers form dense, yellowish cylindrical clusters, which are 1"–2" long. The pods, which follow, are 2"–5"long, ½"–¾" wide, ribbon–like, and slightly twisted. The green pods and seeds have a distinctive onion–like smell.

Distribution

Westward from southern Florida, Acacia angustissima has a patchwork–like distribution. The plant is found through Arkansas, Missouri, and much of eastern Texas, skipping most of New Mexico except for an isolated pocket east of the Rio Grande Drainage's southern expanse. Although the plant does not occur in California, below the Mogollon Rim it is common throughout much of southeastern and south–central Arizona.

From the southern half of Arizona, Acacia constricta is found east to southern New Mexico's Gila River, continuing to the Rio Grande and Pecos River Drainages, finally to Trans–Pecos Texas. A. constricta is found from 2,000'–6,000' in many areas where A. greggii is present. Look to drainages, slopes, and hillsides.

Acacia greggii is found in a large array of vegetation zones throughout the Southwest. From sea level to 5,000', the plant ranges extensively throughout the Mojave, Sonoran, and Chihuahuan Deserts. In low elevation arid areas, look for A. greggii along gullies and washes; in higher elevation areas the plant is more commonly found in Desert Grasslands, open areas, and among rocky hillsides and slopes.

Chemistry

Legume–type condensed and hydrolyzable tannins.

Medicinal Uses

Acacias are simply mild astringents, nothing more, nothing less. Their best use is as a topical wash or powder for redness and skin irritation from insect bites, sunburn, scrapes, and abrasions. Gargled for a raw–sore throat, or swallowed for mild gastric irritation, Acacia proves useful. It is not a major medicine, but it is useful if locally abundant. Along with Mesquite this ubiquitous genus is easily accessed throughout the southwestern part of the country.

Indications

»   Burns/Scrapes/Abrasions (external)
»   Sore throat/Gastric irritation

Collection

From mid–spring through early fall clip the small leafing branch ends. Dry, then garble the leaves from the branches. Discard the branches.

Preparations/Dosage

» Leaf wash/Powder/Poultice: topically as needed
» Leaf infusion: 4–6 ounces 2–3 times daily

Cautions

There are no known cautions with normal usage.

Other Uses

Acacia seeds can be eaten raw in small quantities. The biggest limiting factor is the pseudo onion–like scent that quickly becomes repugnant. Dried, the seeds can be cooked (and eaten in limited quantities) like any other legume, or ground into a meal and eaten alone or mixed with other flours.

Aloe

Liliaceae/Lily Family

Aloe vera (L.) Burm. f. (*Aloe barbadensis, A. chinensis, A. perfoliata var. vera*)
True aloe

Aloe ferox Mill.
Cape aloe, Bitter aloe

Description

Aloe vera is a succulent plant that stands between 2′–4′ tall. At the plant's base form large rosettes of lance–shaped leaves. A well–hydrated leaf is stout and weighty. At maturity, they can reach lengths of 30″ and weigh 2–3 lbs. The leaf skin is smooth, rubbery, and grayish–green with toothed margins. Tall flower racemes originate from the center of the plant. Individual flowers are tubular, yellow, and tend to droop. The lower flowers mature and open first.

In many respects, Aloe ferox and A. vera are very similar. However, A. ferox is a much larger plant, reaching 6′–10′ at maturity. The central stem crown bares a rosette of thick, succulent green leaves. Mature plants develop impressive trunks which become covered by older leaves if they are left unpruned. Reddish–brown teeth are arranged along leaf margins and occasionally on both the upper and lower surfaces. Flower stalks can be branched. The central stalk stands several feet tall and supports a cluster of reddish–orange tubular flowers. Like A. barbadensis, the lower flowers are the first to mature and open.

Distribution

Aloe vera appears to be originally from the eastern Mediterranean area, but like Corn and Cannabis, it has been cultivated and transported for thousands of years making its exact origin difficult to ascertain. Now though, the plant is widely distributed throughout the Middle East, northern Africa, and peninsular India. Here in the West it is found throughout Central America, Mexico, Florida, Texas, and throughout the low–elevation Southwest where it is grown with some extra care. A. ferox is a South African native, but like A. vera, it is extensively grown as an ornamental. In the past, it was widely cultivated for its dried exudate.

Chemistry

Anthraquinones: barbaioin (aloin), which breaks down into aloe–emodin–9–anthrone; isobarbaloin; lignins; saponins; sterols.

Medicinal Uses

There are essentially two different medicines derived from Aloe. Both have diverging physiologic activities, modes of action, and collection techniques.

Aloe leaf exudate, which is yellowish–brown when fresh, is mainly contained within a layer of specialized cells between the rind and inner leaf. Collected and dried, it is the historical Bitter aloe of the old drug trade. Even up to 2002, some over–the–counter and pharmaceutical preparations were comprised mainly of Aloe leaf exudate.

The fresh or dried exudate is useful primarily as a stimulant laxative. If constipated, use it internally for short periods. Aloe exudate stimulates peristalsis and fluid secretion by the large bowel. Curiously, these activities are largely achieved only after colonic bacteria transform the anthraquinone aloin into an active metabolite: aloe–emodin–9–anthrone. Like Senna, the addition of carminative herbs such as Poliomintha or Dogweed will offset potential griping caused by Aloe alone.

Arthritis that is dependent upon poor bowel health and related constipation will also improve under the use of Aloe exudate. Like other stimulant laxatives, Aloe can be habit forming if taken for lengthy periods. Address liver health, stress patterns, and diet before relying on Aloe or any stimulant laxative for regular bowel movements.

Topically Aloe exudate is significantly inhibiting to a number of fungal and bacterial strains. Therefore, as a paint or dust, it is well applied to infections that are non–resolving and tenacious.

Aloe's leaf pulp, really an altogether different medicine, is also used topically for wound healing. Although its mode of action differs from the leaf exudate, the leaf pulp diminishes inflammation through its inhibitory effects on thromboxane and bradykinin. Both compounds are mediators of inflammation. The leaf pulp's polysaccharide content enhances connective tissue synthesis and skin repair. A fresh leaf poultice applied to burns is one of Aloe's foremost applications. Its speed in diminishing pain and redness verges on remarkable.

Secondarily the leaf pulp facilitates wound healing by its absorbent quality. Like all succulent plants, Aloe's internal structure is hydrophilic; it absorbs polar fluids and holds on to them. Placing an open leaf poultice on a damaged area facilitates the absorption of disorganized surface tissue fluids, which speeds healing. To maximize the advantages of Aloe's absorbent qualities, change the leaf poultice often.

The leaf pulp taken internally reduces blood glucose levels. Aloe's array of hydrophilic constituents slows simple carbohydrate breakdown and absorption[1]. To benefit from Aloe's blood sugar lowering effect, take several tablespoons before meals. Relatedly LDL levels are often lowered from Aloe. This is also likely due to the plant's ability of binding – lipids in this case. Lastly the leaf pulp soothes stomach inflammation and is healing to peptic ulcers.

Indications
»   Constipation, chronic, dry feces (leaf exudate)
»   Infections, bacterial and fungal (external–leaf exudate)
»   Burns, heat and sun (external–leaf pulp)
»   Wounds/Injuries (external–leaf pulp)
»   Hyperglycemia/LDL levels, elevated (leaf pulp)
»   Ulcer, peptic (leaf pulp)

1   Due to its pectin content, Prickly pear has a similar mode of action.

Collection

To begin, clip a number of large, hydrated leaves from the lower main stem. Place the clipped leaves, with the cut ends facing down, in a large strainer or colander; pack enough leaves into the strainer as to keep them upright. Place the strainer in a large bowl or pot. Let the exudate drain from the leaves until the flow has ceased. Larger yields will occur if the leaves are well hydrated from recent rains or watering. The collected leaf exudate then can be preserved with 20% alcohol. Alternatively, the exudate can be heated slowly until it thickens. It is then dried and stored. It then can be reconstituted or ground to a fine powder as needed. The overall anthraquinone concentration is greatest throughout the summer months.

After a leaf has been sliced in half, the mucilaginous pulp is scraped out. It can then be stored unpreserved in a refrigerator for 1–2 weeks at a time.

Commercially available gels and juices are refined and usually contain preservatives. Both are derived from the leaf pulp. Most of the anthraquinones and cellulose are removed during processing.

Preparations/Dosage

»   Leaf exudate: 10–20 drops 1–2 times daily or externally as needed
»   DPT (50% alcohol) of leaf exudate: 30–60 drops 2–3 times daily
»   Leaf pulp: 1–2 tablespoons 2–3 times daily or externally as needed

Cautions

Pregnant women should not take the leaf exudate internally – the plant may potentially stimulate uterine contractions. Nursing babies may experience a laxative effect due to anthraquinone's transmission through breast milk.

When used as recommended, the leaf pulp taken internally will not cause gastrointestinal problems. However, *excessive* pulp intake can cause intestinal cramping and diarrhea, which is typical of anthraquinone containing plants.

Other Uses

Aloe (or more specifically its polysaccharide fraction) has a cult–like following among multi–level marketers and the impressionable. Touted as being healing to almost any affliction through its immune system 'modulation', these formulations are expensive and exaggerated.

Antelope Horns
Asclepiadaceae/Milkweed Family

Asclepias asperula (Decne.) Woodson *(Acerates asperula, Asclepiodora asperula)*
Spider milkweed, Inmortal

Description
Antelope horns is a low–growing perennial, 1'–2' tall, by 2'–3' wide. Its stems are herbaceous and radiate outward from a central taproot forming rounded mounds. The leaves, which are creased at the mid–vein, are 3"–4" long and lance–shaped. They have wavy margins, are pointed at the tip, and are alternately spaced but can form in groupings of 2 or 3 around the stems. The globe–like flower clusters are large, solitary, and form at stem ends. Individual flowers are 2–toned in appearance; they are a mixture of greenish–white lobes and purple hoods. The slightly spiny, 2"–4" long seedpods stand upright and contain tufted, light brown, flat seeds.

Distribution
Antelope horns is found over a wide array of elevations. Look for the plant on dry plains, rocky slopes, and openings in Pinyon, Juniper, and Oak habitats from Kansas and Arkansas, west to Nevada and California.

Chemistry
At least four cardenolide–type cardiac glycosides: calotropin, coroglaucignin, uscharidin, and uzarin; preganane glycosides and most likely the flavonoids rutin and quercetin.

Medicinal Uses
Use Antelope horns when upper and lower respiratory tract tissues are dry due to lack of secretion. When it hurts to breath, the lungs feel stuffy and hot, and bronchial mucus is thickened and difficult to expectorate, Antelope horns fits the picture. It is well used in episodes of dry bronchitis with a hacky cough. Relatedly it is well–applied to dry, non–spasmodic asthma and pleuritic conditions. Through Antelope horns' vagus nerve stimulation, similar to Pleurisy root's, bronchial tissue is moistened due to enhanced mucus secretion. This serves to soothe inflamed membranes. Antelope horns works well by itself or in formula for individuals with the

above bronchial conditions that tend to exhibit adrenaline stress patterns. The plant's parasympathetic stimulation can be found sedating by these people. The effect Antelope horns has here is appropriate; often what a sick person needs most is bed rest.

Antelope horns has a moderate cardiac glycoside content, making its use as a mild heart stimulant practical. The plant slows and strengthens the heartbeat, as do the majority of properly dosed cardiac glycoside–containing plants, such as Convallaria and Selenicereus. It is best used when the pulse is weak and fast and cardiac output is diminished. Traditionally Antelope horns is used in heart weaknesses accompanying age, 'tobacco heart', and heart enlargement. In fact, Antelope horns best fits 'old coots' with aging hearts who abhor doctors, pharmaceuticals, and the intrusive nature of that sector. When constrictive breathing is dependent upon heart weakness Antelope horns often seems bronchial dilating, when in fact it simply improves tissue oxygenation through its cardiac stimulation. Also fluid retention, if dependent on heart weakness, is reduced.

Because of Antelope horns' parasympathetic stimulation and its effect on intestinal walls, moderate to large doses of the plant can prove laxative – an attribute of this plant and most Milkweeds that is greatly reduced by drying. Although not very predictable, Antelope horns can stimulate menses if the period is stop and start or is late due to chronic stress or intense episodes of fear or anger. In the past it was used by Hispanic New Mexicans and Coloradoans as a labor stimulant and to assist in the body's full separation and expulsion of the postnatal placenta.

Antelope horns' white–milky sap is antifungal and moderately antibacterial, as is the sap from most other Milkweeds. Although sticky, the fresh latex, when applied daily, is useful in treating athlete's foot, ringworm and other topical fungal infections. The latex, which is also high in proteolytic enzymes, is an effective wart treatment. Apply it fresh daily until the tissue softens enough so the wart can easily be picked off, or falls off by itself.

Indications
» Asthma, dry, non–spasmodic
» Bronchitis, with non–productive cough
» Pleurisy
» Cardiac weakness, from age or tobacco use
» Amenorrhea

» Labor, slowed
» Fungal infections/Warts (external)

Collection

Using the foliage as a locator, dig a hole about 1′ wide and 1′–2′ deep to the side of the plant. Carefully work the ground away from its side. Using this method – digging² from the side – the root can be removed in its entirety.

The taproots of older plants can be several inches thick and up to 2′ deep. They usually descend vertically with some secondary forking. The outside root bark is brownish–tan; the inside is porous and cream–colored.

The last 6″–8″ is the most difficult part to collect; it is the deepest part and has narrowed considerably. Make sure to finish the job by getting the entire root. Discard the foliage. Use the roots within a year, shortly after the oils can become rancid, making the medicine tedious to the gut and liver.

Preparations

If living in an arid environment, split the porous roots several times length–wise, then lay out to dry. If environmental humidity is a factor, chop the roots width–wise every ¼″–½″, or use a dehydrator.

Dosage

» Root decoction/Cold infusion: 2 ounces 2–3 times daily
» DPT (50% alcohol): 5–30 drops 2–3 times daily
» Fluidextract: 5–10 drops 2–3 times daily
» Latex pellets or capsules (00): 1–2, 2–3 times daily
» Latex: externally as needed

Cautions

Do not use Antelope horns internally during pregnancy or while nursing. It is also unwise to mix the plant with heart affecting pharmaceuticals. Antelope horns is not recommended if there is a slow, bounding, forceful pulse, with strong determination of blood (often seen in robust individuals).

---

2   The soils that this plant is found in are typically dry, rocky, and calcrete–laden (at least in the Southwest), so it is usually not an easy root to procure.

Baccharis
Asteraceae/Sunflower Family

Baccharis salicifolia (Ruiz & Pav.) Pers. *(Baccharis glutinosa, B. viminea, Molina salicifolia)*
Seepwillow, Mule–fat, Batamote, Jarilla, Juatamote, Vara dulce

Baccharis pteronioides DC. *(Baccharis ramulosa, Neomolina pteronioides)*
Yerba del pasmo

Baccharis sarothroides A. Gray
Desert broom, Rosin brush

Description
Baccharis salicifolia is a large, fast–growing bush. Its branches are straight and vertical, becoming woody and tan with age. The plant's lance–shaped, green leaves are serrated. When crushed they are sticky and resinous.

Baccharis pteronioides, less dense than B. glutinosa, is a 3'–6' tall bush. The lance–shaped leaves are variable in shape, but generally are toothed and form in stems clusters. The leaves and young stems have visible resin glands, which if crushed become sticky. The flowers develop at branch ends.

Being a pioneer plant, Baccharis sarothroides starts cycles of flora and soil stabilization. It does this by being an advantageous seeder in disturbed soils. Fast–growing and short–lived, after B. sarothroides dies, other longer–lived perennials establish themselves in the recently stabilized ground. If the plant receives adequate water, sizes of 9' by 9' are not uncommon. B. sarothroides' small linear leaves are easily overlooked. The plant is dense and broom–like in appearance.

Distribution
Baccharis salicifolia is a plant of watercourses and streamsides. Up to 5,000' in the western United States it frequently grows among Cottonwoods and Sycamores. Its extensive range stretches from isolated central Colorado pockets to south of the border. Where environmental factors are optimal, in riparian areas, it often grows in dense thickets.

Baccharis pteronioides is found from 3,000'–5,000' from northwestern

Arizona, east through southern New Mexico and to southwestern Texas. Look for the plant growing on rocky hillsides and along drainages throughout Desert Grasslands and Oak Woodlands.

Baccharis sarothroides is commonly encountered in fallow fields, along roadsides, in drainage areas, and in other disturbed soils. At elevations between 1,000'–5,000', it is found from northern Arizona along the Colorado River, south to include much of the lower part of the state, and west to southern California.

Chemistry
Diterpenoids, lactones, coumarins, and saponins.

Medicinal Uses
Use Baccharis when there is spasmodic diarrhea. It lessens intestinal cramping by inhibiting smooth muscle depolarization. Peristaltic waves are diminished, as is transit time of intestinal contents. Baccharis works well to limit intestinal excesses that have inflammatory overtones be them from functional or organic causes. Used in combination with Tree of heaven, its application to intestinal protozoal infections is worthwhile.

Additionally Baccharis diminishes stomach acidity. This has particular value in healing duodenal ulcers. Whether using Baccharis or other plants, such as Bird of paradise, an acidity lowering approach is primary in resolving duodenal ulcers. Establishment of healthier eating habits and stress management is also needed in long–term resolution.

Externally applied to acute physical injuries Baccharis is antiinflammatory. As a fresh plant poultice or liniment, the plant applied to an injured area diminishes redness and inflammation noticeably. It is also mildly antimicrobial.

Indications
»   Spasmodic diarrhea with intestinal cramping
»   Gastritis
»   Ulcer, duodenal
»   Inflammation, intestinal
»   Cuts/Scrapes (external)

Collection
From the branch ends collect the top 4"–6" of new leaf growth.

Preparations/Dosage
»   Leaf infusion: 4–6 ounces 2–3 times daily
»   FPT/DPT (60% alcohol): 30–60 drops 2–3 times daily

Cautions
Research suggests that Baccharis may potentate phenobarbital. Closely
monitor the situation if using the plant with other anticholinergic therapies. Do not use during pregnancy due to the plant's menses stimulating
potential.

Other Uses
Fresh branches of Desert broom were once bound together and used as a
broom.

Beargrass
Liliaceae/Lily Family

Nolina microcarpa S. Watson *(Nolina caudata)*
Sacahuista

Description
Like Agave and Yucca, Beargrass's dense and leafy mass is its most notable attribute. This perennial has numerous, long but narrow leaves with
minutely serrated margins. Dense thickets of the plant are due to underground stem growth and the development of numerous above ground leaf
rosettes. Given ample size, nutrients, and water, Beargrass flowers in the
spring sending 1 or more 3'–6' long stalks into the air. The open inflorescence is approximately 3' long. The compartmentalized seed capsules contain up to 6 small light brown seeds.

Distribution
From several isolated patches in Texas, west of the Pecos River, Beargrass
spreads west through central New Mexico along the Rio Grande and Gila
River Drainages. Through Arizona, Beargrass's range cuts a diagonal
swath from the Colorado River area, below the Mogollon Rim to Pima and
Cochise Counties. The plant is found on rocky slopes, hillsides, in canyons, and along drainages. From 3,000'–6,000' Beargrass inhabits several

diverging vegetation zones making it a common plant in varying areas.

Chemistry
Saponins: nolinospiroside, ruscogenin, and doubtlessly others.

Medicinal Uses
Through a related saponin content, Beargrass's medicinal effect appears similar to (though weaker than) Butchers broom's (Ruscus aculeatus). Applying the ointment, oil, or salve tends to improve varicosities, spider veins, associated leg heaviness, and edema[3]. The effects of these Butchers broom–Beargrass saponins on vasculature are well documented. Apparently, they have an adrenergic–like effect on veins and venules of the lower body, subsequently providing a tightening effect. Similar to other Lily–Agave family plants, there is reason to believe that taken internally Beargrass diminishes arthritic joint pain.

Indications
»   Venous stasis/Varicosities/Spider veins (internal and external)
»   Leg heaviness, fatigue, and fluid retention (internal and external)
»   Arthritis, rheumatoid

Collection
Either the leaf or root can be used, though the root is stronger than the other parts. To gather the root, select a clone from the outer circumference. With a shovel pry it from the ground. Remove and discard the shallow anchoring rootlets (unless succulent) and protective outward layers.

Collect Beargrass's new leaves throughout the spring and summer. The newer leaves originate from the center of the plant and tend to rise vertically from this point. These are long, flexible, and sharp–edged. Paper–type cuts are easily received when harvesting.

Preparations
Cut the root into manageable chunks. The use of a dehydrator will be helpful in order to inhibit mold growth. Dry the long leaves intact, then cut them into 1"–½" pieces for storage.

---

3   Using Beargrass in this capacity is still a work in progress. Being a fairly new application for the plant further study and application is needed.

Dosage

- » Oil/Ointment/Salve: as needed
- » Leaf/Root decoction: 2–4 ounces 2–3 times daily
- » Capsules (00) of root: 1–2, 2–3 times daily

Cautions

Occasionally the tea can cause minor throat–stomach irritation. If this is the case switch to the capsules. For either part, use for only a 2–3 week duration, then switch to other plants. Do not use during pregnancy. There may be possible hemolytic issues with heavy internal use. Stock fatalities have been reported from excessive grazing of the plant.

Other Uses

The immature and flexible, 1'–2' high flower stalks can be clipped at their bases, peeled and eaten either cooked or raw. Being slightly bitter and soapy, they are not the best edible fare, but are at least interesting.

Beebrush
Verbenaceae/Vervain Family

Aloysia wrightii A. Heller ex Abrams
Wright's beebush, Vara dulce, Altamisa, Oreganillo

Description

Beebrush is a small, rounded sub–shrub, often growing next to or under larger shrubs and trees. Beebrush's leaves are small, oval, oppositely arranged, and delicately perched beneath tiny, whitish flower spikes. Younger stems are ridged; older growth lesser so. Bees are quite fond of the plant during the spring and summer when it is in flower. The scent of Beebrush after brushing up against it or crushing a few leaves between the fingers is friendly and disarming. Actually, the plant smells much closer to a cross between Lavender and Lemon verbena – certainly not Oregano with its cutting pungency.

Distribution

From isolated outposts in southern California, Beebrush ranges southeast through Arizona, southern New Mexico, and southern Texas. It is typically

seen growing on hillsides, rocky slopes, and on the edges of drainage areas
between 1,200'–6,000'.

Chemistry

α–pinene, sabinene, limonene, cineole, linalol, β–caryophyllene, neral,
α–terpinyl acetate, geranial, citronellol, nerol, geraniol, caryophyllene oxide, cis–nerolidol, and spathulenol.

This is an essential oil listing for Aloysia triphylla (Lemon verbena)
Beebrush contains similar compounds, but its bitterness also indicates
differences.

Medicinal Uses

The tincture or the tea taken before meals is a functional and aromatic
bitter. Through reflex, in response to bitterness, digestive secretions (particularly pepsinogen and hydrochloric acid) are stimulated. Blood flow is
shifted to the stomach walls by the dilating nature of the plant's aromatics. This activity indicates Beebrush to be taken when there is indigestion
after a meal. Additionally, if a recently eaten meal feels immovable and the
stomach is bloated Beebrush is warranted.

Indications

»   Indigestion with bloating

Collection

If the foliage smells strongly Lavender–like, it will make good medicine.
Strip the leaves and flowers from the upper branches. Dry the herbage for
tea or use fresh.

Preparations/Dosage

»   Leaf infusion: 4–6 ounces 2–3 times daily
»   FPT/DPT (50% alcohol): 30–60 drops 2–3 times daily

Cautions

Due to the plant's potential of stimulating uterine vasculature, do not use it
during pregnancy.

Bird of Paradise

Fabaceae/Pea Family

Caesalpinia gilliesii (Wall. ex Hook.) D. Dietr. *(Erythrostemon gilliesii, Poinciana gilliesii)*
Yellow bird of paradise

Caesalpinia mexicana A. Gray *(Poinciana mexicana, Poincianella mexicana, P. robinsoniana)*
Mexican holdback, Mexican bird of paradise, Mexican poinciana

Caesalpinia pulcherrima (L.) Sw. *(Poinciana pulcherrima, P. bijuga, P. elata)*
Red bird of paradise, Pride of barbados, Peacock flower

Description

Caesalpinia gilliesii is a large perennial bush usually between 4′–6′ tall. The leaves form on stout many–branched stems. They are bipinnate with ¼″–½″ oblong secondary leaflets. The most distinguishing characteristic is the plant's large, yellow flowers, which form in racemes at branch ends. The sepals are larger than the petals. The long red stamens are 2″–4″ long and extend further than the other flower parts. The flattened pods are several inches long. When the seeds mature, the pods pop open and are sent airborne. In the summer, they can often be heard flying into windows and aluminum siding.

Caesalpinia pulcherrima is an ungainly and large perennial bush. In some areas throughout the Southwest, the plant dies back to the ground in response to frost, but if protected it is only deciduous. It is generally between 4′–10′ in height, but grows to be larger in the Tropics.

The bipinnate leaves are feathery and composed of small leaflets. The plant's stems are lined with weak spines. The showy flowers are red–orange and form at branch ends. They are composed of 5 petals, 5 sepals, and 10 stamens.

Caesalpinia mexicana tends to be similar in structure to the others, although the plant's foliage is denser due to larger leaflets. This plant can sometimes reach tree–like proportions in protected areas, but is typically 4′–6′ tall and bush–like. The showy yellow flower clusters form at branch ends. Like C. pulcherrima, this plant is cultivated extensively as an ornamental.

Distribution

All three plants are non–natives from Subtropical or Tropical America. Now though they are planted as ornamentals in warmer locales throughout the Southwest. Caesalpinia gilliesii, originally from Argentina and Chile, is well established in drainage areas and along roadsides from southeastern Arizona, southern New Mexico, to central Texas.

Chemistry

For Caesalpinia pulcherrima: peltogynoids, homoisoflavonoids, caesalpins, diterpenoids, pulcherrimin, bonducellin, and galactomannans; ellagitannins.

Medicinal Uses

Bird of paradise tea is mainly a gastrointestinal tract medicine. Like many other desert Pea family plants, the tea is astringent and antiinflammatory. Internally it has use in irritative conditions such as gastritis and intestinal inflammation. The plant will also prove lessening to diarrhea and dysentery. The plant's range of flavonoids tends to be supportive of tissue structure and healing.

Externally the wash or poultice is soothing to rashes, bites, and stings. The plant has promise in relieving Poison ivy and chemical sensitivity rashes. In combination with internal use of Canyon bursage or Brittlebush it assists in limiting systemic outbreaks of these conditions.

Indications

» Gastritis
» Inflammation, intestinal
» Diarrhea/Dysentery
» Rashes/Bites/Stings (external)

Collection

Gather the flowers, leaves, and smaller stems. Dry all of these parts for tea.

Preparations/Dosage

» Herb infusion/Stem decoction: 4–6 ounces 2–3 times daily
» Wash or poultice: as needed

Cautions

Several varieties of Caesalpinia have traditional use as emmenagogues. It is best not to use these plants during pregnancy.

Bouvardia
Rubiaceae/Madder Family

Bouvardia ternifolia (Cav.) Schlecht. *(Bouvardia glaberrima)*
Smooth bouvardia, Trompetilla, Expatli

Description

Bouvardia is a mid–sized perennial herbaceous shrub. Like Buttonbush (another Madder family plant) its leaves form in whorls of 3–4 and are 2"–3" long. They are shiny, oblanceolate, and have prominent veins. The plant's striking red flowers are its most notable characteristic. They are 1"–2" long, tubular, and widen at the throat. The capsules are pea–sized and rounded. They contain numerous flattened winged seeds.

Distribution

Bouvardia's core range is Mexico. There it is widespread and fairly common to mid–mountain areas. It extends as far south as Central America (to at least Honduras). In the United States it is of limited distribution, however the plant is stable and successful throughout the majority of southeastern Arizona mountain ranges: Baboquivaris, Santa Catalinas, Pinaleños, Santa Ritas, Chiricahuas, etc. Mid–elevation streamsides and canyons are specific areas for the plant. It's also reported for southwestern New Mexico (Peloncillo and Animas Mountains) and West Texas where a few isolated stands are found in the Davis Mountains.

Chemistry

Triterpenes: ursolic acid and oleanolic acid; flavonols: quercetin, rutin, and kaempferol; hexapeptides: bouvardin and deoxybouvardin.

Medicinal Uses

Bouvardia's medicinal use comes to us from Mexico. Although at present it is not a widely employed herb, written ethnobotanical references, a number of scientific studies, and local reports (Tarahumara) shed some light on the plant's usage. From hydrophobia (rabies[4] infection), hyperglycemia, and scorpion stings, to a racing heart and insomnia, indications appear all–over–the–map. In both evaluating the literature and personally collecting and experimenting with the plant, I believe a number of themes are discernible.

Both indigenous use and lab studies (mice) point to Bouvardia being useful for hyperglycemia/type–2 diabetes. Mild to moderate cases, where blood sugar levels are still able to be lowered with proper diet, exercise, and weight loss will see the most benefit from the plant. Drink 2–3 cups daily for best results, however it is important to stress that without lifestyle changes Bouvardia (or any herb) will likely not have a dramatic effect.

Bouvardia's application to scorpion[5] stings is interesting. Both research (mice) and historical usage point to its lessening effect on the venomous symptoms of a sting. One of the more notorious scorpion groups in the Southwest (and Mexico) that Bouvardia has connection to is Centruroides spp. (Bark scorpion). Although usually non life–threatening, its sting is very painful (I can vouch for this), and consists mainly of local nerve hyper–stimulation (spasm and the sensation of shooting electrical pains under the skin). It is postulated that Bouvardia reduces this massive neurotransmitter (principally acetylcholine and a number of catecholamines) surge caused by the scorpion's venom through an interaction between the plant's constituents and either the venom or the body's reaction to the venom (more likely). Secure a tincture–soaked cottonball directly to the sting or apply a fomentation or soak using the tea. Drinking a cup of tea every hour or so until the pain has diminished should further help the situation. A 50/50 combination of Bouvardia and Aristolochia (see Pipevine) can also be applied topically.

Drink a cup of tea before bed if suffering from insomnia, or during the day, if worry and anxiety are common emotional themes. Its mild stress–response sedation is likely connected to its adrenergic–catecholamine antagonism. This is also possibly the mechanism underlying its anecdotal action on the heart (reducing to tachycardia and palpitation).

It's worth noting that Bouvardia is not a particularly strong–tasting

4   If rabies exposure is suspected, do not, I repeat, do not attempt to treat the infection with Bouvardia, or any herb for that matter. Without standard medical treatment (vaccination soon after exposure), a rabies infection is fatal in nearly all cases.

5   Traditional use also includes the plant's application to other venomous bites and stings: snake, spider, and centipede.

herb. Even though taste does not totally quantify/qualify an herb, it is a factor in determining strength. More often than not a bad–tasting plant will
make a stronger medicine than a fair–tasting one. Bouvardia is actually
bland to pleasant tasting and overall a mild plant medicine. Don't expect it
to be drug–like in its medicinal influence.

Indications
» Hyperglycemia
» Scorpion sting, and other venomous bites/stings (internal and external)
» Anxiety/Insomnia

Collection
Prune the upper branch ends, preferably with both leaf and flower, but if
only leaves are available, that is fine too. Once dry, garble the leaves/flow-
ers from the branches. Discard the branches.

Preparations/Dosage
» Herb infusion: 4–6 ounces 2–3 times daily
» External preparations: as needed

Cautions
There are no known cautions for Bouvardia.

Other Uses
It's a favorite of Hummingbirds (red tubular flowers), and has a high ornamental appeal.

Bricklebush
Asteraceae/Sunflower Family

Brickellia californica (Torr. & A. Gray) A. Gray
Prodigiosa, Hamula, Peston

Description
Bricklebush is a semi–herbaceous bush of moderate stature. Normally it is
3'–4' tall by the same dimension wide. The leaves are generally triangular
in shape, covered with small rough hairs, and arranged alternately along

stems. With an oppositely arranged leaf pattern, new herbaceous growth can look deceivingly mint–like. During the winter, at middle and high elevations, the plant loses its leaves entirely. At lower elevations some may remain only to be released as new growth forms in the spring.

Slender flower heads are interspersed with smaller leaves at branch ends. The whole plant is sticky and it is not uncommon for the lower leaves to be dust and debris covered. Crush a leaf: the plant's potency can be partly determined by its sweet smell and stickiness.

Distribution

Bricklebush is a common plant of the West. From coastal California it ranges eastward through southern Idaho to the panhandles of Oklahoma and Texas, south through Arizona and New Mexico. Throughout Bricklebush's lower–elevation habitats, it is usually found in canyons and ravines where at least some seasonal water flows. In areas of greater altitude and/or latitude, Bricklebush becomes a plant of open grasslands and Ponderosa pine forests.

Chemistry

Phenylpropanoid: caffeic acid; sesquiterpenes: caryophyllene, caryophyllene epoxide, costunolide, β–farnesene, d germacrene, α–humulene, kauniolide, spathulenol, and zaluzanin c; flavonoids and pyrrolizidine alkaloids.

Medicinal Uses

Firstly, the tea is a good hypoglycemic agent, being most useful for individuals with NIDDM (non–insulin dependent diabetes mellitus). Bricklebush is best suited for the thin and easily stressed type–2 diabetic who does not take insulin and responds well to newer generation hypoglycemic pharmaceuticals such as Metformin.

Among other unknown mechanisms, Bricklebush is presumed to diminish blood glucose levels by inhibiting the activity of norepinephrine on glycogen breakdown, therefore reducing stress mediated blood sugar elevations. Bricklebush taken before meals can reduce blood sugar concentrations by 15–20%, and potentially more with proper dietary adherence.

As with most bitter herbs, Bricklebush stimulates saliva production, hydrochloric acid, and mucin, all necessary for proper upper gastrointestinal function and food breakdown. Bricklebush suits individuals who are under constant, low–grade adrenaline, fight or flight responses. Existing in this state tends to shift activity and blood movement away from digestion and assimilation to the skeletal muscles and the brain. This pattern is useful if engaged in flight or fight, but not necessarily when stuck in gridlock traffic. Use Bricklebush before meals when long–term stress has caused indigestion, gastritis, and loss of appetite.

Like many other bitters, Bricklebush also has a stimulatory effect on the liver and is a useful cholagogue, increasing the quantity of bile released into the small intestine. Traditionally Bricklebush is used to lessen diarrhea with associated stomach pain and intestinal cramps.

Indications
»   Gastritis, asecretory
»   Dyspepsia
»   Diabetes mellitus, non–insulin dependent
»   Liver congestion
»   Diarrhea with stomach pain and intestinal cramps

Collection
Before the plant flowers, when the leaves are verdant and sticky, prune the herb portion from Bricklebush's upper stems. After drying the herbage, strip the leaves from the stems. Discard the latter.

Preparations
The leaf infusion is the best preparation. Drink the tea between meals for its hypoglycemic action, before meals for its digestive properties, and as needed for diarrhea.

Dosage
»   Leaf infusion: 2–4 ounces 2–3 times daily

Cautions
Bricklebush should not be used by individuals with IDDM (insulin dependent diabetes mellitus), also known as Type–1, juvenile onset diabetes. Like many other Sunflower family plants in the Eupatory tribe, Bricklebush contains various pyrrolizidine alkaloids, but of small quantities. Given the plant's traditional non–toxic history and that the leaves are used, not the flowers (which typically have higher PA levels), consider Bricklebush a

short to intermediate use herb.

Do not use during pregnancy, while nursing or if there is a liver/gallbladder blockage. Although several ounces occasionally for children with diarrhea are fine, consistent use with little ones is not recommended.

Brittlebush
Asteraceae/Sunflower Family

Encelia farinosa A. Gray ex Torr.
Incienso, Yerba del vaso

Description
Depending on the surrounding environment, Brittlebush has differing growth habits. Among rocks and boulders in mid–elevation desert foot-hills, Brittlebush becomes upright, stretching for the sun. Lower in eleva-tion the plant appears as a semicircle mound of leaves hugging the ground. Leaf characteristics can vary depending on water availability. When produced in drier times, they are grayish–white, compact and hairy; the leaves' solar reflective ability increases making the plant more resilient to the intense sun. With rain, the leaves become large and green, enabling the plant to fully utilize the incoming solar energy.

When in bloom, radiant yellow flowers are suspended over the mounded body of the plant. The flower stems are narrow and long, giving the inflorescences a unique suspended appearance. This floral display can usually be seen in early to mid–spring, but it is not unknown for the plant to occasion an off–season bloom if enough water and proper temperatures are present. If the fragile branches of Brittlebush are broken, a fine sap sometimes weeps from the damaged area. After drying the exudate hard-ens into crystallized, yellow bead–like droplets.

Distribution
Sub–freezing temperatures limit Brittlebush in elevation and northward expansion. The plant tops out at about 4,000'. Here it is maintained with the help of sun–charged, heat radiating boulders. At lower elevations, pure stands of Brittlebush can be found growing in huge expanses on open flats and basins. The plant is widespread throughout the Mojave and Sonoran

Deserts. It is also found from the interior valleys of southern California to the southern tip of Nevada, westward through low elevation Arizona.

Chemistry
Sesquiterpene lactone: farinosin; chromenes: encecalin and demethylence-clin; benzofuran: euparin.

Medicinal Uses
The fresh plant tincture works quickly to diminish hayfever reactions. Its drying and antiinflammatory nature is expedient on sinus and ocular membranes. Use it when allergic reaction has caused watery eyes and a runny nose. The plant can also limit isolated Poison ivy outbreaks from expanding into systemic–full body reactions.

Brittlebush tends to be diaphoretic and traditionally has been used in treating arthritic conditions aggravated by cold and damp weather. External preparations of the leaves or resin tend to be pain relieving as well. They can be used in accordance with the internal tea or tincture.

Indications
» Rhinitis
» Poison ivy reactions, systemic
» Arthritis (internal and external)

Collection
After seasonal winter–spring rains but before the plant flowers, collect the hydrated and grayish–green leaves.

Preparations/Dosage
» FPT/DPT (50% alcohol): 30–60 drops 2–3 times daily
» Leaf infusion: 4–6 ounces 2–3 times daily
» External preparations: as needed

Cautions
Though containing no caffeine, occasionally Brittlebush can elicit a caffeine–like nervous system excitability. Because of this it is not recommended before bed. Moreover due to the plant's interesting chemistry, do not take it during pregnancy or while nursing.

Other Uses

Similar to Pine pitch, the collected resin can be used as a patching material. It was also once used as a regional incense in colonial–era churches. When using an 'incense stove' or simply a hot plate to burn the resin, it combines nicely with Elephant tree gum.

Buttonbush

Rubiaceae/Madder Family

Cephalanthus occidentalis L. *(Cephalanthus berlandieri)*
Buttonwillow, Buttonball, Riverbush

Description

Buttonbush is a large and deciduous shrub, usually forming in dense thickets. As the plant matures the blackish–brown trunk bark becomes deeply fissured. Like other Madder family plants, Buttonbush's leaves are situated in whorls of 3 or 4, although sometimes they are found in oppositely arranged pairs. The leaves are shiny, leathery, and oblanceolate. The small trumpet–shaped, cream–colored flowers are arranged densely in ball–like clusters terminating at branch ends, hence the name Buttonbush.

Distribution

Look for Buttonbush along streamsides, pond and marsh borders, and river bottoms, or at least in places where the ground stays consistently moist. From sea level to approximately 6,000', Buttonbush is widely distributed throughout North America.

Chemistry

Cephalanthin, cephaletin, cephalin, and tannin, among other constituents.

Medicinal Uses

Although not used extensively in present–day herbalism, Buttonbush is still used today as an effective gastrointestinal tract strengthener. It best fits chronic states of indigestion with accompanying area weakness and atonicity. Use the plant if after a meal there are oppressive feelings of fullness and general dyspepsia.

Buttonbush is particularly well suited for individuals whom are prone to harmful digestive patterns (worry and rumination while eating) mainly developed through a harried lifestyle. It redirects digestive emphasis back to the belly, where it belongs. Like most bitters, the plant combines well with aromatic herbs such as Ginger, Peppermint, or Fennel. Additionally its stimulatory effect on the liver and gallbladder makes it of use in relieving mild constipation, especially if there is difficulty digesting fat.

Indications
» Indigestion
» Intestinal distress, from high fat meals
» Constipation, dependent on stress and worry
» Congestion, liver/gallbladder, non–organic causes

Collection
Collect the leaves in the spring before the plant flowers or the inner bark in colder seasons.

Preparations/Dosage
» Leaf infusion/Bark decoction: 4–6 ounces before meals 2–3 times daily
» FPT/DPT (50% alcohol): 30–40 drops before meals 2–3 times daily

Cautions
Because Buttonbush is a gastric stimulant, do not use it if there is an over production of hydrochloric acid (which tends to be rare) or if there is an existing duodenal ulcer. Do not use it in pregnancy, while nursing, or if there is an active biliary blockage.

California Poppy
Papaveraceae/Poppy Family

Eschscholzia californica Cham.
Copa de oro

Eschscholzia californica subsp. mexicana (Greene) C. Clark *(Eschscholzia mexicana)*
Mexican poppy, Gold poppy

Description

Eschscholtzia californica is a small, clump–forming annual or short–lived perennial. Its bluish–green, 5"–20" long stems weaken and droop with age. They are smooth and covered with a fine, white–waxy coating that is easily rubbed away. The leaves are finely dissected. Most of them are basal but some are attached alternately along the stems.

The showy 4–petaled flowers are generally orange but are occasionally yellow and even white. The seed capsules are 1–celled, narrow, ribbed, and slender. Contained within them are many small and dark seeds. Although some botanists do not consider Eschscholzia californica subsp. mexicana a different plant, there are some general differences: the plant is smaller and the flowers tend to be predictably yellow–gold.

Distribution

Eschscholtzia californica is found throughout California, usually below 5,000', and in parts of Oregon and Washington. The densest populations occur west and south of the Sierra Nevadas to the Mojave Desert. E. californica subsp. mexicana has a sporadic occurrence across Arizona, Nevada, Utah, southern New Mexico, and southwestern Texas. Both species are dependent upon winter–spring rains and if given sufficient moisture, they will carpet hillsides and rocky slopes with color.

Chemistry

Pavine alkaloids: eschscholtzine and californidine; benzophenanthridine alkaloids: sanguinarine and chelerythrine; protopine alkaloids: protopine and allocryptopine; berberine and other compounds.

Medicinal Uses

Consider California poppy a sub–opiate, meaning its effect is broadly opiate–like, though *much,* weaker than medically used pharmaceuticals. Use the plant when sleep is difficult from anxiousness and physical discomfort. It is mildly lessening to both nerve centered and muscular pain.

The plant can be useful to highly motivated individuals whom need to diminish or eliminate stronger opiate habits or other similar non–opiate pharmaceutical habits used for pain relief. Here it combines well with Golden smoke (another Poppy family plant) and Wild oats. In some sensitive individuals, California poppy may stimulate very subtle euphoric properties. It is a chemically complex plant with diverging effects on adrenergic neurotransmitters.

Topically, the plant is antimicrobial and can be used on a wide array of bacterial conditions that also respond well to Berberis–Mahonia plants. California poppy is useful in diminishing a spasmodic cough when the face and chest are flushed, there is a strong, bounding pulse, and even fever.

Indications
» Pain, from acute injury
» Insomnia/Anxiety
» Cuts/Scrapes (external)
» Spasmodic cough

Collection
When California poppy is fully mature, having both flowers and seed capsules, pull the whole plant from the ground, tap root and all.

Preparations/Dosage
» FPT/DPT (50% alcohol): 60–90 drops 2–3 times daily
» Whole plant infusion: 4–8 ounces 2–3 times daily
» Topical preparations: as needed

Cautions
California poppy may potentate analgesic–sedative pharmaceuticals. Do not use during pregnancy. Long–term use is acceptable, as the plant is generally not considered habit forming. Consider the plant child–safe.

Other Uses
Eschscholtzia mexicana tends to grow abundantly in copper rich soils. It has been used as a visual indicator of the mineral.

Caltrop
Zygophyllaceae/Caltrop Family

Kallstroemia grandiflora Torr. ex A. Gray *(Tribulus fisheri, T. grandiflorus)*
Orange caltrop, Arizona poppy

Kallstroemia californica (S. Watson) Vail *(Kallstroemia brachystylis, Tribulus brachystylis, T. californicus)*
California caltrop

Kallstroemia parviflora Norton *(Kallstroemia intermedia, K. laetevirens)*
Warty caltrop

Description

Caltrop is a ground–hugging herbaceous annual with larger specimens reaching 3'–4' in length. The plant's small leaves are pinnate and arranged in pairs. The flowers are 5–petaled and are greenish–yellow to bright orange. The mature fruit is small and separates into 8–12 nutlets. Caltrop superficially resembles Puncturevine, another Caltrop family plant.

Kallstroemia grandiflora is the largest Caltrop of the three species profiled here. Its many branched stems reach lengths of 4'. They have stiff and prominent yellow hairs as do the leaves (although here the hairs are smaller and isolated mainly to the outer margins). The leaves are 1"–3" long and have 3–7 sets of smaller leaflets. The large orange flowers are prominent and are between ⅔"–1¼" long. They are solitary and are attached to smaller stems originating from the leaf axils. The oval seedpods split into 8–12 nutlets or carpels.

Compared to Kallstroemia grandiflora, K. californica is smaller in size. The stems and leaves are almost completely lacking hairs. The ¼"–½" long leaflets are arranged in 3–7 sets. The orange–yellow flowers have small petals. The seedpods separate into 8–12 wedge–shaped nutlets.

Kallstroemia parviflora is a 1'–3' long plant with few white stem hairs. The leaves are composed of 3–5 sets of leaflets. The flowers, like K. californica, are small; petals are typically a ¼" long. Similar to the others the fruit is small in size.

Distribution

In southern California Kallstroemia grandiflora is often found with Creo-sote bush. In central and southern Arizona, the plant is encountered below 5000', often in disturbed soils, but generally on open slopes, flats, and me-sas. It is also found in similar areas in New Mexico and east to Texas.

Kallstroemia parviflora enjoys a wider range: from 5,000'–6,000' in southern California it is found east to Mississippi. K. californica is found throughout most of Arizona, throughout southeastern California, and north to southern Colorado.

Chemistry

Flavonoids: quercetin, isorhamnetin, and tricin.

Medicinal Uses

Caltrop is an interesting mix of mild astringent and alterative. Internally the tea lessens diarrhea and is mildly sedating to gastrointestinal tract in-flammation. Passive hemorrhaging of the urinary tract as well as menor-rhagia is lessened.

Think of the plant as a diminutive Creosote bush or Guaiacum and be-cause of its mildness it can be used longer–term for many low–grade in-flammatory conditions. It also should be tried for hive outbreaks, rashes, and fevers. Lastly, the isotonic tea used as an eyewash is soothing to con-junctivitis and allergy induced eye irritation.

Indications

»   Diarrhea
»   Inflammation, gastrointestinal
»   Hematuria
»   Menorrhagia
»   Hives/Rashes (internal and external)
»   Conjunctivitis (eyewash)

Collection

Gather and dry the entire plant, including the small taproot.

Preparations/Dosage

»   Herb infusion: 4–6 ounces 2–3 times daily
»   Eyewash: 2–3 times daily

Cautions

To err on the side of caution, do not use Caltrop during pregnancy or while nursing.

Camphorweed

Asteraceae/Sunflower Family

Heterotheca subaxillaris (Lam.) Britton & Rusby *(Inula subaxillaris)*
Telegraph plant, Arnica

Description

When young this annual (occasionally biannual) has distinctly upward–pointing basal leaves. This characteristic of Camphorweed is very different from other herbaceous plants – initial leaf growth is typically parallel to the ground's surface.

Later in the season Camphorweed develops a many–branched top, lending credence to another common name – Telegraph plant. Lower stem leaves are petioled; upper leaves clasp the stem. Generally they are ovoid, irregularly toothed, wavy, and arranged alternately along the stem. In mass, the common–looking yellow flowers appear disorganized. Each is approximately ½" wide by ¼" high. Due to its gland tipped leaf and stem hair, the whole plant is sticky and smells Camphor–like.

Distribution

Camphorweed, like many other weedy plants, does extremely well in disturbed soils. It is found along roadsides, trails, and field margins. Companion plants are Canadian fleabane and Tobacco.

The plant's range is quite extensive (and still expanding) in the United States. From mid–Atlantic states, such as Delaware, it extends to Florida and west to Arizona.

Chemistry

Heterotheca general: flavonoids: galangin, kaempferol, and quercetin; monoterpenoids: myrcene, limonene, and borneol; cadinene and calamenene–type sesquiterpenes; triterpenoids.

Medicinal Uses

Externally applied Camphorweed is diminishing to pain, inflammation, and the fluid build–up of acute injury. The plant's medicinal qualities are well applied to treating numerous acute accidents – sprains, contusions, etc. Specifically, Camphorweed inhibits inflammatory mediators within injured tissues, diminishing subsequent edema and pain.

There are qualitative differences in how to properly use Camphorweed versus true Arnica (Arnica montana and others). Camphorweed is a tissue sedative, lessening the reactive process that brings about inflammation. Arnica actually heightens the body's response locally by increasing white blood cell activity. This is why conventional herbal wisdom calls for Arnica to be applied 'when it hurts to move', not 'when it hurts to be still'. Use Arnica when the condition is subacute or chronic and not when there is acute pain. Inversely, use Camphorweed when the injury is acute and painful, particularly if the pain does not stop when the injured part is at rest.

Indications

»   Acute injury with pain, swelling, and fluid retention (external)

Collection

From late spring through summer, collect the whole herb portion. Leaf, stem, or flower, all parts can be used fresh or dry.

Preparations/Dosage

»   Leaf infusion/Liniment/Oil: as needed

Cautions

There are no known cautions for external use.

Canadian Fleabane

Asteraceae/Sunflower Family

Conyza canadensis (L.) Cronquist *(Conyza parva, Erigeron canadensis, E. pusillus, Leptilon canadense, Marsea canadensis)*
Horseweed, Colt's tail, Pazotillo

Description

Canadian fleabane is a tall and upright annual reaching heights of 5'–6'. From spring through early summer, the plant appears much like an up–turned feather duster: its leaves, which are several inches long, are clustered along the main stems and spread outward. As time passes, nutrient dynamics are shifted to the small inconspicuous whitish flower heads that form in staggered masses at the plant's top. At this point, the lower central stem leaves lose vitality and often yellow. As a prolific seeder, the achenes are wind scattered.

Distribution

Look for this advantageous weed in disturbed places such as roadsides, irrigation ditches, and other moist areas where water tends to collect and linger. Unlike looking for some annuals, Canadian fleabane is predictable in where it is found; year after year it often grows in the same place. Originally indigenous to the eastern part of the country, it is now found throughout the West. Since the early eighteenth century the plant has even crossed the Atlantic Ocean and is now ubiquitous in parts of Europe.

Chemistry

Sesquiterpenes: trans–α–bergamotene, δ–cadinol, α–curcumene, α–farnesene, and farnesol; monoterpenes: carvone and α–thujene; lipids: enoic and diynoic acids; miscellaneous lactone: furanone; flavonoid: syringic acid.

Medicinal Uses

An infusion of Canadian fleabane is highly useful in treating chronic intestinal inflammation, indicated by: diarrhea, attending mucus, and tissue disruption. The tea is also well used in ulcerative colitis. The plant's tonic effect on intestinal walls has use in 'leaky gut syndrome', where immune responses and inflammatory mediators wreak havoc on local tissues. This can result in malabsorption, digestive discomfort, and food allergies. Canadian fleabane's overall astringency and tightening effect on mucus membranes is not derived solely from the plant's tannins. The plant's volatile oil content, which is locally hemostatic, also plays a part.

The essential oil of Canadian fleabane or 'oil of Erigeron' is a systemic hemostatic. In times when modern coagulate pharmaceuticals were non–existent, various herbal preparations did (and still do) work to quell mild to moderate hemorrhaging. Today, the use of oil of Erigeron to staunch internal bleeding is considered antiquated, but there is still merit to the principle. Use oil of Erigeron internally to quell mild hemorrhaging from the lungs, particularly if severe coughing is a contributing factor. Likewise, if there is mild uterine bleeding after childbirth or blood in the urine from acute injury to the kidneys, the essential oil will prove useful. Passive hemorrhaging from the stomach and intestines, likely from ulcerative conditions, physical injury, or the aftermath of viral or microbial exposures can be stopped or at least lessened with oil of Erigeron.

Indications
»   Intestinal inflammation, chronic
»   Diarrhea with mucus and blood
»   Malabsorption with intestinal debility
»   Hemorrhage, passive (essential oil)

Collection
Collect the upper half of the plant before it flowers. After drying the entire portion, garble the leaves from the stems. Discard the woody stem portions since the majority of volatile oils are held within the leaf. The leaf infusion is the choice preparation.

Preparations/Dosage
»   Leaf infusion: 4–6 ounces 3–4 times daily
»   Essential oil: 3–10 drops 2–3 times daily

Cautions
The greatest caution associated with Canadian fleabane or its more potent derivative – oil of Erigeron – is an unrealistic view of its effects. Passive hemorrhaging bet describes oil of Erigeron's main indication. If there is injury resulting in serious blood loss the emergency room is the best place to start. Avoid Canadian fleabane during pregnancy; the plant may exert an unwanted vasoconstricting effect on uterine lining.

Canyon Bursage
Asteraceae/Sunflower Family

Ambrosia ambrosioides (Cav.) W.W. Payne *(Xanthidium ambrosioides)*
Canyon ragweed, Chicua, Yerba del sapo

Description

Canyon bursage is a moderate–sized, perennial shrub. The plant's deciduous leaves are serrated and grow into elongated triangles, 1"–2" wide by 6"–8" long. In the spring, the pistillate flowers mature into burs resembling a small cocklebur, and similarly they stick to clothing and animal fur. Of all the Ambrosias, Canyon bursage is the most tropical in appearance and requirements. It is dependent on summer monsoon rains and warm temperatures to survive in the southwest deserts. The name Ambrosia refers to the fragrance the leaf aromatics emit when the plant is crowded in canyons and the summer air moves through. It may not be the nectar of the gods, but it certainly is not rank as described by many botanical authors.

Distribution

Look for Canyon bursage growing along washes, canyons, and draws where rainfall deeply saturates the ground. From central Arizona it ranges south.

Chemistry

The foliage contains sesquiterpene lactones: damsin, damsinic acid, franserin, parthenolide, and psilostachyin c; flavonoid: hispidulin.

Medicinal Uses

Due to Canyon bursage's interesting chemical makeup it is a unique plant medicine. Considering that its uses are both varied and strong, it is no wonder that this species of Ambrosia is generally thought of as the most medicinally active of the genus (and most likely of longest traditional use throughout its range in Mexico). Both root and leaves are useful, yet medicinal qualities of each part slightly differs.

Canyon bursage root is a valuable remedy for the relief of menstrual cramps. In addition to being a reliable menstrual stimulant, the root is also useful when menses has become sluggish and there are corresponding pelvic feelings of inertia and congestion. Root preparations are additionally quieting to stomach and intestinal cramps. Its spasmolytic activity is especially well suited in diminishing rapid intestinal movement from acute viral or stress initiated diarrhea.

Although not an entirely different medicine, the leaves of Canyon bursage elicit other therapeutic responses. They tend to diminish allergic reactions that are head centered. Rhinitis from pollen, dust, and animal hair is abated through the leaves' use. Whole body allergic reactions that manifest as general itchiness or even hive breakouts are diminished. It is proposed that Canyon bursage is broadly antiinflammatory and specifically is diminishing to IgE antibody responses that play a central role in the allergy process.[6]

Indications
» Cramps, menstrual with pelvic congestion
» Menstruation, tardy, with stop and start bleeding
» Cramps, gastrointestinal
» Rhinitis/Sinusitis, allergy derived
» Allergy, body–wide

Collection
Harvest Canyon bursage leaves when they are dark green and aromatic, usually in mid–spring or during summer monsoon rains. Collect the roots throughout the winter or spring when available moisture has enlivened them, rather than in the fall when they are in a dry stupor. The plant's taproots may reach downward 3′–4′ so it is wise to collect in a wash where digging is easy.

As long as the roots are somewhat flexible they will make for good medicine. They should smell aromatic and earthy. Discard the more woody sections.

Several other species, namely Ambrosia deltoidea, A. artemisiifolia, and A. trifida have similar leaf uses. In comparing root qualities, these

6   Chemically, Burrobrush (Ambrosia monogyra and A. salsola) and Canyon bursage are closely allied. Medicinally there are many similarities between the two plants, though I believe Burroweed to be the weaker of the two. Traditional use in Mexico indicates Burrobrush be used in reducing sensitivity and pain in joint inflammations. Otherwise use Burrobrush leaf as a weaker analog of Canyon bursage leaf.

species are woody and less aromatic, therefore less therapeutic.

Preparations/Dosage

» FPT/DPT (60% alcohol): 20–60 drops 2–3 times daily
» Leaf infusion/Root decoction: 2–4 ounces 2–3 times daily

Cautions

Allergy suffers beware: this is a variety of Ragweed. Using the leaf or root poses little caution, but gathering the plant when in flower may cause a reaction due to pollen sensitivity. Considering Canyon bursage's stimulating effect on the uterus, it is not an herb to use during pregnancy. Consider it a short–term use medicine, not a long–term tonic.

Canyon Walnut
Juglandaceae/Walnut Family

Juglans major (Torr.) A. Heller *(Juglans microcarpa var. major, Juglans rupestris var. major)*
Arizona walnut, Arizona butternut, Black walnut, Nogal

Description

Canyon walnut is a hardwood deciduous tree, not unlike in form and character Black walnut (Juglans nigra) of the East. A mature tree can reach 50' in height and develop an impressively broad canopy. The trunk can span several feet in width; the bark is dark and becomes deeply fissured with age. Canyon walnut's leaves are composed of 5–7 pairs of large, lanceolate, and serrated leaflets with 1 terminating each bunch. Being monoecious, this tree has separate male and female flowers grouped on the same tree. The staminate flowers hang catkin–like, while the pistillate flowers, once pollinated, form fruit. As the fruit or walnut matures, the skin around the hull turns from green to brownish–black. The whole plant has a unique pungency, particularly when the leaves or fruit is bruised.

   In the spring, when Canyon walnut saplings are beginning to leaf out, they look very similar to Smooth sumac (Rhus glabra). Often the two plants can be found growing next to each other in mountain drainages. Crush a leaf and smell: the distinct Walnut family pungency is a definite give away, helping in plant identification.

Distribution

Canyon walnut is found along waterways and in canyons throughout central and southeastern Arizona. In New Mexico, it is predominant along the Gila River and southern Rio Grande Drainages. It is also found in isolated pockets in the southern part of the state. The tree as well can be found in southwestern Texas. Juglans californica, a closely allied species is found in drainage areas among foothills and valleys in warmer coastal–inland California.

Chemistry

Juglone, α–hydrojuglone and β–hydrojuglone, ellagic acid, gallic acid, caffeic acid, neochlorogenic acids, and germacrene d.

Medicinal Uses

One hundred years ago Juglans cinerea, or Butternut, was the most popularly used Juglans. Today it is Black walnut. Fortunately Canyon walnut, and nearly all other varieties can be used in similar ways.

In small, sub–laxative doses, Canyon walnut is tonifying and soothing to the gastrointestinal tract. It is mainly useful in quieting gastritis, irritative diarrhea, and intestinal inflammation with associated ileocecal irritation. Use the tea or tincture when chronic intestinal inflammation is causing nutrient malabsorption, particularly of fats.

Canyon walnut is moderately antispasmodic. It is called for when there is intestinal spasm with flatulence. Internally the plant also clears the skin of acne–like eruptions particularly when there is fat malabsorption dependent on poor diet.

In larger doses, Canyon walnut is laxative and is indicated in constipation when there is liver sluggishness. Equally, the plant is called for if constipation easily ensues when attention is not diligently maintained in keeping elimination regular. It is also of note that constrictive respiratory disturbances and systemic inflammatory issues sometimes are benefited by Canyon walnut through its tonifying effect on intestinal walls. Through this influence metabolites and toxins are less apt to enter the systemic circulation where they are likely to cause harm.

Although not systemically useful in limiting Candida infections, Canyon walnut can be helpful if the issue is limited to the gastrointestinal tract. Even though the plant is somewhat antifungal, berberine–containing plants such as Barberry or Oregongrape are more so, making Canyon walnut overrated in this area.

Sometimes recommended in diminishing fungal infections, the fresh plant applied topically as a poultice, whether from the green hulls, bark, or leaves, is rather caustic and can cause redness and blistering in even short exposures. Canyon walnut's juglone content is largely the causative factor – when the fresh plant is crushed larger juglone–like complexes are oxidized and reduced to juglone, which is responsible for both Canyon walnut's characteristic brown pigmentation and smell.

The plant is often touted as a vermifuge. Like so many other semi–laxative herbs with unique aromatics, in large amounts Canyon walnut occasionally gives positive results (pinworm or tapeworm), but all too often its influence is widely exaggerated.

Indications
» Inflammation, gastrointestinal
» Malabsorption, nutrient/lipid
» Cramps, intestinal
» Candida albicans infection, gastrointestinal tract involvement

Collection
Collect the green leaves when they are available. The hulls of the fruit should be harvested when they are just starting to turn brown. Collect the bark in long strips from secondary branches with no thickened fissured layer. Be aware that juglone will temporarily stain the skin brown.

Preparations/Dosage
» FPT/DPT (50% alcohol): 30–60 drops 2–3 times daily
» Infusion: 4–6 ounces 2–3 times daily

Cautions
Do not use Canyon Walnut during pregnancy or topically on abraded or sensitive tissues.

Other Uses
The kernels of the ripe fruit, like English walnut, are edible. As a stain or dye, the tincture or tea is only rivaled by Wild rhubarb in its impermeability.

Chaste Tree
Verbenaceae/Vervain Family

Vitex agnus–castus L.
Monk's pepper, Indian spice, Safe tree

Description
Chaste tree is a large and deciduous bush or small tree capable of obtaining heights of 20'–25'. The plant's 5–7 lance shaped leaflets are palmately
arranged and are supported on long leaf stems. Each leaflet is dark green
above and much lighter beneath. Like other Vervain family plants the
leaves are oppositely arranged along ridged upper stems. The spike–like
racemes form at branch ends. Individual flowers can be a variety of colors
– lavender, blue, and white are typical. They are tubular with 5 fused petals, which curl under at the flower's opening. The fruit are surrounded by
a hardened layer and resemble peppercorns. They are green when young
but dry to a purplish–grey. When crushed their smell is distinctly aromatic
and spicy.

Distribution
Originally a plant of the Mediterranean region, northern Africa, and western Asia, Chaste tree is now found throughout warmer parts of the United
States. The plant is extensively naturalized through the Southeast and is
found as a thriving ornamental in warmer southwestern regions.

Chemistry
Iridoid glycosides: agnuside, agnucastoside (a, b, and, c), aucubin, and mus-
saenosidic acid; flavonoids: casticin, orientin, isovitexin, luteolin, artemetin, and isorhamnetin; diterpenes: vitexilactone, vitexlactam, and rotun-
difuran; phenylbutanone glucoside: myzodendrone; α–pinene, β–pinene,
limonene, cineole, and sabinene.

Medicinal Uses
Chaste tree is best used by women whom suffer from premenstrual breast
tenderness and heavy menstrual bleeding associated with longer than 28–
day menstrual cycles. The plant is doubly indicated if lifestyle stress and
moderate to heavy caffeine use is present. While inhibiting excess prolactin

levels, Chaste tree supports proper corpus luteum function and therefore progesterone level. The plant is effective in rectifying anovulatory cycles, corresponding infertility, secondary amenorrhea, uterine fibroids, and excessive menstrual bleeding dependent upon excessive cellular proliferation of the endometrium – all essentially issues of progesterone deficiency.

Because of Chaste tree's alignment with the Vervain family, the plant tends to be a mild sedative, even outside of its diminishing effect on stress mediated prolactin release. This makes Chaste tree useful in premenstrual discomforts with associated anxiety, mood swings, and irritability. The plant is equally indicated in beginning stages of menopause. It combines well with Motherwort in reducing hot flashes and associated irritability.

Chaste tree is of use in reestablishing coherent menstrual cycles after prolonged estrogen–based contraception. Moreover, an important distinction between Chaste tree and oral or topical pharmaceutical–grade progesterone use is necessary: progesterone, as it naturally occurs, is a reproductive hormone that is dependent upon a healthy corpus luteum and proper levels of FSH (follicle stimulating hormone) and LH (luteinizing hormone). Chaste tree supports correct corpus luteum function and therefore is pro–progesterone. Oral or topical use of progesterone only affects tissues that respond to that hormone but does little for the corpus luteum. The use of progesterone for PMS or associated corpus luteum deficiency issues is a superficial approach to an underlying constitutional tendency. Additionally, it is important to note that the reproductive effect of Chaste tree may not be perceived immediately. Often several months of use is needed to notice the plant's benefit.

Traditionally Chaste tree, as its name implies, has been used as a male anaphrodisiac. I have observed several cases where amorous sensations have diminished under its influence. Lastly Chaste tree has been found to increase milk production in lactating women. It especially combines well with Verbena particularly if stress is a factor.

Indications
» Premenstrual syndrome
» Menstruation, heavy
» Anovulatory cycles
» Fibroids, uterine, subserous
» Perimenopause
» Lactation, insufficient

Collection
Strip the mature fruit from the branch ends. Dry normally.

Preparations/Dosage
» DPT (60% alcohol): 30–40 drops 2–3 times daily
» Fluidextract: 10–25 drops 2–3 times daily
» Capsule (00): 2–3, 2–3 times daily

Cautions
Do not use during pregnancy.

Chinchweed
Asteraceae/Sunflower Family

Pectis papposa Harv. & A. Gray
Manybristle chinchweed

Description
No more than a foot high, this small and mounding annual often rests on
the ground forming tidy circles. Its leaves are notably verdant in relation
to the tan–yellowish sandy soils in which it is found. Chinchweed's oil–
gland dotted opposite leaves are linear and 1"–2½" long by ¼"–½" wide.
The small yellow flowers form at stem ends and are comprised of both disk
and ray florets with the latter being the most prominent. They are also dotted with oil glands. When crushed the whole plant is strongly aromatic.
Its peculiar odor is not at all unpleasant. The plant's growth is signaled by
summer rains and is usually seen from mid–summer to early fall.

Distribution
Look for Chinchweed from 6,000' and lower. The plant is common to sand
and clay rich soils, mostly occurring on desert flats with Creosote bush and
Joshua tree yucca. It is found from Utah and southeast California through
to Arizona and New Mexico.

Chemistry
Specific constituents for Chinchweed are not known but the plant at least
contains flavonoids and volatile oils.

Medicinal Uses

Chinchweed is closely allied with Poreleaf, Dogweed, and Mountain marigold. Due to this botanical and chemical similarity, medicinal uses generally overlap. Chinchweed's principle area of influence is the gastrointestinal tract. The tea or tincture of Chinchweed is of use in relieving gas, bloating, and related indigestion. Its carminative effect often makes for an efficient hiccup remedy. The plant diminishes intestinal cramps and will lessen diarrhea in associated conditions. Colicky babies will find several teaspoons of the tea soothing. Chinchweed's volatile oils, when in contact with gastrointestinal tissue, tend to sedate, lessen spasm, and therefore provide relief. Mixed with a bitter tonic herb such as Tarbush or Rayweed it will enhance gastric stimulation by bringing more blood to the stomach walls through topical vasodilation.

Indications

» Indigestion with gas and bloating
» Hiccups
» Cramps, gastrointestinal, with diarrhea

Collection

Gather the whole plant – preferably pre–flower (so the flower's achenes do not develop and expand as a 'fuzz' after drying). The plant's aroma can become overwhelming after an hour or so of gathering.

Preparations

If using for tea, after drying, garble the leaves and smaller twigs from the larger stems. Discard the stems and roots.

Dosage

» Herb infusion: 4–6 ounces 2–3 times daily
» FPT/DPT (60% alcohol): 30–60 drops 2–3 times daily

Cautions

There are no known cautions with normal usage.

Other Uses

The Zuni rubbed Chinchweed on themselves as an aromatic perfume. It is a traditional dye plant of the Hopi. Both tribes used the plant as a seasoning.

Clematis
Ranunculaceae/Buttercup Family

Clematis drummondii Torr. & A. Gray *(Clematis dioica subvar. incana, C. dioica subvar. ochracea, C. dioica var. drummondii, C. nervata)*
Texas virgin's bower, Drummond's clematis, Old man's beard

Clematis ligusticifolia Nutt. *(Clematis brevifolia, C. neomexicana)*
Western virgin's bower, Western clematis

Clematis pauciflora Nutt. *(Clematis lasiantha var. pauciflora, C. nuttallii)*
Ropevine clematis

Description
Clematis is a perennial climbing vine, often exceeding 40′ in length. It is frequently seen clambering over trees, bushes, and fences. The older stem sections, closest to the ground, are woody and often have thin and fissured bark. Clematis attaches itself by tendril–like petioles, which wrap around supporting plants or structures.

The leaves are usually opposite and deeply cleft, entire, pinnate, or bipinnate. With the exception of Clematis hirsutissima, which has purple flowers, the flower sepals are petal–like and typically cream–colored. The mature fruit are small with attached long feathery tails. Actually they are converted styles, which lends descriptiveness to one of the plant's common names: Old man's beard.

Clematis drummondii can reach upwards of 30′ in length. Its lower stem bark is striated and tawny or light gray. Leaves are composed of sets of 3–5 leaflets and are cleft, lance shaped, or ovoid. They are grayish–green and covered with an ashy pubescence.

Clematis ligusticifolia has 5–7 toothed leaflets per leaf. The green leaves are hairless, except in southern California where the plant has wool-ly leaf surfaces.

Clematis pauciflora has 3–5 roundish leaflets that are toothed or lobed and sparsely hairy. Another California species appearing similar to the others is C. lasiantha or Pipestem clematis, and like its relatives, when chewed it is very peppery–hot.

Distribution

From 3,000'–4,000' look for Clematis drummondii along washes, canyons, and streamsides. This plant is found from Arizona eastward to southern New Mexico and central–southern Texas.

At various elevations C. ligusticifolia is widely found throughout the West. From British Columbia and North Dakota it ranges southward through much of the coastal and interior West. Look for the plant in moist places, bottomlands, and along streams.

Clematis pauciflora is largely found throughout southern California. From Los Angeles County to the Little San Bernardino Mountains, it ranges south. It is found, as are most species profiled here, in moist drainage areas, and along canyon sides, streams, and gullies.

Chemistry

Anemonin, protoanemonin, β–sitosterol, campesterol, chlorogenic acid, caffeic acid, and other compounds.

Medicinal Uses

The medicinal potency of Clematis can be largely rated by its acridity when chewed. It is in these acrid Buttercup family volatiles (anemonins and related constituents) that Clematis musters its array of effects.

A most telling use of Clematis is a Nez Perce application: if a horse had collapsed from exhaustion from being raced too hard a peeled section of Sugar bowls root (Clematis hirsutissima) was placed in its nostril. If the horse was revived by this, it would then be led to water, bathed, and (as the account declares) after a short time appear to suffer no ills from the experience – an equestrian herbal smelling–salt.

Many varieties of Clematis have traditionally been used to relieve headaches. Use the fresh plant tincture or leaf infusion to relieve congestive–type headache pain, particularly the pain of migraines. Since Clematis has a relaxing and dilating effect on brain lining vasculature, it is best used in beginning stage episodes. Applied as a preventative, use Clematis to abort a migraine when visual and auditory disturbances are first noticed, before the intense pain of an episode fully develops. If a strong cup of Coffee (or Periwinkle) has no effect on the migraine (or makes it worse) try Clematis.

Second to Clematis' dilatory effect, the plant is moderately antiinflam-matory when taken internally. It provides cyclooxygenase and interleukin inhibition. Certainly, this plays a role in its effect on headaches, but it is of value also in its application to rheumatoid arthritis, especially if aggra-vated by cold and damp weather. Relatedly, the freshly crushed plant or fresh plant tincture applied topically is rubefacient. As a counter–irritant it is well applied specifically to areas where the above description of joint pain fits.

Indications
» Migraines and migraine–like headaches, as an abortive
» Arthritis, rheumatoid
» Arthritis, as a counter–irritant (external)

Collection
After finding a sizable stand of Clematis, chew a leaf. If it is hot and ac-rid then it will make for good medicine; if not, then move on (new spring growth is usually the most acrid). Also it is common for acridity to vary from species to species. Prune and collect the leafing vine ends, with or without flowers.

Preparations
Drying diminishes Clematis' potency. The recently dried herb has some value, but even sealed it degrades quickly. The fresh plant tincture is the choice preparation.

Dosage
» FPT/DPT (50% alcohol): 10–40 drops 2–3 times daily
» Leaf infusion: 2–4 ounces 2–3 times daily
» Fresh plant poultice: use as needed, remove if the skin begins to redden

Cautions
As with most Buttercup family plants, do not use Clematis during preg-nancy. Although Clematis is useful in reducing the pain and inflamma-tion of rheumatoid arthritis, the plant is contraindicated in vasculitis, immunologically derived or otherwise. For some individuals even chew-ing a leaf can paradoxically usher in a headache. If this is the case, due to

idiosyncratic vascular dynamics, Clematis is not for you.

Cocklebur
Asteraceae/Sunflower Family

Xanthium strumarium L.
Common cocklebur

Xanthium spinosum L.
Spiny cocklebur

Description

Xanthium strumarium is a stout stemmed, 2'–3' tall annual. The plant's reddish–purple stem blotches are distinctive. The leaves are suspended on long petioles. They are heart shaped, or sometimes triangular, lobed, and irregularly toothed. Their stout leaf hair makes them rough to the touch. Both male and female flowers emerge from the upper leaf axils. Male flowers are small, inconspicuous, and situated above the bur–like female flowers. After being pollinated 2 flattened seeds mature inside each bur. These brown, oblong, and spiky pods have 2 prominent spines that stand apart from the other 400+ smaller spines. Each spine is recurved making the burs extremely efficient at attaching to anything – clothes, hair, and fur – which assists in its habitat expansion.

Xanthium spinosum is distinguishable from X. strumarium by its large, 3–pronged, and stiff spines protruding from the base of each leaf. The leaves are deeply lobed, narrow, covered with small white hairs, and have a distinctive white mid–vein.

Distribution

Although in the past Xanthium strumarium was limited in distribution, it is now found throughout many parts of the world. In our area, it is commonly found in the moist soils of drainages, roadsides, fields, and other areas where water tends to stand and is slow to drain. Although less common, X. spinosum is found in areas similar to where X. strumarium is encountered.

Chemistry

Sesquiterpene lactones: xanthinin, xanthatin, xanthanol, isoxanthanol, xanthinosin, and tomentosin.

Medicinal Uses

Cocklebur is primarily a plant affecting the urinary tract. As a soothing astringent diuretic, it is particularly useful in painful urination with corresponding mucus and blood tinged urine. Cocklebur even proves useful in injury–initiated hematuria. Whether recovering from prostrate, kidney stone, or other regional issues, the tea is usually found effectively astringent. Internally the plant also checks diarrhea and can be useful in diminishing sweating with attending weakness in non–infectious states (called colliquative sweating).

Topically Cocklebur is moderately antimicrobial. Applied to cuts, scrapes, and like it retards bacterial growth, and therefore facilitates the healing process. Like Canyon bursage and Brittlebush, Cocklebur tends to be drying to the sinuses, making it well used in allergic conditions of the area.

Indications

» Cystitis, with cloudy urine
» Hematuria, passive
» Diarrhea
» Sweating, colliquative
» Rhinitis/Sinusitis
» Cuts/Scrapes (external)

Collection

Gather the burs when they are fully mature, usually between mid to late summer. Be sure to wear gloves, as they are spiny. Fortunately, where there is one plant there are others, so finding an adequate amount of collectable material is usually not a problem. In the spring, the young bur–forming, leafing tops can be collected. Both parts of the plant are then dried.

Preparations/Dosage

» Herb infusion/Bur decoction: 2–3 ounces 2–3 times daily
» DPT (60% alcohol): 20–30 drops 2–3 times daily
» Oil/Salve/Wash: topically as needed

Cautions
Cocklebur should not be used continuously over 2 weeks. Large doses can irritate the kidneys and liver. Do not use during pregnancy or while nursing.

Copperleaf
Euphorbiaceae/Spurge Family

Acalypha lindheimeri Müll. Arg.
Three seeded mercury

Acalypha neomexicana Müll. Arg.
New mexican copperleaf

Description
Most species of Acalypha are either shrub–like or herbaceous. The leaves are petioled and arranged alternately along stem branches. The species profiled here are monoecious with either male and female flowers arranged separately in shorts spikes or staminate flowers in groupings above the pistillate flowers, both grouped on the same flower spike. The small seeds are contained in 3–celled capsules.

Acalypha lindheimeri is low–growing, deciduous, and shrub–like. The plant's weak branches often lay on the ground, only to be terminated by upright red flower spikes. The leaves are wedge–shaped, toothed, hairy, and have a mid–vein fold. Stem growth can be reddish–brown and is ridged and hairy.

Acalypha neomexicana is a small and weedy annual standing between 1'–3' tall. Its leaves are thin, light green, and ovoid with serrated margins. They often turn reddish–brown in response to cold stress. The female flowers have 3 distinctive red styles that are long and threadlike.

Distribution
Acalypha boasts over 250 species throughout both hemispheres, though they are primarily limited to the Tropics. Look for A. lindheimeri throughout the mid–elevation mountains of southeastern Arizona, then east to New Mexico and Texas. It usually is found in drainage areas and tucked around boulders.

From 2,400'–7,500', Acalypha neomexicana is found from central Arizona to New Mexico. It frequents disturbed sites such as ditches, roadsides, and over grazed rangelands. It also is found in more pristine areas like canyons sides and shaded rocky slopes.

Chemistry
The genus contains anthraquinones, cyanogenic glycosides, tannins, and other polyphenols.

Medicinal Uses
Copperleaf is best used topically to speed the resolution of slowly healing wounds and ulcers. It is particularly beneficial to skin afflictions that linger due to lack of regional vitality. Where it is applied topically, Copperleaf stimulates phagocytosis, cellular mediators, and general oxidation, literally delivering more biological activity to the area.

Acalypha indica, popularly used throughout India and Africa, is an effective snakebite remedy. Applied as a poultice it speeds venom detoxification and limits tissue destruction. Our varieties may have similar uses.

Use the tea or tincture as a modest lung medicine. Most will find it soothing to dry–irritating coughs, as well as mildly expectorating. It combines well with Wild cherry or Chokecherry bark.

Indications
» Wounds/Ulcers, poorly healing (external)
» Cough/Bronchitis, mild

Collection
When collecting Acalypha neomexicana, pull up the entire plant. Prune the flowering branch ends from A. lindheimeri. Dry normally.

Preparations/Dosage
» Oil/Salve/Poultice: use as needed
» FPT/DPT (60% alcohol): 30–60 drop 2–3 times daily
» Infusion (cold or standard): 2–4 ounces 2–3 times daily

Cautions
Although largely non–toxic, taken internally Copperleaf does have uterine stimulating effects, so it is not recommended during pregnancy.

Individuals with G6PD (glucose–6–phosphate–dehydrogenase deficiency) are advised not to orally use Copperleaf. The plant has been shown to cause intravascular hemolysis in these individuals.

Cottonwood
Salicaceae/Willow Family

Populus fremontii S. Watson
Fremont cottonwood, Alamo

Description
At maturity, Cottonwood is one of the largest trees in its habitat. It has a broad crown and can reach heights of 80'–90', though usually it is 50'–75' tall. A 2'–4' thick trunk is common and the trunk bark is grayish–brown and deeply furrowed. Younger limbs have a thin and grayish–white outer bark coating. The sticky–resinous leaf buds form into leathery and thick leaves. They are deltoid and taper to a terminal point.

Like all other Willow family plants, Cottonwood is dioecious. Each tree is either male or female; the flowers of both sexes form in catkins. The 'cotton' of Cottonwood is from the fibrous tufts that surround the mature fruit. In the spring the cottony–seed containing fuzz is carried easily by the wind. Cottonwoods are very fast–growing and in only several decades, are able to reach monstrous proportions. The upper limit of its lifespan is about 100 years.

Cottonwoods are not known for their strength. Their light and brittle wood makes for relatively weak branches. In strong winds these trees are notorious for dropping large branches, sometimes at the great inconvenience of campers sheltering beneath them. Similar to Aspen, another Populus, in a breeze the leaf patter is serene and peaceful.

Distribution
Cottonwood can be found along streamsides and washes where there is reliable underground water. From 6,500' and below the tree is found throughout the Sonoran and Mojave Deserts and generally from Trans–Pecos Texas, the southern half of New Mexico, through to Arizona, central Nevada, southwestern Utah, and central–southern California.

Chemistry

Phenolic glycosides: isoferulic acid, ferulic acid, caffeic acid, prenylferulate, prenylcaffeate, pinocembrin, pinostrobin, pinobanksin, chrysin, benzyl–(e)–caffeate, galangin, isosakuranetin, phenylethyl–(e)–caffeate, kaempferol, salicin, salicortin, salireposide, populin, temuloidin, and tremulacin.

Medicinal Uses

Although Cottonwood's phenolic glycoside content differs slightly from Aspen (Populus tremuloides) and Balsam poplar (Populus balsamifera), the tree's uses are very similar. The bark tea is a reliable, broadly acting antiinflammatory agent. Whether the pain is from an acute sport's injury or long–standing arthritis, Cottonwood's cyclooxygenase inhibition will prove relieving. If feverish, the plant lowers body temperature without potentially elevating it first, unlike Elder or many Mint family plants. The bark tea taken before meals is a useful gastric stimulant. Its tonic activity is mainly imparted through its bitterness.

Like many Willow family plants, Cottonwood is a urinary tract medicine. The bark tea is mildly diuretic and is indicated in chronic disturbances of the area. Use it in long standing kidney inflammation and prostatitis.

Externally the poultice, liniment, salve, or oil made with the leaf buds[7] is curbing to headache pain or the inflammation and swelling from contusions, sprains, arthritic joints, and the like. Topical preparations are soothing to burns and scrapes. These applications also retard infection due to being antimicrobial.

Indications

» Rheumatic conditions/Injuries (internal and external)
» Fever, mid to high
» Indigestion, asecretory
» Nephritis, chronic
» Prostatitis, chronic
» Burns (external)

Collection

In the spring, when new leaf buds are starting to develop find a secondary branch with light, non–fissured, smooth bark. With a saw cut the branch

7   Although Balsam poplar is the stronger topically applied Populus, use Cottonwood as a weaker substitute.

from its attaching point. Clip all of the small branchlets less than a finger–width from the collected branch and discard. With a knife, peel off the bark starting from the cut end. Once started the bark strips easily. Dry the bark in the open, out of direct sunlight.

Preparations/Dosage
» Bark decoction: 4 ounces 2–3 times daily; externally as needed
» External applications of leaf bud: as needed

Cautions
Use Cottonwood with prudence if taking anti–coagulant pharmaceuticals. The chance of Cottonwood triggering Reye's syndrome in feverish children is remote, but it is best to err on the side of caution and not use Cottonwood internally is these situations.

Creosote Bush
Zygophyllaceae/Caltrop Family

Larrea tridentata (Sessé & Moc. ex DC.) Coville *(Larrea divaricata var. triden-tata, Covillea tridentata)*
Chaparral, Greasewood, Little stinker, Hediondilla, Gobernadora

Description
At maturity Creosote bush is approximately 8'–10' tall by the same dimension wide. Flexible and ash–colored stems rise vertically, or nearly so, from the ground. When growing on desert flats it has a distinctive funnel–like appearance with the top section of the plant having the widest radius. Most of the leaves are collected in groupings among the upper branches. The leaflets are fused in pairs and resemble a 'packman'. The younger leaves are particularly resinous and shiny; with age, their luster diminishes. The yellow flower petals have a particular way of twisting perpendicularly to the reproductive center, making the arrangement fan–like. When mature the small and fuzzy seed capsules separate into individual wedges, called mericarps.

Beyond normal seed germination, Creosote bush has a relatively unique way of reproducing. The plant is very adept at cloning. If the root crown of Creosote bush is imagined as a circle, clones are created on the circumference, increasing the root crown's diameter. After a time the center roots die of old age, leaving numerous, physically independent, genetically identical clones spread out in a localized area. Eventually as this process continues plants spread outward like ripples in water created from a dropped stone. Some extremely old plants have been dated in southern California to be approximately 12,000 years old. The ages of these ancient plants were determined by calculating the known outward growth rates with the furthest distance genetically identical clones were apart from each other.

Distribution
Creosote bush can be found throughout the Sonoran, Mojave, and Chihuahuan Deserts. Huge expanses are found in valley bottoms and basins. It more sparsely occupies slopes and rocky hillsides.

Chemistry
Lignans: nordihydroguaiaretic acid, dihydroguaiaretic acid, isoguaiacin, and norisoguaiacin; flavonoids: apigenin, gossypetin, herbacetin, kaempferol, luteolin, morin, myricetin, and quercetin; saponins: larreagenin a, larreic acid, and erythrodiol; monoterpenes: α–pinene, limonene, camphene, linalool, borneol, camphor, and bornyl acetate; sesquiterpenes: α–curcumene, calamine, β–santalene, edulane, α–bergamotene, cuparene, β–eudesmol, farnesol, and α–agarofuran.

Medicinal Uses
If just one hallmark plant medicine of the southwestern deserts had to exist, it would be Creosote bush. When traditional perspectives are combined with science–based evidence, it is clear that the plant is a medicinal powerhouse. Creosote bush has three main spheres of influence: that of a unique antiinflammatory, antioxidant, and antimicrobial agent.

Creosote bush is sedating to pro–inflammatory mediators. Specifically leukotriene and leukocyte activities are diminished, as are histamine and prostaglandin release. This translates to Creosote bush being useful in lessening rheumatoid arthritis pain and soreness. For the above problem it combines well with Yucca or Turmeric. Many also find relief by soaking in a Creosote bush bath. Likewise, in asthmatic conditions the plant reduces bronchial airway stuffiness through diminishing the 'heat' of the autoimmune process. For other systemic autoimmune hypersensitivities, Creosote bush is often found helpful, as it is also profoundly antioxidant in nature.

Topically it has been used with success in resolving psoriasis and eczema, particularly in combination with deeper liver therapies – removing dietary and environmental allergens are also important steps.

Creosote bush inhibits several prominent sexually transmitted viruses. HPV (Human papillomavirus), the cause of genital warts (and cervical dysplasia), is sensitive to Creosote bush's NDGA (nordihydroguaiaretic acid) content as is HSV (herpes simplex virus) types 1 and 2. A sitz bath of Creosote bush tea applied twice daily or a suppository used before bed are both effective approaches for either virus affecting vaginal and/or cervical tissues. For men, topical use of the oil or salve is efficacious. Cold sores respond very well to external salve application.

Studies suggest the plant is both antimicrobial and antifungal. Moreover, observable results have been positive, particularly in the topical application of Creosote bush to infected cuts and skin punctures. It can be applied successfully to a wide array of fungal/yeast and bacterial infections. The salve is also a 'must–have' when living in venomous spider/cone–nose insect territories. Continually applied, Creosote bush is remarkable in reducing the deleterious effects of these varmints.

Although internal use of the plant as a cancer therapy is controversial at best, external preparations are useful in resolving a particular form of premalignant squamous cell carcinoma, called actinic keratosis. These reddened and sometimes scaly patches arise on sun–damaged skin. A topical pharmaceutical preparation of NDGA, called Actinex, is currently used in the treatment of the condition. By dry weight Creosote bush contains 2–10% of NDGA – whole herb preparations are adequate and chances of adverse skin responses are limited.

Indications
» Arthritis, rheumatoid (external and internal)
» Asthma
» Psoriasis/Eczema (external)
» HPV (external)
» HSV–1 and –2 (external)
» Cuts/Abrasions (external)
» Infection, bacterial/fungal
» Insect bites, venomous and non–venomous (external)
» Actinic keratosis/Sun–damaged skin (external)

Collection

Collect Creosote bush when new leaf growth is apparent. Using the thumb and forefinger, strip the leaves that form in clumps towards the outer–most branch ends. They are easily pulled from their branchlets. If the flowers and seeds are collected this also is fine. The application of a high proof alcohol will help in the removal of accumulated resins that often adhere to the hands though collection.

Preparations/Dosage

» DPT (75% alcohol): 20–40 drops 1–3 times daily
» Leaf infusion (cold or standard): 2–4 ounces 1–3 times daily (1 teaspoon of herb to 1 cup of water)
» Ointment/Oil/Salve: as needed
» Douche: 1–2 times daily

Cautions

Do not use Creosote bush while pregnant or nursing. The plant (internally) is also not recommended if there is existing liver impairment or inflammation. Do not use Creosote bush with other drug therapies that may affect the liver, be they over–the–counter or prescription.

There were a number of cases, particularly in the early nineties that implicated Creosote bush in triggering liver inflammation. Most cases were self–resolving after discontinuing Creosote bush. The two individuals who required liver transplants took the plant for over a year and either drank regularly an undisclosed amount of alcohol or took a cocktail of pharmaceutical and over–the–counter drugs. In summation Creosote bush is therapeutic if used properly by healthy individuals. Nevertheless, when used as a cure–all for long periods, Creosote bush can be problematic. There are no cautions for the plant's external use.

Crownbeard

Asteraceae/Sunflower Family

Verbesina encelioides (Cav.) Benth. & Hook. f. ex A. Gray *(Verbesina australis, V. scabra, Ximenesia encelioides, X. microptera)*
Anil de muerto

Description

Crownbeard is an herbaceous annual reaching several feet in height. Its grayish–green triangular leaves alternate along slender stems. The small sunflower–like flowers are yellow; each disk petal is 3–notched. Being an aggressive seeder, it is very adept at self–propagation. One distinctive characteristic of Crownbeard is its odor. When the plant is brushed against or when downwind from a stand, it exudes a distinctive smell. It is both difficult to describe and unique.

Distribution

Crownbeard enjoys a large range throughout the West. Look to disturbed roadsides, embankments, culverts, and low–lying ditches. Occasionally it can be found in relatively pristine areas, often under Mesquites or on wash banks. In urban areas look to the undeveloped city block with low–lying land.

Chemistry

Triterpenes: amyrin, taraxastanone and taraxasterol; flavonoids: quercetin and hyperoside; steroidal glycosides: campesterol, daucosterol, and β–sitosterol.

Medicinal Uses

Crownbeard is used externally to reduce inflammation from a variety of causes. It works well to diminish swelling from contusions, bruises, insect bites and stings, burns, and other similar injuries. Alone or combined with St. John's wort, use it topically on chicken pox, shingles, and cold sore outbreaks. Rashes from allergic reaction are quieted. Additionally through its application, tissues more quickly heal from cuts and incisions.

In combination with Tobacco or Datura, it makes a good hemorrhoid treatment. Traditional Mexican use calls for the plant's application in gastritis and ulcerative conditions of the stomach. Indicated through research, Crownbeard's inflammatory mediating effects on troubled mucosa and dermal tissues, have promise when applied to a wide array of topical problems.

Indications

»   Injuries, acute (external)
»   Shingles/HSV, type–1/Chicken pox (external)

» Hemorrhoids (external)
» Gastritis
» Ulcer, gastric

Collection

Collect the upper half of the plant when it is in flower. In the Southwest this will be after the plant has responded to summer rains. Dry loosely arranged in paper bags or on a cardboard flat. When harvesting the plant be mindful of various insects and worms – it seems to be a favorite food source for a wide array of creatures.

Preparations/Dosage

» Herb infusion: 2–4 ounces 2–3 times daily
» External applications: as needed

Cautions

There are no problems for external use. Internally in excessive amounts, Crownbeard may slow respiration and decreases blood pressure. Do not use Crownbeard while pregnant or while nursing. To be on the safe side, use the plant internally for two weeks at a time, and then rotate to another plant.

Crucifixion Thorn

Simaroubaceae/Quassia Family

Castela emoryi (A. Gray) Moran & Felger *(Holacantha emoryi)*
Burro thorn, Corona de Cristo

Castela texana Torr. & A. Gray *(Castela erecta subsp. texana, C. nicholsoni var. texana)*
Goatbush, Allthorn, Mexican bitterbush, Bisbirinda, Chaparro amargo, Chaparro amargoso/a

Description

Castela emoryi is a leafless large shrub or small tree capable of displaying intricately branched (and formidable) forms. Branches are composed of stoutly pointed thorn–appearing branchlets. A fine–felty pubescence covers the younger light–green branches. Both male and female flowers are greenish–yellow, somewhat insignificant, and form separately on each plant – making this species and others dioecious.

Fruit clusters persist on female plants for years[8]. From a distance these clumps appear deceivingly like Mistletoe infestations. Upon closer inspection Castela emoryi's 'drupes' become apparent. When each matures they separate and spread star–like; each wedge or carpal contains a single seed. Growth of established adult plants is slow, with sporadic spurts likely dependent upon adequate rainfall.

Slightly more tame and less stout in appearance, Castela texana is also a thicket–forming shrub. Branchlets are light in color and form thorns at growth ends. Unlike C. emoryi, which is basically leafless, C. texana develops linear, 1" by ¼" leaves, often with reflexed margins. Upper leaf surfaces are shiny; lower surfaces are fine hair–covered. Flowers are small, showy, and red to orange. C. texana's fruit are berry–like, red, and about the size of a large pea.

Distribution

The bulk of Castela emoryi is relegated to Arizona's Sonoran Desert. Widely dispersed throughout low–elevation silty bottomlands and flat plains between mountain ranges, individual plants are often isolated or exist in small pockets. In California, the largest colony on record exists in the designated 'Crucifixion–thorn Natural Area' – just north of the Mexican border in Imperial Valley. Look for C. texana in the Chaparral–brush zones of central–to–southern Texas to northeast Mexico.

Chemistry

Lactones for Castela nicholsoni (other species are similar): chapparin, glaucarubol, glaucarubol 15–isovalerate, glaucarubolone, and chaparrinone.

Medicinal Uses

Nearly all of our uses for Crucifixion thorn originate from traditional Mexican use of Castela texana or better known south–of–the–border as Chaparro amargo or Chaparro amargosa. Since the beginning of the 20th century it has successfully been used for diarrhea and associated distresses from

---

8   It is hypothesized that this reproduction characteristic is a remnant of an ancient time when the plant relied upon large herbivores (sloth, horse, and/or camel) for seed dispersal.

drinking 'bad water' or eating 'bad food'.

Like Tree of heaven, Crucifixion thorn is best used to quell diarrhea and dysentery caused from protozoal infections. Additionally, like most Quassia family plants, these shrubs are active against an array of gastro-intestinal tract pathogens, particularly Entamoeba histolytica (the cause of traveler's diarrhea) and Giardia. Crucifixion thorn is doubly beneficial because the plant is also tonic and rebuilding to weakened or damaged intestinal wall mucosa (which can easily result from these types of infections). Use Crucifixion thorn when diarrhea has become chronic and has caused a general state of weakness. It combines well with Silk tassel (Garrya spp.) or Wolfberry (Lycium spp.) if there is accompanying intestinal spasm or cramping.

Preparations are of use in combination with conventional medications for malaria. The quassinoids found in Crucifixion thorn have modest anti-malarial activity. The plant's use may prove beneficial with drug-resistant/tenacious strains.

Lastly, a little-known use for Crucifixion thorn is its application to vaginitis, especially if caused from Trichomonas vaginalis. This protozoon is responsible for trichomoniasis, considered in some circles to be the most common sexually transmitted disease. Daily internal doses in combination with the external sitz bath of Crucifixion thorn tea is nearly as effective as Flagyl (Metronidazole). At the very least, use Crucifixion thorn in tandem with the antibiotic if resistance issues are a problem.

Indications
» Diarrhea and dysentery from amebic and protozoal infections
» Vaginitis, from Trichomonas vaginalis

Collection
With pruners clip the outer 6"–12" of spiny tips from extended branches. Often only 3–4 clippings from one large plant is all that is needed for an adequate supply. To protect against skin punctures while collecting, wear gloves and a thick long-sleeved shirt. Be sure to leave fruit-bearing branches intact for future seed dispersal.

Preparations/Dosage
» FPT/DPT (50% alcohol): 30–60 drops 3–4 times daily
» Branch decoction: 4–6 ounces 3–4 times daily

» Sitz bath: 2–3 times daily

Cautions
Excess amounts of Crucifixion thorn are apt to cause nausea – a common complaint with large quantities of most bitter plant medicines. The use of the plant for several days at a time is not a problem during pregnancy, but longer use may be: quassinoids are biologically active and may have unwanted effects on the reproductive environment if used longer–term.

Cudweed
Asteraceae/Sunflower Family

Pseudognaphalium leucocephalum (A. Gray) Anderb. *(Gnaphalium leucocephalum)*
Lemon cudweed, Everlasting, Gordolobo, Manzanilla del rio, Lampaquate

Description
In the Southwest Cudweed is one of the first plants to show new leaf growth in the late winter. The woolly, grayish–green, and lance–shaped leaves form tidy mounds under the previous year's dried flower stalks. At this stage, they appear as strange, sand–loving sea anemones. Older perennials can send up 30–40, 1'–2' high stems upon which in the late spring, small, white, and papery flowers appear. The inflorescences look to be roundish buttons; numerous bracts surround the reproductive flower parts at the center. As the flowers age the bracts radiate outward giving the inflorescence a disk–like appearance. The entire plant is sticky and smells like a mixture of Lemon verbena and freshly crushed pine needles.

Distribution
Cudweed can be found from 2,000'–5,000' in and around sandy gullies and wash bottoms where water flows seasonally. It ranges from southern Arizona to southern California.

Chemistry
A similarly used Cudweed, Pseudognaphalium oxyphyllum, contains diterpenoids, flavonoids, acetylenic compounds, and carotenoids.

Medicinal Uses

Use Cudweed in the initiatory stages of bronchitis particularly if there is a dry and painful cough. The tea is useful in dislodging mucus that is difficult to expectorate. Its mild diaphoretic properties are excellent in dry feverish states when the body is hot and flushed. Lending credence to Cudweed's beneficial effect on the pneumal environment are its genus–wide, mild antimicrobial properties: a number of Cudweed species have been found to inhibit several Staphylococcus and Streptococcus strains making it a good fit for bacterial associated bronchitis.

Most other species of Cudweed not profiled here, particularly the aromatic varieties, can be used in a similar fashion. Though slightly less stimulating, the Antennaria and Anaphalis genera are closely related to Pseudognaphalium and can be used in associated ways.

Indications

» Cough, dry and painful
» Bronchitis with difficult expectoration
» Bronchitis with dry fever

Collection

From early to mid–summer collect the herb just before flowering. Dry either loosely or in bundles. It is a pleasing plant to collect – paper bags, hands, and pruners all become lemon scented. Pruner blades will sometimes stick together from the buildup of lemon waxy–aromatics...the hardships.

Preparations/Dosage

» Herb infusion: 4–8 ounces 3–4 times daily

Cautions

It is best not to purchase Pseudognaphalium/Gnaphalium or Gordolobo as it is locally known in the Southwest and northern Mexico, in commerce. Confusion starts in that Gordolobo is also a common name for Mullein (Verbascum thapsus) in the area, which is not necessarily a major problem for the uses of both plants are somewhat similar. The more important issue is Pseudognaphalium's/Gnaphalium's occasional adulteration with Senecio longilobus, a rather toxic pyrrolizidine alkaloid–containing plant. In Mexico where the bulk of this plant is collected, it is occasionally mistaken for this look–alike Senecio. This mix–up was responsible for the tragic death of a 6–month year–old baby in Tucson during the late 70's. Cudweed on the other hand is completely non–toxic and can be used freely.

Cypress
Cupressaceae/Cypress Family

Cupressus arizonica Greene *(Callitropsis arizonica)*
Arizona cypress

Cupressus sempervirens L.
Italian cypress

Description
Standing 50'–90' tall, Arizona cypress's crown is stately and pyramidal. Like Alligator juniper, the outer brownish–gray bark is often cross–fissured in a checkerboard pattern, but can also be thin, fibrous, and vertically layered. In the case of Cupressus arizonica var. glabra the outer branch and tree bark typically sheds leaving a smooth, brownish–red exposed under–layer.

Arizona cypress's leaves form as small scales. Collectively the branchlet groupings are fan–like. Although not visible, universally each leaf has a small, central pitch–secreting gland that appears as a small white dot. Pollen bearing cones are small and form at branch ends. At full development the seed bearing cones are large. Normally they are between ½"–1" across, round, and formed of 6–8 flattened scales. At maturity, the surrounding cone scales open and extend, thereby releasing the seeds.

In its native environment Italian cypress is a large tree reaching 75'–100' in height. Planted as an ornamental in foreign climates it is usually smaller. The common variety cultivated in the West is conical to columnar shaped. The bark is smooth and gray when young, though with age it becomes vertically furrowed. Each scale–like leaf, like Arizona cypress, has a small resin gland on one side. The cones are brownish–gray and are about an inch across.

Distribution
From 3,000'–6,000' Arizona cypress is found from central–eastern Arizona, southwestern New Mexico, to Big Bend National Park in Texas. Look for

the tree in mid–elevation canyons and along streamsides. It particularly gravitates to northern facing exposures. Typical plants found in proximity are Manzanita and Canyon walnut.

Italian cypress is native to the Mediterranean area. Due to the fact that the tree has been cultivated for thousands of years, its original distribution is impossible to determine with accuracy. It is planted as an ornamental throughout parts of the Southwest. Large, mature trees can still be found around remnant homesteads, farms, and old churches.

Chemistry

For Cupressus sempervirens: volatile constituents: pinene, fenchene, camphene, myrcene, carene, terpinene, limonene, phellandrene, terpinolene, cymene, cubebene, copaene, caryophyllene, humulene, muurolene, germacrene d, cadinene, and calamenene; sesquiterpenes: cedrene, elemene, carvacrol, acoradiene, selinene, acoradine, curcumene, cuparene, calamenene, and cedrol.

Medicinal Uses

Due to Cypress's aromatic composition the plant's main area of influence is over the genitourinary and bronchial systems. Secondly, as a topical medicine it is well applied to numerous microbial involvements. Part stimulant and part astringent with bacterial–fungal inhibiting overtones, the plant is worthy of note.

Suffers of chronic bladder and urethra infections will surely benefit from Cypress tea or tincture. It is best applied to long–standing infections that come and go and seem to be dependent upon general weakness of the area. Corresponding urinary tract pain and irritation will likewise be soothed. If the Heath family group of plants (Uva–ursi, Cranberry, or Manzanita) don't have an impact on the area, most likely Cypress will.

Urinary incontinence, again from tissue weakness (not organic disease), should lessen under the plant's use. For bed wetting children, Cypress combined with Mullein root, is often useful. An emotional component usually needs to be addressed in such cases. In older individuals with poor bladder control Cypress's tonic effect often has perceivable results, particularly when small amounts of urine are uncontrollably voided due to coughing, sneezing, or laughing. If in older men prostate enlargement or irritation of the area is the cause of dribbling of urine, the plant should be reached for first. Cypress's benefit here is due, not any shrinking of prostrate tissue per se, but to its antibacterial/tonic properties.

Cypress's aromatics are inhibiting to Giardia lamblia and the ameba group of organisms, particularly Entamoeba histolytica. The tea or tincture can be used alone, or more successfully with Castela emoryi or Ailanthus altissima.

Externally Cypress is a valuable treatment for a number of fungal involvements. Various nail and skin fungi are inhibited by the plant. Application of the undiluted essential oil should be used several times a day. The same is well applied to both common (Verruca vulgaris) and genital warts (Condyloma acuminatum). Be the growths upon the genital or anal region, continual application is important. Dilute the essential oil with olive oil for more sensitive tissues. Alone or in combination, Cypress makes an excellent vaginal suppository for cervical dysplasia[9]. Over time (6 months) I have observed class 2 and 3 cases resolve completely.

Women will find a douche or sitz bath made with the leaves resolving to vaginal Candida infections. Other areas typical of Candida growth are around the mouth, under arms, and between mid–section rolls of skin. Although more rare, intestinal/systemic infections can result in more severe cases. For such situations combine Cypress with Desert willow or Pau d'arco. Use it both externally and internally. Babies whom suffer from thrush (oral Candida infections) will additionally benefit from external application of the tea or ointment.

Similar to Cypress's fungicidal properties, the plant is also distinctly antibacterial. External preparations are well applied to poorly healing wounds, bedsores, and other slow–to–heal afflictions. As a mouthwash, Cypress is beneficial to the oral environment due to its inhibition of plaque–forming enzymes. Used twice a day in this way, especially before bed, the plant is one of our best for gingivitis prevention.

Alone or in combination with Marshmallow, Cypress makes an excellent stimulating poultice. Applied to abscesses it certainly will encourage their resolution – through coming to a head or resolving internally. This effect is due not so much to the plant's antibacterial overtone, but to its stimulation of innate immunity.

9   The majority of cases are caused by HPV (human papillomavirus) infection, a viral group responsible for common and genital warts and most cases of cervical cancer. Cervical dysplasia is used to describe pre–cancerous tissue alterations usually caused by HPV. Detectable through a 'pap smear' (papanicolaou test) results are ranked in classes: class 1 – normal to class 5 – cancerous.

Although not a systemic immune stimulant like Echinacea, Cypress does stimulate innate immunity, and to a lesser degree, acquired immunity (T–cell activity) within contacted surface tissues. Doubtlessly this is one reason why the plant has such a noted effect on the urinary tract. This is one region where Cypress's aromatics are excreted as waste products to be eliminate from the body. To our benefit these compounds affect the surrounding urinary tissues.

Like the urinary tract, the bronchial environment is also influenced by Cypress's aromatics. Used as a potent antimicrobial agent, as well as a local immune stimulant, successful application will be seen in a number of respiratory–centered distresses. In chronic bronchitis when expectoration is copious, mucus is green or yellow, and the lungs feel weakened, Cypress will be of great value. Lingering coughs, as a symptom of a chronic or sub–acute bronchial condition, usually will cease or lessen.

Specifically the plant stimulates resident macrophages or dust cells within the alveoli. These specialized cells are at the center of the lung's infection–fighting process. Like the plant's involvement with the urinary tract, Cypress's aromatics, which are excreted and therefore dispersed throughout the lungs, serve to inoculate the area with antimicrobial/immune–stimulating constituents.

Steam applications of Cypress also affect the respiratory tract. In many ways, this method is more direct, and ultimately more effective than internal preparations. With it, topical exposure is achieved. It is as if an ointment is being applied to pneumal mucus membranes. For chronic sore throats (pharyngitis), laryngitis, and even bacterial oriented strep throat, Cypress–based stream inhalation will be most beneficial. Both the recently dried leaf and the commercially purchased essential oil are fine articles that will produce a medicated steam.

Cypress has been used with success in treating valley fever, or coccidioidomycosis, caused by the soil mold Coccidioides immitis, commonly found in alkaline soils throughout the hot and dry Southwest. It is responsible for flu–like symptoms of fatigue, fever, headache, aches and pains, and cough. Susceptibility is largely dependent upon immune system condition, overall vitality, and racial/genetic disposition.

The isotonic tea as an eyewash is applied several times a day for the elimination of styes. Both budding and mature styes will be affected by treatment, but early–stage styes will more reliably resolve. If the eyewash gives negligible results, try applying a small amount of ointment directly to the stye.

Cypress is best used as an emmenagogue when menses is slowed from uterine laxity or illness/stress.

In conclusion, Cypress shares many of its therapeutic qualities with other Cypress family plants, in fact consider them all more–or–less interchangeable.

Indications

» Infection, urinary tract, chronic
» Urinary incontinence/Bed wetting
» Prostrate irritation
» Traveler's diarrhea (Amebiasis)/Giardiasis
» Infection, fungal (external)
» Cervical dysplasia/HPV/Common warts/Genital warts (external)
» Infection, Candida (external)
» Wounds/Bedsores, poorly healing (external)
» Gingivitis (external)
» Abscess (external)
» Bronchitis, chronic
» Pharyngitis/Laryngitis/Strep throat (gargle)
» Valley fever
» Ocular styes (eyewash)
» Menses, to stimulate

Collection

Gathering Cypress is fairly straight–forward. Collect new spring–summertime growth by snipping off outward leafing branch tips. Prepare fresh, or dry first by laying out well spaced.

Preparations

Most methods of Cypress delivery are commonly known – tea, tincture, etc. The steam inhalation technique, lesser so: in a large pot bring 1 gallon of water to a boil, add 4 ounces of Cypress leaf (or 10–15 drops of the essential oil), reduce to a simmer, and inhale the volatile oil infused steam.

Dosage

» FPT/DPT (60% alcohol): 20–40 drops 2–3 times daily
» Leaf infusion: 4–6 ounces 2–3 times daily

» Inhaled steam from the infusion or essential oil: 5 minutes 2–3 times daily
» Spirit: 10–20 drops 2–3 times daily
» Essential oil, topically applied: as needed
» Oil/Salve/Ointment/Poultice: as needed
» Suppository: 2 times daily, once before bed
» Eye wash: 2–3 times daily

Cautions

Do not use during pregnancy or while nursing. Excessive doses of internal and steam derived preparations can irritate the lungs, upper respiratory tissues, and kidneys. Italian Cypress has the tendency to pick up heavy metals in its bark. The leaves may or may not exhibit the same tendency, but since no plant should be collected next to industrial sites or roadways, this should not pose a problem.

Datura

Solanaceae/Nightshade Family

Datura wrightii Regel. *(Datura inoxia subsp. quinquecuspida, D. metel var. quinquecuspida, D. meteloides)*
Sacred Datura, Toloache

Datura discolor Bernh. *(Datura thomasii)*
Desert thornapple

Datura stramonium L. *(Datura tatula)*
Jimsonweed, Jamestown weed

Description

Datura wrightii is a large, herbaceous, 2'–3' high perennial. Often mound–like in growth it has large, grayish–green, and alternating leaves. They are ovoid in shape, can be toothed and deeply lobed, and are narrowed at the tip and wider at the base. Flowers are folded into compact swirls before they fully form. After unfurling the large funnel–form flowers are white and sometimes suffused with violet. They originate from forks in the upper branch stems. Each flower does not last long: they open in the evening and typically wither by the middle of the next day. The green circular seedpods droop (as opposed to D. stramonium's, which remain upright) and are covered with coarse and slender spikes. After drying the brown pods contain numerous, compact, small kidney–shaped seeds that are light brown. With the exception of the flower, as with most species, the whole plant smells like rancid peanut butter.

Datura discolor is a smaller, 1'–2' high annual with grayish–green, several inch long, ovate leaves. The flowers, which emerge from a 2"–3" long calyx, are trumpet–like. The floral tube is constricted, opening widely at the very end. The corolla is white, tinged with violet, and is 10–toothed. The spiny, drooping seedpods contain numerous black seeds.

Datura stramonium is a leggy annual sometimes reaching 5' in height. Its coarsely lobed–toothed leaves are dark green and prominently veined. Depending on variety D. stramonium's trumpet shaped flowers are 3"–5" long and are either white or purplish. The upright seedpods are situated between the upper stem branches. The seeds are dark brown to black at maturity.

Distribution

Datura wrightii is widely distributed throughout the Southwest. It is found from central California, east to Colorado and Texas, and south through Arizona and New Mexico. Creosote Bush Scrub, Coastal California Sage Scrub, and mid–elevation Grasslands are just some of the numerous vegetative zones it frequents. From sea level to nearly 6,500' look for the plant along slopes, washes, and other drainage areas. Fond of disturbed soils, it is often found along roadsides, the sides of washes, and over grazed rangelands.

Datura discolor is limited to elevations below 2,000', but on occasion it has been reported up to 4,000'. The plant is found from southeastern California to southern Arizona. Disturbed soils, washes, and other drainage areas are places where the plant is found.

Datura stramonium, native to Tropical America or North America (no one is sure), is sporadic in distribution. Look for it in vacant lots and waste areas throughout the country.

Chemistry

Tropane alkaloids for Datura discolor (D. wrightii is very similar): hyoscine (scopolamine), apohyoscine, norhyoscine, hyoscyamine, meteloidine, tropine, atropine, littorine, and cuscohygrine; flavonoids: quercetin and kaempferol.

Medicinal Uses

Datura is one of the strongest analgesic herbs we employ. Its influences are strong, drug–like, and potentially toxic. The leaf poultice, oil, or liniment will give symptomatic relief to swollen and painful sports injuries, contusions, sprains, and the like. The freshly pureed leaf, alone or mixed with Prickly pear or Aloe leaf pulp, is soothing and will relieve pain from burns. Datura's broad antimicrobial activity keeps infection from setting in damaged and susceptible tissues. Datura oil applied to hemorrhoids reduces swelling and associated discomfort. A liniment soaked cloth applied to a throbbing headache is pain relieving. The same external preparations are applied over the lower abdomen for menstrual and intestinal cramps. It is also of use in diminishing back or leg muscle spasms from over work, injury, or stress.

The dried foliage of Datura can be crushed and rolled to make a cigarette, packed into a pipe, or simply lit on a small tray. Several inhalations of the smoke are taken for the bronchial constriction of asthma or severe allergies from pollen or insect stings. It by no means is safer or more effective than regular medications, but it works in a pinch when the latter are not available. In lieu of the inhaled smoke a small piece of leaf (½″ x ½″) can be chewed and eaten. This will help to keep the respiratory passages open until regular medical help becomes available. Datura exerts an anticholinergic effect on bronchial passageways, opening the area so air can be more fully inhaled and exhaled.

Indications

» Injuries, acute, unbroken skin (external)
» Burns (external)
» Hemorrhoids (external)
» Cramps, menstrual/intestinal (external)
» Spasm, muscle (external)
» Bronchial constriction (smoke)

Collection/Preparations

The entire plant is medically active, although the leaves and/or seed capsules are the most practical part to collect. Dry the leaves and seed capsules for storage or tincture fresh for the liniment.

Dosage

» Liniment: topically 2–3 times daily
» Oil/Salve/Wash: topically 2–3 times daily
» Smoke: several inhalations 2–3 times daily in acute situations

Cautions

Apart from smoking small amounts, Datura should not be used by the in-experienced internally, though in small amounts the plant does have thera-peutic uses. Regularly ingested the plant is toxic and can lead to a number of nervous system derangements, temporary or permanent blindness (in extreme cases) not being the least of them. Do not use if pregnant or nurs-ing. Prolonged external application can affect the central nervous system. Remember, exposed surface area plus duration equals dosage. Stop exter-nal application if dizziness or altered vision develop.

Desert Anemone
Ranunculaceae/Buttercup Family

Anemone tuberosa Rydb.
Desert windflower

Description

Desert anemone is a small, thin–stemmed, and herbaceous perennial. The divided, semi–succulent leaves are few and mostly originate from the base and mid–stem. The 1½″ diameter flowers are positioned at stem ends and are composed of approximately 10 modified sepals, appearing as petals. The sepals are often white but can also have pink or purplish twinges. Seeds are woolly and form in dense and cylindrical heads. Throughout much of Desert Anemone's western expanse, the plant is dependent upon winter–spring rains to sprout above ground. In dry years, it is common for the plant to forgo rising from its small tuberous roots.

Distribution

From 2,500′–5,000′ Desert anemone is found on slopes and hillsides crowd-ed around rocks and boulders and occasionally under shrubs and trees.

The plant is found from the southern California Desert to southern Nevada and Utah, through much of Arizona to New Mexico.

Chemistry
Lactones: anemonin and protoanemonin; triterpenoid glycosides; flavonoids.

Medicinal Uses
The understanding of Desert anemone comes to us largely from the associated use of Anemone patens or Pulsatilla by 19th and 20th century Eclectic and Homeopathic physicians. For all practical purposes, Desert anemone is just as useful as Pulsatilla and can be used in similar ways.

The plant is both an emotional and physical medicine. Use small doses of the fresh plant tincture in episodes of fear, gloom, and depression. The plant works well if there is also restlessness, insomnia, and nervous system debility from substance abuse or too much cerebral work. Desert anemone has the ability of lifting the spirits and making needed rest possible. It is of particular use to individuals whom are thin, cold–bodied, and tend to have reactive skin allergies.

The plant is not to be underestimated in calming premenstrual mood fluctuations and first or second day period cramps. In addition, slowed menses tends to be stimulated particularly if there is congestion of the pelvic area and the lower back. Ovarian pain during ovulation or otherwise is sedated by Desert anemone.

For men, the plant proves relieving to epididymitis, idiosyncratic orchitis, and varicoceles. For both men and women, through its restorative influence on venous circulation, relief is provided to most chronic inflammations of the genital/urinary systems. Use it also if there is decreased libido and lack of sexual interest from stress, overwork, and nervousness.

Like Clematis, Desert anemone is useful as a migraine abortive. Use it as a cerebral vasodilator when visual disturbances and the classic migraine aura is noticeable. 5–10 drops directly on the tongue can stop the progression almost immediately, although if in the advanced pain of a migraine Desert anemone may worsen the episode (try Coffee, Kola nut, or Guaraná in these cases).

In small amounts, Desert anemone is a gastric stimulant: through a dilatory effect it provides more blood to the stomach walls. For indigestion and digestive atony combine the plant with bitters and take the combo before meals, particularly if the emotional picture fits as previously described.

The plant reduces cerebral spinal fluid and intraocular pressure: it is of value in mild cases of glaucoma. An eyewash made with the fresh plant tincture is of use in chronic conjunctivitis, ocular irritation, and styes. Topically, Desert anemone, like Clematis, is rubefacient. It will cause vasodilation, bringing more blood to surface tissues in a matter of minutes. A fresh plant poultice is well-applied to chronic arthritic conditions. Be sure to remove the poultice at the first sign of redness.

Indications
- » Depression
- » Debility, genital/urinary system
- » Libido, decreased
- » Dysmenorrhea/Amenorrhea
- » Migraines, beginning stages
- » Indigestion
- » Glaucoma
- » Conjunctivitis/Styes (eyewash)
- » Arthritis, as a counter-irritant (external)

Collection
Gather the foliage – leaves, flowers, and stems – in early spring. Chew a small piece of leaf to better understand the plant's medicinal effect. There is no need to dig the tubers since the above ground portion is medicinally potent.

Preparations
Desert anemone's potency tends to degrade through the drying process (and storage) so it is best to tincture a fresh batch every year or two. For an eyewash mix 10 drops of fresh plant tincture in 2 ounces of isotonic water; make fresh daily.

Dosage
- » FPT: 10–20 drops 2–3 times daily
- » Fresh poultice: apply as needed
- » Eyewash: 3–4 times daily

Cautions
Desert anemone can be mentally unsettling for some people (mesomorph body type). Too much of the plant will cause gastric irritation and diarrhea. Do not use it in acute vascular conditions that are inflammatory. In addition, like most other Buttercup family plants do not use Desert anemone during pregnancy due to its dilatory effect on the uterine environment.

Desert Barberry
Berberidaceae/Barberry Family

Berberis fremontii Torr. *(Mahonia fremontii)*
Fremont barberry, Holly–grape

Berberis haematocarpa Wooton *(Mahonia haematocarpa)*
Red barberry

Berberis trifoliolata Moric. *(Mahonia trifoliolata)*
Algerita

Berberis nevinii A. Gray *(Mahonia nevinii)*
Nevin's barberry

Description
The species profiled here are large, spiny–leaved shrubs with 6–petaled yellow flowers, mostly juicy fruits, and deeply yellow inner roots. Berberis fremontii is often a large shrub, occasionally reaching 12'–15' in height. The stiff bluish–green leaves have 3–7 pinnately arranged, spiny leaflets. The developing fruit are yellow or sometimes red. At maturity they are bluish–black.

Berberis haematocarpa is a large many–branched shrub obtaining 12' in height. Each leaf is comprised of 3–7 lanceolate leaflets with 1 terminating the group. Flowers are yellow and 6–petaled. At maturity, the berries are pea–sized, red, and juicy. Berberis trifoliolata can reach heights of 10'. This dense shrub has stiff, grayish–blue and spiny leaves that are composed of 3 leaflets. After flowering, the red, tart, and juicy fruit develop.

Berberis nevinii is also a large rounded shrub. Although not as stiff as the others, the holly–like leaves are comprised of 3–5 spiny, lanceolate leaflets. The yellow flowers form in loose racemes. The fruit are yellowish–red to red and are succulent.

Distribution

Berberis fremontii is found between 4,000'–7,000', mostly throughout Desert Grasslands and Juniper–Pinyon Woodlands. Occasionally it is found lower in elevation in isolated pockets in southern California. From these holdouts the plant is found east through southern Nevada, central–northern Arizona, Utah, Mesa and Delta Counties in Colorado, to the Sandia Mountains of New Mexico.

From 3,000'–7,500' Berberis haematocarpa ranges from Arizona where the bulk of the plant cuts a diagonal swath across the state just below the Mogollon Rim, east to central–south New Mexico and finally to Trans–Pecos Texas. The plant is commonly found in Desert Grasslands and in Oak Woodlands.

Berberis trifoliolata's most significant range is along the Pecos River Basin in New Mexico and south and east through most of western Texas. The plant is prominent on hillsides and slopes overlooking drainages. Below 2,000' in southern California, M. nevinii is found in Coastal Sage and Chaparral Scrub habitats. Look for the plant in arid sandy valleys.

Chemistry

For Berberis general: isoquinoline alkaloids: oxyacanthine, berberine, columbamine, corydine, isocorydine, glaucine, jatrorrhizine, magnoflorine, obaberine, obamegine, palmatine, thaliporphine, and thalrugosine; lignan: syringaresinol.

Medicinal Uses

Desert barberry's medicinal activity is mainly defined by its isoquinoline alkaloid (berberine) content and even though the plant does contain other compounds, it is this group that remains the most important. As other berberine containing plants, consider closely related Oregongrape (Berberis aquifolium) and Common barberry (Berberis vulgaris) identical in use.

There are not many other botanicals that rival Desert barberry's broad antimicrobial activity. Dozens of bacterial and fungal strains are inhibited by the plant. Some of the more common ones that are known to present clinical symptoms that call for Desert barberry's use are: several Bacillus varieties (known to cause food poisoning), Escherichia coli (urinary tract and intestinal infections), numerous Staphylococcus and Streptococcus strains (responsible for a myriad of systemic and local infections), and at least four Salmonella varieties (also a causative factor in food poisoning and intestinal infections). Candida albicans, Trichophyton mentagrophytes, and Microsporum gypseum are several fungal strains that Desert barberry inhibits.

For systemic infections Desert barberry combines well with Echinacea or Myrrh. For local or topical involvements, the same applies, though the plant can be used solely with good results. Of course serious infections (systemic infections usually are) will be most efficiently treated with conventional antibiotics (barring allergy or bacterial resistance).

Although bitter, it makes an effective gargle for bacterial–derived pharyngitis. The nasal wash or repeated gargle is a sound treatment for sinusitis as well. Combined with internal use (along with Echinacea or Myrrh) its upper–respiratory cold–fighting power should not be underestimated.

Although not an exact match to Goldenseal, Desert barberry is similar enough to serve as a decent replacement for this overused, yet potent plant. Combined with Bayberry or Yerba mansa, Desert barberry's influence will be found nearly identical to Goldenseal's.

Desert barberry will be found effective as a sitz bath or douche for vaginal Candida infections. Likewise thrush in babies and children will be remedied with topical application. Fungal infections that affect the skin and nails respond particularly well to long soaks in the root decoction.

Food poisoning from a variety of pathogens will be remedied. Not only is Desert barberry, like Oregongrape, directly inhibiting to these microbes, it also reduces the harmful effects of related endotoxins. Combine Desert barberry with Peppermint or Ginger if there is nausea or intestinal cramping and with Slippery elm or Marshmallow if irritative diarrhea is evident.

Although Simaruba family plants such as Castela emoryi or Ailanthus altissima, due to their array of quassinoids and tannins, prove better medicines for traveler's diarrhea (amebiasis) and even giardiasis, Desert barberry is a worthy second choice. The plant is inhibiting to both Entamoeba histolytica and Giardia lamblia.

The tea or tincture is a simple bitter tonic. Being of use in simple indigestion, it is best taken several minutes before meals. Like many other bitter herbs, Desert barberry is overtly a hepatic stimulant. As a chologogue/choleretic the plant triggers bile manufacture. This activity provides more of this digestive substance for lipid breakdown and assimilation. If plagued by general feelings of sluggishness, frontal headache, and nausea, all upon eating a high–fat meal, the tea will particularly be of use. Occasionally the plant will benefit suffers of anorexia by enlivening the gastrointestinal tract, therefore promoting hunger sensations. Of course psychological issues should be addressed in tandem.

Underlying the plant's bile augmentation is an interesting hepatic anti-inflammatory activity. This reduction of cellular inflammation is decidedly useful to hepatitis sufferers. Elevated hepatic enzyme levels tend to lower with the plant's use. Although Desert barberry's hepatoprotective influence is not as strong as Milk thistle's, the plant can still be used with therapeutic results in many situations if there is liver distress.

Due to Desert barberry's effect on the liver, it has a marked influence over inflammatory skin conditions. Poorly healing skin, reactive dermatitis, including eczema, and acne are the plant's main indications. Most likely Desert barberry's healing effects are due to its influence over hepatic detoxification pathways – the plant neutralizes hepatic/systemic/local metabolites and toxins. Topical use of the ointment/oil/salve will compound the plant's benefit to these conditions. Even psoriasis with its related scaly skin patches of dermis over–proliferation responds well to Desert barberry application.

Another interesting effect of the Berberis–Mahonia group of plants is their influence over liver suppression in mild cases of hypothyroidism[10]. Use Desert barberry as a stimulant when thyroid and hepatic activities are both depressed. It can be used with conventional thyroxin therapies. Lastly, as an eyewash the isotonic tea is useful for bacterially–derived conjunctivitis.

Indications

» Food poisoning
» Infection, bacterial/fungal (external and internal)

10   In overt and particularly sub–clinical hypothyroidism liver functions are often slowed due to insufficient or ineffective T3 (triiodothyronine) and/or T4 (thyroxine) levels. Proper activity upon the liver by these thyroid hormones are important for normal hepatic function. Any number of liver–centered metabolic insufficiencies run hand–in–hand with thyroid deficiency. Poorly healing skin and nails, slowed intestinal movement, and increased allergic reaction, are several of the more common presentations.

- » Pharyngitis
- » Sinusitis/Common cold
- » Infection, Candida (external and internal)
- » Thrush (external and internal)
- » Amebiasis/Giardiasis
- » Indigestion/Poor protein and fat digestion, assimilation
- » Hepatic sluggishness or inflammation
- » Poorly healing skin/Dermatitis/Eczema/Psoriasis (external and internal)
- » Hypothyroidal induced hepatic deficiency
- » Conjunctivitis, bacterial (eyewash)

Collection

Desert barberry, being a substantial woody bush, will have similar semi–woody roots. Its subterranean mass is composed of 1 or several larger tap roots and many secondary spreading lateral or semi–lateral roots. On larger bushes lateral roots should be gathered, ensuring the plant's continuation and future harvest.

Drier locales will produce roots with less water content. These should be dried and used for tea and/or the dry plant tincture. Hydrated roots, collected in wetter seasons/soils, can be dried and used in the aforementioned ways, or prepared through tincturing fresh.

Preparations/Dosage

- » Root decoction/Cold infusion: 4–6 ounces 2–3 times daily
- » FPT/DPT (40% alcohol): 30–60 drops 2–3 times daily
- » Capsule (00): 1–2, 2–3 times daily
- » Fluidextract: 10–30 drops 2–3 times daily
- » External preparations: as needed

Cautions

There are few cautions considering Desert barberry's significant therapeutic activity. Normal doses will not create any problem. One obscure exception is Berberine's possibility of causing hemolysis in babies with G6PD (glucose–6–phosphate–dehydrogenase) deficiency. Also extremely high doses may erratically affect blood pressure, and common sense tells us – do not use if there is a biliary blockage.

Other Uses
Desert barberry is commonly planted as a hedge–divider shrub. The fruit is mildly sour–sweet and very refreshing. It is a useful edible and jam/jelly base.

Desert Cotton
Malvaceae/Mallow Family

Gossypium thurberi Tod. *(Thespesia thurberi, Thurberia thespesioides)*
Wild cotton

Description
As a many branched, moderately sized shrub, Desert cotton can reach heights of 12′, although 3′–5′ is more common. Its petioled leaves are palmately 3–5 parted; each lobe is pointed. The large, showy, and white flowers are occasionally crimson spotted. They exist in groups of 2–3, are 5–petaled, and 2″–3″ across. The seed capsules are round and 3–parted. Look closely for the small cotton fibers after the seed capsules split open from age.

Distribution
In the United States, Desert cotton is limited in distribution to central and southeastern Arizona. Look for the plant along washes, streamsides, and canyon bottoms – at higher elevations, look to draws, among foothills, and rocky slopes. Although limited in range it is a fast–growing, successful plant. It sprouts easily and is not difficult to propagate.

Chemistry
Phenolic acids, condensed tannins and the sesquiterpene: gossypol.

Medicinal Uses
Desert cotton is primarily an emmenagogue. Use the fresh plant tincture (the most active preparation) when menses is slow to start and there is pelvic and lower back pain. In larger doses, the plant may even cause mid–cycle spotting. Alone or in combination with other herbs that address constitutional imbalances, Desert cotton is of help in resolving uterine and breast fibroids. In combination with Wild peony or Hopbush, it is well suited in

diminishing first and second day period cramps. Modern day use of Desert cotton primarily originates from the Eclectic Doctors, traditional Mexican use, and the associated use of Gossypium spp. by slaves throughout cottonlands in the Southeast.

In recent years, gossypol's physiological effects have become better known. The compound is largely present in the seed and in smaller amounts throughout the whole plant. Initially discovered in China where the poor in times of scarcity eat cottonseed meal cakes, the plant disrupts fertility in men. In at least one study funded by the World Health Organization it was determined that proper sperm formation in the testes was inhibited. Apparently, spermatogenesis is negatively affected by gossypol's disruptive effect on the testes' sertoli cells. In a small percentage of men taking the isolated compound, fertility was impaired permanently. In conclusion, men are ill advised to use Desert cotton.

Indications
»   Menses slow to start with back and pelvic pain
»   Fibroids, breast and uterine

Collection
In the spring when Desert cotton is beginning to develop leaves, dig the slender and woody taproots. On older plants they become forked and are larger.

Preparations
Clip the fresh roots into small ¼"–½" sections and tincture fresh. A more potent tincture of Desert cotton is made by peeling and then tincturing just the outer root bark. The color of the tincture is a striking dark red.

Dosage
»   FPT: 20–40 drops 2–3 times daily

Cautions
Do not use while pregnant or nursing. Men are advised not to use Desert cotton and additionally should avoid foods containing cottonseed oil.

Desert Lavender
Lamiaceae/Mint Family

Hyptis emoryi Torr.
Bee sage

Description
Desert lavender is a medium to large–sized shrub. As a member of the Mint family, it has the typical square stem–opposite leaf arrangement. Both the leaves and young stems are covered with a woolly pubescence. The flowers are purplish–blue and are arranged in clusters among the upper leaves or in terminal spikes. When in flower it attracts a whole assortment of pollinators, particularly bees. When the plant is in full bloom the lavender scent is heady.

Distribution
From 4,000' and below Desert lavender is found from southern parts of the California Desert, north to southern Nevada, and east throughout much of southwestern Arizona and southern New Mexico. At lower elevations Desert lavender is commonly found along washes and on alluvial fans. Where it is slightly colder at higher elevations, the plant prefers rock and boulder strewn foothills. The rocks warmed by the sun during the day act as atmospheric heating blankets enabling Desert lavender and other warmth loving plants such as Brittlebush to thrive.

Chemistry
General essential oil content for the genus: α–pinene, β–pinene, thymol, and rosmarinic acid; lignans; flavonoids.

Medicinal Uses
Desert lavender is a sedative of mild strength. Like Verbena, a distant cousin, its sedation on the central nervous system makes usage appropriate in times of emotional stress and anxiety. It is particularly useful as a sudorific in febrile states when the skin is hot and dry and the mind and body are tired and agitated. A cup or two of the hot tea is a sure way to break a mild to moderate fever.

Topical application of Desert lavender makes an excellent injury dressing. Many Mint family plants contain aromatic oils that are antimicrobial and anti–inflammatory. Desert lavender being no exception to this, limits bacterial growth, capillary bed inflammation, and subsequent leakage. A salve or poultice applied to burns, contusions, cuts, and other injuries speeds healing.

For Candida infections, the leaf infusion applied as a wash to involved tissues will help speed resolution. Sitting in a warm sitz bath of tea for 15–20 minutes is one of the better methods of directly limiting Candida growth affecting vaginal and urethral tissues.

For inflammatory conditions of the stomach such as gastritis and peptic ulcer, Desert lavender has the distinct effect of not only reducing inflammation (through several mechanisms, but notably by inhibiting pro–inflammatory prostaglandin synthesis) but also of reducing hyper–secretions of the stomach. Hydrochloric acid secretion is lowered with internal usage of the plant making these overly acidic, hyper–secretory conditions more apt to heal.

Indications
» Anxiety/Tension/Sleeplessness
» Fever, dry, moderate temperature
» Gastritis/Peptic ulcer
» Burns/Cuts/Scrapes (external)
» Infection, Candida (external)

Collection
Gather the plant in the spring or summer when new growth is apparent. Crush a leaf – it should be hydrated and lavender scented. Collect the leaves and flowers since these parts have the greatest concentration of medicinal aromatics.

Preparations/Dosage
» Leaf infusion: 4–8 ounces 2–3 times daily
» FPT/DPT (60% alcohol): 30–60 drops 2–3 times daily

Cautions
Due to Desert lavender's array of uterine stimulating aromatics, it is unwise to use it during pregnancy.

Desert Milkweed
Asclepiadaceae/Milkweed Family

Asclepias subulata Decne.
Rush milkweed, Leafless milkweed

Description
Desert milkweed is a large, 4'–6' tall, clump–forming perennial. Its green-ish–white stems are rush–like, slender, and form in numerous clusters that rise up from a central root crown. Its leaves, which are small and thread–like, are ½"–1" long and usually fall away quickly in response to drought or cold temperatures. The light yellow flowers form in umbels at branch ends and have a typical milkweed structure: 5 united sepals and 5 petals, which generally appear dumb–bell like. The seedpods are 2"–3" long by a ½" wide and upon opening release densely tufted seeds to the wind. When any part of the fresh plant is broken, a white–milky sap exudes from the wound.

The form of Desert milkweed's roots is variable in relationship to the soil types in which it grows. In fine sandy soils it often has one main tap-root reaching depths of 3'–4'. Roots with tortuous secondary rhizomes oc-cur in soils that are composed of gravel and larger sediments.

Distribution
From nearly sea level to 2,500' Desert milkweed is found from Clark Coun-ty, Nevada, south along the Colorado and Gila River Basins in Arizona, to lower portions of the California Deserts. The plant is commonly found next to washes, sandy and gravely plains, and on dry and rocky slopes. Desert milkweed is cold sensitive, a factor that limits its range in more northerly locations.

Chemistry
At least three cardenolide–type cardiac glycosides; lignan: lariciresinol.

Medicinal Uses
The medicinal quality of Desert milkweed dovetails nicely with most of the other Milkweeds: they all tend to have more usage similarities than differ-ences. More specifically, Milkweed species are unified by their stimulation

of the heart, skin, uterus, and gastrointestinal tracts.

Desert milkweed (and other closely related species such as Asclepias erosa, A. albicans, and A. linaria) is known to have a high cardiac glycoside content. Therefore Desert milkweed will affect the heart more profoundly than other commonly used Milkweeds, i.e. Pleurisy root (A. tuberosa) and Antelope horns. Think of Desert milkweed as Antelope horns plus more 'heart'. Unlike Antelope horns, the plant does not have a coherent history of traditional use, or at least one that has been recorded or revealed, so approach its use with prudence.

The plant's lung and skin centered attributes are predictable; its influences on the heart, uterus, and intestines, lesser so. For a general overview of medicinal uses and indications, see Antelope horns.

Collection

Gather the roots in the fall or winter. Sandy soils will make for easy digging, but that luxury is not always available. After picking a large and robust plant, dig a hole to one side, 1' or so out and 1'–2' deep. Slowly work in to the main root mass; collect any secondary rhizomes that are encountered. When the main root mass is reached take a pound or two while being careful as not to disturb the entire root complex.

The latex of Desert milkweed can be harvested by chopping ½" sections from the stems starting at the top of the plant. After several minutes, the latex will harden. Scrape it off with a razor blade or knife; chop another piece from the same branch ½" lower, repeat. Like harvesting Wild lettuce latex, the process is very time consuming. If the plant is flowering leave at least half for seed reproduction. After drying to a glue–like consistency, the latex can be tinctured or rolled into pellets and swallowed.

Preparations

Clean the roots of any debris and embedded stones. Chop them into ¼"–½" pieces; then dry and store. It is good to use the dried roots within a year's time. After this point the root oils tend to oxidize and become rancid.

Dosage

- » Infusion (cold or standard): 2–3 ounces 2–3 times daily
- » DPT: (50% alcohol) 5–20 drops 2–3 times daily
- » Fluidextract: 5–10 drops 2–3 times daily
- » Latex tincture: (50% alcohol) 5–20 drops 2–3 times daily

127

» Latex pellets or capsules (00): 1–2, 2–3 times daily

Cautions

Desert milkweed has the same cautions as Antelope horns, with possibly additional heart concerns. Until more is known, I caution against its combing with heart–affecting pharmaceuticals.

Desert Willow
Bignoniaceae/Bignonia Family

Chilopsis linearis (Cav.) Sweet *(Bignonia linearis, Chilopsis glutinosa, C. saligna)*
Mimbre, Sauce

Description

Desert willow[11] is a small deciduous tree with alternate drooping leaves. The tree's conspicuous funnel–like white, pink to purple flowers are of note due to their size and pleasant fragrance. Like Trumpet flower, the narrow and elongated seedpods hold numerous seeds that take to the air by way of their winged outer coating.

Distribution

Desert willow needs ample water supply to thrive, making it is a reliable indicator of permanent underground water. Most often the tree can be seen growing along washes, gullies, and other drainage areas. It is found from southwestern California, north to Kansas, where it has been added recently to the state's flora, south through Oklahoma and Texas.

Chemistry

Unknown, besides typical cyanin flavonoids in the flower.

Medicinal Uses

A leaf infusion of Desert willow applied externally, like other Bignonia family plants (Pau d'arco), is antifungal. It is useful in treating various skin and nail fungi and Candida infections. A douche or sitz bath of the tea is an excellent localized application for vaginal Candida infections, especially if from antibiotics or steroid use. Additionally, the internal tea can be

11   Desert willow is completely unrelated to true Willow – Salix spp.

systemically useful in the above–mentioned issues.

Desert willow has promise in treating valley fever or coccidioidomy-cosis. The responsible organism, Coccidioides immitis, is a soil mold common in the arid American Southwest. Exposure in susceptible individuals is usually self–resolving but can manifest fever, malaise, cough, and skin rashes among other symptoms. In immune compromised and dark skinned individuals, deeper pulmonary and systemic infections are more apt to result. Allopathic intervention is warranted in these advanced cases. Desert willow in combination with pulmonary inoculating herbs such as Ligusticum or Lomatium is of use in mild to moderate cases of valley fever infections.

Indications
» Candida albicans and other fungal infections (internal and external)
» Valley fever

Collection
In late spring to early summer when Desert willow is in bloom collect the last 8″–12″ of branch ends, as these will have the newest leaves and developing flowers. The bark can be collected, as it is also medicinally active (this only being necessary in colder times of year when the leaves are absent).

Preparations/Dosage
» FPT/DPT (50% alcohol): 30–60 drops 2–3 times daily
» Leaf infusion/Bark decoction: 4–6 ounces 2–3 times daily
» Douche/Sitz bath/Wash: 2–3 times daily

Cautions
There are no known cautions with normal usage.

Other Uses
Being a fast grower, adaptable to various planted conditions, and ascetically appealing, Desert willow is often cultivated as an ornamental throughout the Southwest.

Dogweed
Asteraceae/Sunflower Family

Dyssodia pentachaeta (DC.) B.L. Rob. *(Thymophylla pentachaeta)*
Golden fleece, Golden dyssodia, Parralena

Dyssodia acerosa DC. *(Thymophylla acerosa)*
Needle leaf dogweed, Prickleleaf dogweed

Dyssodia papposa (Vent.) Hitchc. *(Tagetes papposa)*
Fetid marigold, Pagué

Description
Dyssodia pentachaeta is a small plant, usually standing no more than 8"–
10" high. This perennial forms in clumps and has opposite and pinnatifid
leaves arranged in 5–7 linear divisions. The yellow flowers are ½" across
and form on slender stalks above the foliage clumps. When crushed (as
with most Dogweeds) the leaves emit a pleasant scent.

Dyssodia acerosa is another small perennial. It has a woody base and
stands approximately 1' tall. The dark green linear leaves are attached to
the main stems either oppositely or alternately. Small circular glands are
noticeable on the leaf surfaces. The yellow flowers are ¾" across and form
at branch ends.

Dyssodia papposa is a small 4"–16" tall annual. Its leaves are 1"–2"
long, pinnatifid, and linearly divided. The flowers are small and tend to be
surrounded by inconspicuous rays. All Dogweeds are aromatic. Judge the
medicinal potency of various species by their pungency.

Distribution
Dyssodia pentachaeta is found from 2,500'–5,600' sporadically throughout southern California, southern and western Arizona, and parts of New
Mexico to Texas. Roadsides are a typical favorite of the plant. Otherwise, it
is found in washes and on dry slopes and hillsides. D. acerosa ranges from
western Texas to southern and central New Mexico, southeast and central
Arizona, and finally to the Grand Canyon area. Look for this Dogweed on
limestone soils between 3,500'–6,000'. D. papposa inhabits a wide range of
territory: from Illinois to Montana, then south to Louisiana and Arizona.

Throughout the arid Southwest, it is often found in waste places – ditches, field sides, etc.

Chemistry
Flavonoids, acetylenic thiophenes, and monoterpenes.

Medicinal Uses
Dogweed, like closely related Mountain marigold and Chinchweed, is used as a tea to settle an upset stomach and to relieve bloating and fullness. It serves as a useful carminative, working nicely to relieving gas pains from poorly digested food dependent upon stress or general debility of the area. A small amount of the tea is likewise good for colicky babies. Additionally, when the stomach lining is inflamed from an over production of hydrochloric acid, an excess of alcohol or other gastric insults, Dogweed tea will be found soothing.

Indications
»   Gastritis
»   Indigestion/Gas pains/Colic

Collection
Prune the upper herbage just before or during flowering. Throughout the Southwest, Dyssodia papposa is best collected between late July and August, after it has responded to Monsoon rains. The other perennial Dogweeds are collected throughout the spring and summer.

Preparations/Dosage
»   Leaf infusion: 4–8 ounces 2–3 times daily

Cautions
There are no known cautions with normal usage.

Elder

Caprifoliaceae/Honeysuckle Family

Sambucus canadensis L. *(Sambucus caerulea var. mexicana, S. nigra subsp. canadensis, S. mexicana, S. oreopola)*
American black elderberry, American elder, Mexican elder, Flor sauce, Flor de saugua, Saúco

Sambucus nigra subsp. cerulea (Sambucus cerulea, S. caerulea var. neomexicana, S. glauca, S. neomexicana)
Blue elderberry

Description

Sambucus canadensis is a small tree reaching 15'–35' in height. Given the tree's propensity for dropping branches in favor of conserving water (a common survival mechanism of desert trees) its appearance can be unruly and non–uniform. The branches have an erratic way of growing and can be angled, arched, drooping, or nearly horizontal. Upon maturation, the crown is wide and rounded. The bark is finely fissured and yellowish–brown. The leaves are composed of 3–9 ovoid, thickened leaflets which are smooth above, occasionally hairy beneath, and have finely serrated margins. When crushed they are strong–scented, almost unpleasant. The small cream flowers form in flat–topped clusters 6"–8" across. The fruit that follow are clustered, pea–sized, sweet, and very edible.

The closely allied Sambucus nigra subsp. cerulea is smaller, at least at higher elevations. The leaves are composed of 3–9 lanceolate leaflets and like S. canadensis has edible fruit.

Distribution

Sambucus canadensis has a significant distribution throughout the country. Its main territory is from the Rocky Mountains east to the coast. Although missing throughout the northwestern states and the Great Basin Desert, the tree is found from coastal mountainous regions of southern California to central–eastern Arizona, the Gila River and Rio Grande Drainages in New Mexico, and finally to the Nueces River area of western Texas. In the Southwest it is common to drainages at elevations of 2,000'–4,000'.

Sambucus nigra subsp. cerulea is common throughout the coastal and inter–mountain West. It is typically a tree found with Douglas fir and other conifers.

Chemistry

Sambucus canadensis: triterpenes: α–amyrin palmitate, balanophorin, oleanolic acid; flavonoids: cyanidin, cyanin, quercetin, rutin; monoterpene: morroniside; sterols: campesterol, β–sitosterol, stigmasterol; sambucine.

Medicinal Uses

Elder's use as a diaphoretic is as old as it is reliable. Its application to low to moderate fevers, when the skin is hot and dry is its most specific indication. Though Elder does reliably promotes sweating, timing and preparation are also important factors. It is best if the tea is hot and drunk during the latter part of the day[12] and before bed. Keeping the body warm with a hot bath and/or blankets will also promote sweating. Once the fever breaks, usually in the middle of the night, it is important to change perspiration soaked clothes and bedding. Depending on the severity of the infection, this cycle may repeat itself several times before finally resolving. Well–applied diaphoretic therapies work in accordance with the body's innate intelligence. In essence, elevated body temperate, or fever, serves to stimulate immune system activity. Fever is not an illness, but a natural infection–fighting defense. Modern conventional approaches typically strive to suppress a temperate through Tylenol, etc., truly opposing the body's proven infection–fighting approach.

Children will certainly benefit from Elder, and other diaphoretics such as Spearmint and Ginger. Fevers dependent upon wintertime viral infections: common cold, sinusitis, bronchitis, and even the flu, will be dealt with efficaciously. If the fever resolves the infection has as well. Depending on secondary symptoms Elder will combine well with Echinacea, Wild indigo, or other immune stimulants.

There are times when diaphoretic approaches to an infection are inadequate. In these times, when fevers are dangerously high, or when other threatening symptoms delineate a severe infection, the usefulness of pharmaceuticals outweighs their drawbacks.

Elder has been found to inhibit varieties of Salmonella and Shigella

---

12   Body temperate tends to naturally rise throughout the day and into the evening, so using Elder in accordance with the body's innate rhythm only makes sense.

dysenteriae, so its application to gastroenteritis coincides with traditional use for the plant in Guatemala. The leaf and flower tea are somewhat similar in effect to now popular Elder fruit or Elderberry preparations, which relatively speaking are recent in application.

External preparations are mildly antimicrobial and antifungal. Elder is well applied to these situations particularly if the affected tissues are edematous, slow to heal, and tend to ulcerate.

Indications

» Fever, dry, low to moderate temperature, with lung centered viruses
» Fluid retention
» Wounds, edematous, ulcerated, slow to heal, with or without bacterial or fungal involvement (external)

Collection

Prune the last foot or so from the flowering branch ends or collect the flowers and leaves separately. The fruit clusters can be collected in bunches and then separated from their respective small stems.

Preparations

The flowers are simple enough to dry; the leaves though can be problematic. If they are not dried quickly they often mildew, turn black, and become unusable. Dry quickly in a warm and arid environment or use a dehydrator.

Dosage

» Leaf/Flower infusion: 2–4 ounces 2–3 times daily, though often less of the leaf tea is needed as it can be more stimulating

Cautions

Although species and populations within species can differ markedly in concentrations of sambucine and cyanogenic compounds, it is best to use flower and leaf preparations, versus the bark which tends to contain higher amounts of these compounds. The berries of Red elderberry (Sambucus racemosa), common to the higher-elevation western mountains, contain large amounts of these compounds and therefore should generally be avoided, though they were once rendered safer to eat by various American

Indian tribes by applying heat[13], through boiling, steaming, or roasting.

Some sensitive individuals may find the flower and especially leaf preparations mildly laxative. Like any vasodialating herb, Elder can potentially increase body temperature very briefly before promoting diaphoresis. Be mindful of this when using it in higher febrile states.

Other Uses
Any fruit of blue–black Elder types are sweet and edible raw. Jams, jellies, and wines are made from them.

Elephant Tree
Burseraceae/Torchwood Family

Bursera microphylla A. Gray
Torote, Copal

Description
A distinctive plant, Elephant tree grows from small tree to large bush sizes. Its best–known characteristics are its inflated, disproportionately large trunk and tortuous lower limbs. These inflated areas are covered with a thin papery–peeling white bark of sorts. Thin inner green and reddish layers are found intermingled with the exfoliating outer whitish layer. Newer branch and twig growth is reddish–brown.

Elephant tree's leaves are comprised of 8–16 pairs of small linear to linear–oblanceolate leaflets. The inconspicuous small flowers give rise to ½″ diameter ovoid capsule. When crushed the fruit has a distinct aromatic–citrus scent. On close inspection of Elephant tree's branches, depending on the season (or in response to injury), hardened or semi–hardened sap nodules are often visible. All parts of Elephant tree are pleasantly balsamic–aromatic.

Distribution
The bulk of Elephant tree is found throughout lower elevation southwestern Arizona. A number of sizable stands are also located in California just west of the Salton Sea Basin to Anza–Borrego State Park.

The tree is almost always found on rocky slopes and hillsides, above

13   Heat has been shown to reduce cyanogenic compounds significantly.

drainages and washes, where nighttime temperatures are slightly warmer. Being extremely frost sensitive this positioning allows for optimal growth, especially when on the edge of its range in more northern latitudes.

The epicenter of 'New World' Bursera, is found within Mexico which hosts around 85 species of the 90–100 found from Peru to the United States' Southwest. B. microphylla, covered here, is the northern–most grower of the group.

Chemistry
Essential oils, triterpenes, sterols, lignans, and flavonoids.

Medicinal Uses
Due to Elephant tree's medicinal potency it should be considered a 'top–tier' southwestern plant medicine, on–par with Creosote bush, Yerba mansa, and Ligusticum. Moreover, Elephant tree's therapeutic activity can be thought of as a combination of Myrrh (Commiphora) plus Boswellia[14].

The gargled (then swallowed) tea or tincture in a little water is a superb treatment for immune deficiency related canker sores, sore throats, and even regional swollen lymph nodes. The tea, tincture, or powdered gum is also useful for spongy and bleeding gums that tend to recede – Elephant tree's astringing effect is well put to use in these conditions. Due to the plant's antiseptic qualities it also is effective against a number of harmful oral bacteria responsible for gingivitis and periodontal disease.

Use Elephant tree tea as a nasal wash or spray if suffering from difficult–to–resolve sinus infections. Like Myrrh, the plant's indications here (and with other tissues) are pallid and lax mucus membranes that tend to ulcerate – denoting lack of vitality and circulatory strength. For these issues it combines well with Echinacea or even Yerba mansa or Bayberry if some extra tissue stimulation is needed.

For chronic bronchitis with an accompanying nagging cough, the internal tea or tincture is surprisingly effective. Sufferers of chronic asthma, where long–standing tissue inflammation is interlinked with bronchial constriction, will feel unobstructed after a strong dose of the tincture.

Elephant tree is also of benefit to long standing bladder and urethra infections that are non–resolving due to area weakness. The plant's affect over the kidneys should not be underestimated. In chronic nephritis, when

---

14   With overlapping medicinal similarities, these plants are closely related botanically, chemically, and therapeutically.

there is no active inflammation, Elephant tree can be used like Juniper – in small amounts to stimulate a healing response in atonic tissues.

Lesser known is Elephant tree's influence over systemic inflammations affecting the joints, muscles, and connective tissues. Undoubtedly here, its chemical relation to Boswellia is at the heart of the matter. Most forms (with the exception of severe osteoarthritis) of chronic joint, connective, and soft tissue pain see some degree of relief with internal tincture/tea applications. Try it for long–standing tendinitis, bursitis, arthritis–like situations, and even fibromyalgia.

Topically the ointment, salve, or oil makes a useful antimicrobial (and antifungal) application for poorly healing cuts, scrapes, and superficial wounds. Even insect stings and bites are soothed by the plant's continued application. Poorly healing ulcers and bed sores are almost always benefited by the ointment, salve, or oil. As long as the situation is sub–acute to chronic Elephant tree will likely do good. Some interesting successes with Bursera simaruba (Red gumbolimbo) topically applied to eczema and psoriasis are worth noting. Likely our Bursera microphylla is of equal use to this Central American grower.

Most species of Bursera are or have at one point in time been utilized as medicines – from Bursera microphylla by the Seri and B. simaruba by the Mayans and Aztecs, to Bursera tonkinensis by Vietnamese. The genus serves as an important plant medicine, capable of numerous applications, some that we know of and others which await our detection.

Indications

» Spongy/Bleeding gums (external)
» Periodontitis/Gingivitis (external)
» Pharyngitis with swollen tonsils (external and internal)
» Sinusitis (external and internal)
» Bronchitis with debility
» Cystitis/Urethritis, chronic
» Nephritis, chronic
» Inflammation, chronic, related to joint/connective/muscular pain
» Poorly healing ulcers/Bed sores (external and internal)
» Cuts, abrasions, wounds, poorly healing (external)
» Eczema and psoriasis (external)

Collection

Elephant tree's branch ends are best collected a week or two after a decent rain when leaf growth has been initiated. Like Ocotillo the plant is capable of numerous leaf growth–shed cycles depending on rainfall.

With pruners snip 4"–6" inches from leafing branch tips. Move around from tree–to–tree, taking a little from here–and–there. Occasionally resin–gum nodules are found at trunk/branch junctures or seeping–crystallized around (insect/mechanical) damaged areas. These nodules can usually be gently removed from the tree with no ill effects to the area. When in season it's a nice treat to eat a fruit or two – pleasantly piney–lemon tasting and semi–sweet. But it's best to leave the majority of them for the plant's reproduction.

Do try to 'go–lightly' with Elephant tree – there are abundant stands in California and Arizona, but still the species is of limited quantity. Keep in mind in both states the plant is protected – not endangered, but due to its isolated range it is designated as a sensitive species.

Preparations

Grind the resin–gum nodules to a coarse powder before tincturing. Tincture the leafing branch ends fresh (best) or dry for later use. A leaf tea (infusion) comes in third place for serviceability; be sure to keep the infusion covered while brewing – this will keep the aromatics from dissipating.

Dosage

» DPT (80% alcohol) of gum: 10–20 drops 2–3 times daily
» FPT/DPT (80% alcohol) of Leaf/Twig: 30–60 drops 2–3 times daily
» Leaf infusion: 4–6 ounces 2–3 times daily

Cautions

The gum tincture can be a little tortuous on the stomach if used in excess. Keep dosages small but frequent. Elephant tree is likely not the best plant to use liberally during pregnancy – its exact influence over reproduction is still unexplored.

Other Uses

The resin from this and other Buseras (or really any sap–resin–gum used as an incense) is known as Copal. Its ceremonial application predates recorded history with traditional Mesoamerican use. Today, it is still occasionally used in regional Catholic churches.

Use an incense stove or simply place a small piece on an electric stove burner turned on low–medium. Coming from someone who is not a big incense fan, I can attest Elephant tree Copal is able to turn a naysayer into a follower. It also combines well with Brittlebush resin.

Filaree
Geraniaceae/Geranium Family

Erodium cicutarium (L.) L'Hér. ex Aiton (*Erodium millefolium, E. moranense, E. praecox, Geranium cicutarium*)
Storksbill, Alfilerillo, Alfilaria

Description
Filaree is a small herbaceous annual (rarely biennial) with spreading basal leaves which radiate out to form compact rosettes. Lobed leaflets form in alternate pairs along the stems. They are hairy and can reach several inches in length. Later Filaree's growth is more erect and in ideal conditions reaches 1′–1½′ in height. Its stems are reddish and branched. The small, 5–petaled, and purplish–pink flowers are clustered in small groupings on slender stalks and originate from the leaf axils. Another common name, Storksbill, applies to the massed pointed fruit. The fruit clusters separate into 5 individual seeds, all having a tail–like appendage that coils and uncoils in corresponding dry and wet conditions, thereby assisting the seed's placement in the ground.

Distribution
This non–native, European originator is found throughout the West and much of North America. From practically sea level to 9,000′, look for Filaree along roadsides, vacant lots, fallow fields, gardens, and other areas where the ground has been disturbed. This allows for the easy seeding of the plant.

Chemistry
Flavonoids: quercetin, kaempferol, luteolin, and ellagic acid.

Medicinal Uses

Filaree is used as a mild astringent in various external and internal conditions. Internally the tea is soothing to the urinary tract. Use it when tissues are inflamed and it hurts to urinate. In addition, the plant is mildly hemostatic, lessening regional passive hemorrhages. Filaree has a reputation as a reliable diuretic. It is particularly indicated when there is rheumatic pain and associated fluid retention around the joints.

Like Geranium, Filaree often reduces heavy menstruation. It has no hormonal effect, but if the episode is due to idiosyncrasies or defunct biorhythms, the plant will make a difference. Regional passive hemorrhaging will also lessen under its use. Use the internal tea and sitz bath to tone vaginal tissues after childbirth. It is also well–applied to general vaginal/cervical irritation.

Similar to Geranium, Filaree is a soothing gargle for sore throats. Additionally, the tea or fresh plant poultice can be applied topically to diminish redness and sensitivity from sunburn, scrapes, and rashes.

Indications

» Inflammation, urinary tract/Hematuria
» Fluid retention with accompanying rheumatism
» Menstruation, heavy
» Inflammation, vaginal/cervical (external)
» Sore throat (gargle)
» Burns/Rashes (external)

Collection

When the herbage is still fresh and verdant, unearth the entire plant, root and all. The slender taproot should come up easily especially if the plant is in moist, non–compacted soil. Larger roots may have to be split lengthwise as to insure their proper drying. It is acceptable to mix the herb and root together in storage as they complement each other well; the root's lack of density makes the infusion method fine.

Preparations/Dosage

» Herb/Root infusion: 4–8 ounces 2–3 times daily
» Sitz bath/Douche: 2–3 times daily

Cautions

Filaree growing in the desert occasionally is a host for Synchytrium papillatum, a fungus that causes the plant to produce a burgundy pigment. Do not gather and use infected plants.

Other Uses

The young green leaves are edible and can be added to salads and the like.

Flat–Top Buckwheat

Polygonaceae/Buckwheat Family

Eriogonum fasciculatum Benth.
California buckwheat

Description

Flat–top buckwheat is a compact and dense sub–shrub growing 2'–3' wide and high. Its initial appearance is often larger since the plant is occasionally found in clump–forming colonies. The main stems are woody and around the plant's circumference they tend to lay partially along the ground, where some varieties aggressively root at stem nodes.

The leaves are bunched in crowded groupings along the stems and point upward. They are linear and are approximately ½"–¾" long, greenish above, and lighter underneath. The flowers are white to pink and form in dense flattened clusters at branchlet ends where they appear to hover over the body of the plant.

There are a number of varieties of Eriogonum fasciculatum that overlap in range and appearance. For simplicity, the varieties here are described as a whole. Besides the Flat–top buckwheat types, which are uniform in growth, dense, and bushy, there are also Skeletonweed morphologies (E. deflexum). They tend to be annuals, but not always, and have basal rosettes of petioled leaves that are often kidney shaped. They tend to have 1 or several central, sometimes inflated, leafless or nearly so, vertical stalks on which spreading and tiny inflorescences are borne. Another biotype is that of Desert buckwheat or E. wrightii. These are bushy perennials similar to E. fasciculatum but they lack the stoutness of the latter. New growth tends to be non–uniform and weak–branched. The elliptical leaves are approximately a ½" long, downy, and spread alternately along the stems. The flowers also form in clusters at branch ends.

Distribution
Flat–top buckwheat can be found from Santa Barbara and Monterey Counties, California, east through southern Nevada and western Arizona. Look for the plant on bluffs and cliffs overlooking the ocean in southern California, on disturbed soils, the edges of washes and occasionally on desert flats throughout the rest of its range. Overall, the genus contains 200+ species throughout the United Sates. They are particularly abundant across the West.

Chemistry
Buckwheat family array of hydrolyzable and condensed tannins; other flavonoids.

Medicinal Uses
All Eriogonums can essentially be used the same way. The bushier perennials, because of their mass and subsequent collectability, are better suited for therapeutic use.

The plant's mild astringency can be applied to a number of situations. When the lower urinary tract is inflamed and it is painful to urinate, possibly from urine pH changes or from the throes of a lower urinary tract infection, Flat–top buckwheat will be found soothing.

The tea will check diarrhea, be it from dietary or stress reactions. Similarly, the plant has use in diminishing simple intestinal inflammation. Externally the crushed plant applied fresh or the strong infusion used topically is soothing to burns, rashes, and other outbreaks that tend to be weepy and inflamed.

Indications
» Pain/Irritation, lower urinary tract
» Diarrhea with intestinal inflammation
» Inflammation, skin (external)

Collection
In the spring when new leaf growth is apparent, collect Flat–top buckwheat by pruning its upper growth. After drying, garble the leaves and flower from the stems. Discard the stems.

Preparations/Dosage
Herb infusion: 4–8 ounces 2–3 times daily

Cautions
Due to Flat–top buckwheat's potential vasoconstriction of the uterine lining, it is not recommended during pregnancy.

Globemallow
Malvaceae/Mallow Family

Sphaeralcea spp. A. St.–Hil.
Desert hollyhock, Desert mallow, Sore eye poppy, Yerba de la negrita

Description
Although several species are in fact smaller annuals, Globemallow is a 1'–4'
tall, short–lived, perennial bush. These plants are covered with small star–
shaped hairs making them fuzzy to the touch. Due to species' differences
and environmental conditions, the leaves are of varying size and shape, but
most are lobed or at least shallowly dentate. When crushed they are mucilaginous. Thickened leaves alternate along the main stems. The flowers
form in racemes or panicles. They are 5–petaled and showy. Orange and
red are usually the predominate colors but varieties can be white, lavender, or pink. The seedpod is wheel–shaped, composed of 5 or more carpels,
and surrounded by a persistent calyx. Kidney–shaped and pubescent seeds
are held within each wedge–shaped carpel. Globemallow is notorious for
inter–species crossbreeding. This often makes individual classification
difficult.

Indian mallow or Abutilon spp. and Hibiscus spp. are other regionally
available native plant genera in the Mallow family that can be used in a
similar fashion. Depending on species, Indian mallow is a small, deciduous shrub or herbaceous plant. The leaves, like Globemallow, are covered
with small hairs and alternate along the stems. They are petioled, entire, or
toothed and often cordate, at least towards the base. The 5–petaled flowers
are usually yellow or orange, but sometimes according to species, they can
be white, pink, or red. The seed capsules are cylindrically shaped and composed of seed containing carpels.

Hibiscus denudatus and H. coulteri are perennial and herbaceous multi–stemmed small plants. H. denudatus's leaves are ovoid or obovate, with prominent teeth. The large lavender flowers contrast the light green leaves. H. coulteri's mature leaves are deeply 3–lobed; the lower leaves are lesser so. The plant's large flowers are yellow and have a red basal spot. There are several seeds in each wedge–shaped carpel.

Distribution

Globemallow is abundant throughout the interior West and can be found in a wide array of elevations and climates. Sphaeralcea coccinea, one of the larger distributed species, stretches from Arizona and New Mexico, north to Saskatchewan and Alberta. Look to dry hillsides, roadsides, trailsides, and disturbed soils.

Indian mallow is generally a plant of the southwestern Deserts. Southern California, Arizona, New Mexico, and Texas contain the bulk of the plant. It is found from 1,000'–5,500' on rocky slopes, streamsides, and canyon bottoms. From sea level to 4,000', Hibiscus denudatus is found from southeastern California, east through much of southern Arizona (skipping the bulk of New Mexico), to southern Texas, west of the Pecos River. A disjointed pocket exists in Clark County, Nevada. H. coulteri is found from 2,000'–4,000' throughout Arizona's Sonoran Desert and southeast Cochise County to the Big Bend area of Texas.

Chemistry

Various polysaccharides (pectin, mucilage, and starch), namely arabinogalactans; tannins: similar to Mallow.

Medicinal Uses

Use Globemallow in beginning stages of bronchitis when the lungs and throat feel hot and irritated. Also if there is an unproductive cough the tea sipped throughout the day will gently diminish the cough reflex. Most find it soothing to inflamed bronchial and throat tissues.

Globemallow's pharmacological activity provides a slight immunologic boost to the lung environment. Dust cells[15] or macrophages that reside in the alveoli are stimulated by Globemallow's polysaccharide content. These immunologic mucilages – mainly arabinogalactan and other related

15   The dust cells reside deep within the lungs, beyond the larger bronchi, in the air sacs (alveoli). They engulf and eliminate foreign particles that are small enough to become deposited within the alveoli.

compounds – serve as stimulators of the area. Globemallow amplifies lung immunity, making the local respiratory environment more resilient and active.

Urethral and bladder irritation responds well to this soothing plant. Surrounding urinary tract tissues are soothed through contact with these Malvaceae constituents, which are eliminated through the urine. If there is an infection, extra benefit will be seen from the addition of an appropriate urinary tract antibacterial herb such as Manzanita or Juniper.

Externally Globemallow makes an excellent emollient poultice. It is very useful in reducing swellings from injury, bringing abscesses to a head, and getting splinters to slowly gravitate to the skin's surface. Globemallow's immunological stimulation quickens the tissue's natural process of resolution[16].

Indications
» Bronchitis, with an irritative cough
» Irritation, urinary tract
» Abscess/Splinters (internal and external)

Collection
Collect Globemallow in the spring after it has been enlivened by winter–spring rains. Its growth will be full and new, as opposed to early summer collection where the leaves are smaller, more condensed, and a bit more astringent (but still good medicine). Snip the upper herbage that consists of the stem, flower, and leaf. Dry normally.

Preparations
Globemallow has a pleasantly sweet, mucilaginous, and astringent taste. When making the foliage infusion, strain it well to remove the very small leaf hairs. Use a cloth for best results. If left in the tea they can be irritating to the throat.

To prepare a poultice, slowly stir enough hot water into the dried and powdered leaf so a thick, pudding–like consistency is obtained. Place this glob in several folds of cheesecloth or flannel and then place it on the

16   The body naturally encapsulates spent phagocytes, damaged tissue cells, and other cellular wastes. This mass is then slowly resolved from the inside or comes to a head on the outside and is released. Copperleaf or Leadwort can be added for an additional stimulating effect.

affected area after it has sufficiently cooled – but is still warm. Cover with a warm damp towel. Repeat the process as needed.

Dosage
» Herb infusion: 4–8 ounces 2–3 times daily
» Poultice: as needed

Cautions
The small stem and leaf hair of Globemallow is irritating to the eyes, throat, and sinuses. Be sure to wash hands after collecting the plant and strain the tea well.

Golden Smoke
Papaveraceae/Poppy Family

Corydalis aurea Willd.
Scrambled eggs

Description
Golden smoke is a small, weak–stemmed biannual or short–lived peren-nial. The plant is bluish–green, glaucous, and 4"–16" tall. The distinctively yellow and spurred flowers tend to form in racemes at the branch ends. These little clump–forming plants have deeply lobed (almost feather–like) leaves. The seedpods are elongated, slightly curved, and scimitar–like. They are approximately 1" long and contain numerous small black seeds.

Distribution
Although the plant is sporadic in local distribution, it is found commonly throughout much of the West (at most elevations). Look for it along stream-sides, in washes, and other drainage areas beneath larger shrubs and trees or next to boulders. It also frequents disturbed areas and is occasionally seen along road and trail sides. In arid, lower elevation areas, it is one of the first plants to bloom in the spring. Golden smoke's reoccurrence (in the same place) from year to year is unpredictable. It is more often discovered than visited.

Chemistry

Berberine, bulbocapnine, corpaverine, corybulbine, protopine, sanguinarine, and other isoquinoline alkaloids.

Medicinal Uses

As a moderately–strong sedative, Golden smoke is particularly useful when
nervous system distress manifests as muscular twitching, tics, and mild
seizure activity. Use it when these symptoms are accompanied by pain.
Another interesting application of the plant is to cognitive issues. Most species show mild to moderate AChE (acetylcholinesterase) inhibition; meaning with its use acetylcholine remains as a neurotransmitter a little longer
in CNS/PNS synapses. Alzheimer's and dementia suffers should notice an
improved mental state from regular use of the plant.

Chronic skin conditions that are of a low–grade and allergic nature
respond positively to Golden smoke. The plant seems to be particularly
suited to thin individuals whose skin and nervous systems are hypersensitive. If prone to lymph node enlargements, general lymph sluggishness,
and blood dyscrasias then Golden smoke will prove corrective.

The plant positively influences digestion. It is used when the tongue is
chronically coated, and there is stomach distention and sluggishness upon
eating. As an alterative or sedative, Golden smoke is best used in combination with other herbs. Think of Golden smoke as a combination of Desert
barberry, California poppy, and Red root (Ceanothus spp.). It is a complex
plant worthy of revitalization in modern–day herbalism.

Indications

» Seizure activity, mild/Tremors/Tics
» Irritability, nervous system
» Alzheimer's disease/Dementia
» Skin conditions, chronic, from allergy/autoimmune disturbances
» Enlargements, lymph node
» Digestion, atonic
» Poorly healing tissue with tendency towards ulceration

Collection

Collect the whole plant when flowering in early spring.

Preparations/Dosage

» FPT/DPT (50% alcohol): 10–30 drops 2–3 times daily
» Leaf infusion: 2–4 ounces 2–3 times daily

Cautions

Pharmacologically Golden smoke is a complex plant. It has been shown to inhibit platelet aggregation, so is not recommended if taking medications that affect blood viscosity. Used alone, Golden smoke can be taken for 2–3 weeks at a time; longer at lower doses in combination with other herbs. Do not use Golden smoke during pregnancy or while nursing.

Greenthread

Asteraceae/Sunflower Family

Thelesperma megapotamicum (Spreng.) Kuntze (*Bidens leyboldii, B. megapotamica, B. paradoxa, Thelesperma gracile, T. scabiosoides*)
Navajo tea, Hopi tea, Cota, Pampa tea

Description

Greenthread is a deep–rooted perennial. The plant usually stands 2′–3′ tall and has numerous long and narrow stems, which are smooth, bluish–green, and glaucous. The leaves, of similar characteristic, are opposite and either entire or divided into 1 or 2 linear divisions. The nodding yellow flower heads sit atop long peduncles – they seem too large to be properly supported by the thin stems. The flowers fade to a tannish–brown with age. Other species of Thelesperma are similarly formed. T. subnudum is a smaller plant also with large yellow flower heads. T. longipes′ flowers are smaller. Its delicate leaves are prominently divided.

Distribution

Greenthread has a large distribution throughout the interior West. From Nebraska and Wyoming, the plant is found south through most of the Great Plains and finally to Arizona, New Mexico, and Texas. From 4,000′–8,000′ look to open woodlands, grassy flats, mesa tops, on the edges of gullies, and along secondary roads.

Chemistry
Stigmasterol, phenylpropanoids, and flavonoids: luteolin and marein.

Medicinal Uses
In the past the Hopi, Navajo, and Hispanic New Mexicans used the plant as a beverage tea. Today though soft–drinks have come to replace Green–thread tea. That said, it can still be drunk simply for the taste. The tea is non–bitter, pleasant tasting, and sweetens well with a little honey or sugar. Aside from being mildly diuretic, Greenthread is not significantly medicinal.

Collection
For easier identification, gather Greenthread while it is in flower. Snip the above ground foliage and bundle loosely or dry normally.

Preparations/Dosage
»   Herb infusion: as desired

Cautions
There are no known cautions with normal usage.

Other Uses
The foliage and roots have been used as a traditional dye. They provide a yellow, brownish–orange pigment.

Hopbush
Sapindaceae/Soapberry Family

Dodonaea viscosa Jacq. (*Dodonaea angustifolia, D. burmanniana, D. dombeyana, D. spatulata, Ptelea viscosa*)
Switch sorrel, Jarilla

Description
Hopbush is a 4′–8′ tall perennial shrub. Its evergreen leaves are several inches long, much less wide, and generally lanced shaped. If crushed, the leaves are resinous and slightly sticky. The male and female flowers are insignificant and are dwarfed by the 3–4 winged, yellowish–green, and

occasionally pink–tinged fruit. Although they do not really resemble true Hops flowers (Humulus), the coloration is similar and they are relatively papery. The winged fruit clusters are noticeable during mid–spring and are showy.

Distribution

Hopbush is primarily found in central–southern Arizona and parts of Florida. Variants are found throughout much of the tropical and subtropical world – it is a far–reaching genus that is even dominant in parts of Australia.

Look for Hopbush from 2,000'–4,000' among rocky hillsides and boulder strewn slopes. The plant is one of the first to begin repopulation of burned and disturbed land in upper desert areas.

Chemistry

Diterpenoids: dodonic acid and hautriwaic acid; flavonoids: pinocembrin, viscosol, santin, and penduletin; dodonones: methyldodonate and dodonolide; saponins: dodonosides a and b.

Medicinal Uses

As a traditional plant medicine, Hopbush has a striking alignment of use even by unrelated cultures existing oceans apart. The correspondence of American Indian, Mexican, and South African application is just too similar to ignore.

The plant is used extensively in sedating the smooth muscle contractions of spasmodic diarrhea and stomach cramps. It also is of value in diminishing uterine cramps and additionally, gallbladder colic, whether from gallstone formation or an adverse response to dietary fat, is lessened. All of these areas – upper and lower gastrointestinal tract, gallbladder, and uterus – can be further affected by an externally applied poultice of fresh leaves or a paste made of the moistened leaf powder. It has been suggested that Hopbush exerts this spasmolytic effect by interfering with ionic calcium uptake in smooth muscle cells, thereby subsequently inhibiting contraction.

Externally Hopbush applied as a wash or poultice is soothing to any number of rashes and inflammations. The plant is mildly antimicrobial and has been found to inhibit numerous pathogens, namely Escherichia coli, Staphylococcus aureus, and Candida albicans. For lessening Candida flare–ups use a topically applied tea, sitz bath, or soak.

It is interesting to note that various Dodonaea species growing in different parts of the world show differences in antimicrobial activity on the same pathogens. As with most plants, environmental conditions greatly influence internal chemistries, even plants of the same species.

Indications
» Cramps, gastrointestinal
» Colic, bilious
» Cramps, uterine (internal and external)
» Rashes and inflammations, allergy and/or mechanically induced (external)
» Infection, bacterial (external)
» Infection, Candida (external)

Collection
From spring through summer, collect Hopbush leaves when they are green and sticky. Dry normally for tea.

Preparations/Dosage
» Leaf infusion: 4 ounces 2–3 times daily
» FPT/DPT (60% alcohol): 30–60 drops 2–3 times daily
» Wash/Fomentation/Poultice/Oil/Salve: apply as needed
» Sitz bath/Douche: 2–3 times daily

Cautions
Do not use during pregnancy due to the plant's effect on uterine musculature.

Jojoba
Buxaceae/Boxwood Family

Simmondsia chinensis (Link) C.K. Schneid.
Goatnut

Description
Jojoba is a many–branched shrub reaching 3'–6' in height. The ovoid leaves are entire, leathery, and arranged oppositely along the stems. They

are ¾"–2" long, grayish–green, and tend to yellow with age or stress. The leaves are positioned upright so most of its exposure to the sun occurs in the morning and late afternoon. This orientation minimizes sun–stress.

Jojoba is divided between male and female plants. Both flower types are inconspicuous. The seed produced from the female, the famed 'goat-nut', is shaped like an acorn, dark brown when mature, and surrounded by a lighter husk. At any given time, it has been placed in the Boxwood, Spurge, or Jojoba families.

Distribution
Between 1,500'–5,000' look for Jojoba growing on rocky slopes and hillsides throughout the Sonoran Desert and Chaparral Scrub regions of Arizona and southern California.

Chemistry
Glycosides contained within fruit: simmondsin, d–pinitol, and galactinol; leaf tannins: both condensed and hydrolyzable types.

Medicinal Uses
One of the most persistent groups of medicinal compounds found within the plant world are tannins. And like so many other southwestern natives, Jojoba contains an abundance of these phenolic glycosides. Topically applied to the skin the plant is simply astringent. The fresh leaf poultice, tea, or dried leaf powder will lessen surface inflammation from scrapes, rashes, and burns. The plant's tightening effect will diminish blood flow from minor cuts and discharge from weepy rashes.

Jojoba is also slightly antimicrobial. Surface tissues are helped to heal more quickly with its application. The tea used as a mouthwash or gargle will help to resolve mouth sores, lessen bleeding from gums, and soothe sore throats. If swallowed the tea will diminish diarrhea through its astringing effect on the intestines.

Indications
» Cuts/Burns/Rashes (external)
» Mouth inflammations/Sore throats (gargle)
» Diarrhea

Collection

Trim the upper branches when new leaf growth is apparent. The leaves should be light green and hydrated.

Dosage

» Leaf decoction: 4–6 ounces 2–3 times daily
» Topical preparations: as needed

Cautions

Jojoba's array of tannins can be disrupting to sensitive mucus membranes that line the gut and intestines, so keep use short term: 5–7 days at a time. Like other tannin containing plants caution should be applied if taking Jojoba while pregnant due to its vasoconstricting effects on uterine lining. In some individuals kidney irritation may develop if used in excess.

Other Uses

Jojoba seeds are fully mature and –somewhat– edible from late summer through fall. It's best to consider them more of an accent food rather than a subsistence food. Most people can eat a small handful of the raw seeds without any stomach upset...but much more than that and they tend to be tortuous on the digestion. After roasting or parching they do become more flavorful but still are a 'difficult' food. Occasionally the roasted and ground seeds are listed in older references as a coffee substitute. There is merit to this – the percolation is rich and bitter. The liquid wax (called Jojoba oil in commerce) extracted from the seed is used widely in the natural cosmetic industry.

There is some speculation based on research that eating Jojoba seeds produces satiation through its influence of CCK (cholecystokinin); eating several seeds before meals may reduce the amount of food needed to feel full.

Jumping Cholla
Cactaceae/Cactus Family

Cylindropuntia fulgida (Engelm.) F.M. Knuth *(Opuntia fulgida)*
Chain–fruit cholla, Cholla brincadora, Velas de coyote

Description

Jumping cholla is a tree–like cactus that in rare circumstances reaches 12' in height, though normally it is between 3'–9' tall. This cactus has a thickened and branching trunk upon which joints of varying lengths form and radiate outward. The green fruit are oval and uniquely form in hanging chains. As these cacti age the fruited chains become quite long. They are easily broken and seem to 'jump' to anyone lightly brushing against them.

The flowers are rose–purple with pink and yellow tinges. The larger thorns, which cover the trunk, are surrounded by papery sheaths that tend to glisten with bright sunlight. Most of the fruits are sterile, which does not affect the plant's successfulness, for it excels at asexual reproduction. Any joint or seedless fruit that falls to the ground will almost invariably take root.

Distribution

From sea level to 3,600', Jumping cholla is found on gravely and sandy soils. It inhabits flats as well as rocky foothills. From central Arizona, it ranges south to Mexico.

Chemistry

Similar to Prickly pear, Jumping cholla has carbohydrate–containing polymers, consisting of a mixture of mucilage and pectin; calcium oxalate.

Medicinal Uses

Like many plant medicines in the southwest, Jumping cholla is a traditional Mexican remedy geared towards the urinary tract. It principally is a soothing diuretic used to treat urinary tract pain and irritation. The root also has a widespread reputation in diminishing kidney and bladder gravel. It seems to be of better use with uric acid/low pH urine deposits, though using the root tea as a kidney stone preventive is its optimal application.

A tea made from Jumping cholla gum is soothing to gastrointestinal inflammation. Like Prickly pear pulp, the gum serves as a protectant making its application useful in healing peptic ulcers, gastritis, or soothing intestinal irritation associated with diarrhea. Topically the gum mixed with water is soothing to burns, bites, and rashes.

Indications

» Irritability/Pain, urinary tract

» Urinary gravel, preventive/Uric acid stones
» Gastritis/Ulcers, peptic
» Diarrhea with intestinal inflammation
» Burns/Skin irritation (external)

Collection

When digging Jumping cholla roots start at least 1' out from the central trunk as the plant sends out secondary horizontal roots close to the surface for rainfall absorption. As you dig closer to the central roots, collect the secondary roots. The main anchoring roots will be directly under the cactus trunk. These tap roots are thicker and reach deeper into the ground. The ideal sized plant to collect is 2'–3' in height: the bigger the plant the more spines and branches there are to navigate. After finishing, spread the fruit and branches around the area, this will insure a plentiful recovery in the future.

The gum, which occasionally exudes from injuries along the trunk and joints, dries in varying sized nodules. After dislodging the gum from its anchoring point, scrape off any embedded thorns or debris.

Preparations

Cut the roots into ¼"–½" sections and dry normally. The gum can be stored as is or broken into smaller chunks for future use. In preparing the gum tea, use ½ ounce (weight) of material in 1 pint of water. Simmer, stir, and strain well.

Dosage

» Root/Gum tea: 4–8 ounces 2–3 times daily
» Gum tea: apply as needed

Cautions

Consuming an excess of Jumping cholla for medicine or food, like Prickly pear, may cause stomach upset and usher in chills and attending elevated temperature.

Other Uses

Occasionally very large gum nodules can be found on the cactus. If relatively recent in formation, the nodule's center part maybe somewhat soft and pliable. This can then be cut into pieces and eaten. The Seri Indians of northwest Mexico once considered it a supplemental food.

The most recently developed fruit at the end of the chain can be peeled and eaten. Some will be seed filled, others not. Whether eaten raw or cooked, they are mild tasting and mucilaginous. Be mindful of the very small thorns, (glochids). They cover most parts of the plant.

Juniper
Cupressaceae/Cypress Family

Juniperus monosperma (Engelm.) Sarg. *(Juniperus gymnocarpa, J. mexicana var. monosperma)*
One seed juniper

Juniperus deppeana Steud. *(Juniperus foetida, J. gigantea)*
Alligator juniper

Juniperus scopulorum Sarg. *(Juniperus occidentalis var. pleiosperma, J. virginiana var. scopulorum, Sabina scopulorum)*
Rocky mountain juniper

Description

Depending on species Juniper is a small shrub or medium–sized tree, often rounded or conical in shape with stringy or checkerboard–like bark. These evergreen plants have either branchlets covered by short scale–like leaves clustered in pairs (sometimes in groupings of 3) or branchlets supporting needle–like leaves in groupings of 3. Usually there is a resin gland situated on the back of each scale–like leaf.

When crushed all Junipers are aromatic. Male and female flowers tend to develop on separate trees, although in rare circumstances both types can be found on the same tree. Both male and female flowers are small and un-remarkable. The berries are actually specialized cones and take one or two seasons (depending on species) to mature fully. They are blue to copper in color, fleshy, sweet, and contain 1–12 hard seeds.

Juniperus monosperma is a small tree or large shrub that branches from the ground. Typically, it has no main trunk to speak of, but if so, it is short. Its bark is light gray and tends to shred. The leaf groupings of 2 or sometimes 3 are scale–like and are pressed against the branchlets. The

mature fruit is dark blue with a fine bluish–white and waxy powder covering its surface. Normally they each contain 1 seed, but on rare occasions
they may have up to 3. They are brown and oval.

Juniperus deppeana is a small tree reaching 30' in height. This species
is remarkably long–lived – some are ascertained to be 1500 years old. The
grayish checkerboard bark lends credence to the common name: Alligator
juniper. Trunks on older trees can be thickened and somewhat tortuous,
with sometimes only small strips of living bark enliven a full canopy. On
the back of each leaf there is a noticeable resin gland. The fruit are reddish–
brown and are covered by a grayish waxy coating. Each berry contains 3–4
angled seeds.

Juniperus scopulorum is a large bush or small tree reaching 35' in
height. Its slender crown and drooping branches gives it a weeping appearance. The bark is brownish–gray and pulls away in narrow strips. The
small pointed leaves are scale–like and arranged in pairs. Each has a small
resin gland. The fruit are blue and are covered by a whitish coating that is
easily rubbed away. They are juicy, sweet, and contain 1–2 seeds.

Juniperus scopulorum is very closely related to J. virginiana or Red cedar of the eastern part of the country. Morphologically the two trees are
almost identical. The most significant variation is that it takes one season
for J. virginiana's fruit to mature, while it takes two for J. scopulorum to do
the same.

Distribution

Juniperus monosperma is found from western Kansas and central Colorado to the Texas Panhandle, through much of New Mexico and central–
eastern Arizona to southern Nevada. Throughout the bulk of its range look
for the tree between 3,000'–5,500'. To the north and east it can be found also
at lower elevations. It is commonly found in rocky soils with Pinyon pine.

Juniperus deppeana is found throughout middle mountain elevations
of 4,500'–8,000'. Look for it in canyons and drainage areas and on hillsides.
It ranges from west Texas through New Mexico to Arizona. J. scopulorum is distributed from Alberta south to western Texas. From there it is
found west to British Columbia, Washington, eastern Oregon, Nevada, and
northern Arizona. It is found throughout a great array of elevations – from
nearly sea level along the northwest coast, to almost 9,000' throughout the
Southwest.

Chemistry

Prominent volatile content includes: α–pinene, β–pinene, sabinene, myrcene, δ–2–carene, α–phellandrene, β–phellandrene, δ–3–carene, limonene, bornyl acetate, (e)–caryophyllene, α–humulene, α–muurolene, germacrene a, germacrene d, germacrene d–4–ol, γ–cadinene, δ–cadinene, and α–cadinol.

Medicinal Uses

Juniper has centuries of cross–cultural usage supporting its application as a urinary tract medicine. A stimulant to the area, it works best to alleviate low–grade, long–standing, subacute, or chronic urinary tract irritability and discomfort. Use it in chronic cystitis and painful urination accompanied by mucus in the urine. Although alcoholic preparations tend to extract Juniper's volatile constituents more completely, the leaf/berry tea is just as useful as a urinary tract antiseptic (both fungal and bacterial strains are inhibited). Small amounts of the tea are also useful in imparting cellular stimulation in low–grade, on and off again nephritis, particularly if used in formula.

Due to its aromatics, Juniper tends to be moderately carminative. Several ounces of the tea or 30–40 drops of the tincture can lessen stomach bloating and cramping. Topically Juniper oil or salve can be helpful in resolving long–standing episodes of eczema and psoriasis. Through the plant's interesting mix of antiinflammatory qualities and stimulating aromatics, it often is the right plant for long–standing problems of the urinary tract and skin.

Indications

» Infection, urinary tract, chronic
» Nephritis, chronic
» Dyspepsia
» Eczema/Psoriasis (external)

Collection

Collect the leaves and/or fruit alone or together. Both parts are equally potent. Dry them normally.

Preparations

For internal use, Juniper's essential oil fraction can be prepared as a spirit, or the essential oil can be added to ointment and oil bases.

Dosage
» Leaf/Berry infusion: 4–6 ounces 2–3 times daily
» FPT/DPT (75% alcohol): 30–40 drops 2–3 times daily
» Spirit: 20–30 drops 2–3 times daily
» Ointment/Oil/Salve: as needed

Cautions
Due to the plant's potential uterine stimulation, do not use it during pregnancy. Also do not use Juniper in acute kidney inflammation.

Other Uses
Though the percentage of Juniper is so small that it adds no medicinal component, the berries are a traditional flavoring agent in the making of Gin.

Kidneywood
Fabaceae/Pea Family

Eysenhardtia orthocarpa (A. Gray) S. Watson *(Eysenhardtia amorphoides var. orthocarpa, Viborquia orthocarpa)*
Palo azul, Bura dulce

Description
Kidneywood is a large bush or small tree. Occasionally it reaches 18′ in height, but usually it is less. The outer bark on older sections is gray and checkerboard formed. Kidneywood's leaves, which are deciduous in response to drought stresses and low temperatures, are pinnate and are composed of numerous, small leaflets. Upon closer examination, small dot–like resin glands are apparent on leaflet undersides, young stems, and flower calyxes. A unique resinous odor is noticeable when the foliage is crushed. Terminal spikes are composed of small, white, and delicate flowers. They appear in response to warm temperatures and rainfall from early spring to late summer. They are followed by equally small, linear, and clustered green seedpods. Within each pod is 1 flattened seed.

Distribution
Kidneywood is found from 4,000'–5,000', from Pima County, Arizona, east to southern Hidalgo County, New Mexico. Typically, the plant grows on hillsides and canyons of Desert Grasslands and Oak Woodlands.

Chemistry
At least several florescent isoflavones; chalcones: coatline a and b.

Medicinal Uses
As the name Kidneywood implies, the tea made from the small branches affects the kidneys and lower urinary tract. If prone to acidic and overly concentrated urine, associated kidney stones, and urinary tract sediment then Kidneywood will be of use. Because of the plant's alkalinizing effect, acidic precipitants tend to dissolve back into the urine. Pain and urinary tract irritability associated with lithic deposits will therefore be reduced. Kidneywood is also mildly diuretic, generally soothing to the area, and moderately antimicrobial.

Indications
» Deposits, urinary tract
» Urine, acidic, overly concentrated
» Irritability/Pain, urinary tract

Collection/Preparations
After pruning a number of small secondary branches from several large plants, cut them into small ½"–¼" sections. The leaves also can be used. The branch/twig decoction makes a pleasant tasting, slightly astringent tea.

Dosage
» Branch/Twig decoction: 4–8 ounces 2–3 times daily

Cautions
The heartwood should not be collected in the United States given its limited (but locally abundant) population. Moreover, there is not a great medicinal advantage between these parts and the smaller branches.

Other Uses

16th and 17th century Western Europe imported great quantities of a closely allied Eysenhardtia (then called Lignum nephriticum) for the above mentioned issues. During the same period, chemist Richard Boyle used heartwood preparations as an acid – base indicator. Considered a scientific breakthrough, the process gained wide acceptance as a method of measuring pH.

Leadwort

Plumbaginaceae/Plumbago Family

Plumbago zeylanica L. *(Plumbago scandens)*
Doctorbush, Wild leadwort, Pitillo, Hierba de alacran

Description

This perennial is often found along the ground or weakly growing up through near–by bushes. The leaves form alternately along stems. They are entire with wavy margins. The flowers cluster in spike–like racemes at branch ends. They are white, tubular, and have 5 petals. The small seed capsules have surfaces covered by numerous thickened hairs. They easily stick to clothes and animal fur. Plumbago capensis, which is cultivated as an ornamental in warmer parts of the country, has sky–blue flowers. It serves as a substitute for our own native variety.

Distribution

This species is found world–wide[17] in topical and semi–tropical environments. In southern Arizona Leadwort is mainly isolated to Pima and Pinal Counties, where the summer monsoons play an essential part in its growth cycle. It is also found in southern Florida. Between 2,500'–4,000', look for the plant in ravines, canyons, and gullies where rain run–off frequently courses. Ideally, Leadwort grows under larger shrubs and trees where it gains some protection from intense sunlight. Look under Acacia, Mesquite, and Hackberry trees. The plant does not have a wide range in the United States but it is locally abundant, robust, and is easily propagated.

17   Some botanists label this plant as Plumbago scandens when growing in the New World and P. zeylanica when growing in the Old World. Side–by–side specimens are virtually identical and were botanically split due to geography.

Chemistry

Plumbagic acid, naphthoquinones: plumbagin, chitranone, maritinone, elliptinone, isoshinanolone, and epiisoshinanolone; coumarins: seselin, 5–methoxyseselin, suberosin, xanthyletin, and xanthoxyletin.

Medicinal Uses

There are numerous species of Leadwort currently used in TCM (Traditional Chinese Medicine) and Ayurveda. Throughout Tropical America, these plants are also used medicinally. Although internal uses differ to some degree according to what therapeutic system is used, external uses coincide and are practical and safe.

Topical preparations stimulate tissue healing. The plant has an augmenting effect on parenchymal and connective tissue cells, collagenation, and other related factors. Tissue macrophage activity is also stimulated, which not only accounts for the plant's indirect antimicrobial activity but also further complements its wound healing properties.

Use Leadwort much like Copperleaf. Apply it topically when wounds, ulcers, cuts, and abrasions have become subacute. Use it when inflammation has diminished somewhat and tissues are lax and slow to heal. Topically Leadwort also speeds the time it takes abscesses to come to a head. Moreover it is of use in splinter removal.

Internally Leadwort has a long history of traditional use (India and Africa). Useful for an array of issues, its most clear application is to gastrointestinal infections, particularly involving Helicobacter pylori. Several cups of the tea daily will assist in the healing of gastric and duodenal ulcers.

Indications

» Wounds/Ulcers/Cuts, that are slow to heal (external)
» Edema, from injury (external)
» Abscesses/Splinters, to bring to a head (external)
» Ulcer, gastric/duodenal

Collection

Gather the whole plant, then dry it normally.

Preparations/Dosage

» Poultice/Fomentation/Salve/Oil: topically as needed
» Herb/Root infusion: 2–4 ounces 2–3 times daily

Cautions

Since Leadwort is a cellular stimulant there is a slight possibility of external preparations causing redness and inflammation. Discontinue if this occurs. Do not use during pregnancy or while nursing. Do not use concurrently with pharmaceuticals affecting blood viscosity.

Limberbush

Euphorbiaceae/Spurge Family

Jatropha cardiophylla (Torr.) Müll. Arg. *(Mozinna cardiophylla)*
Heartleaf limberbush, Sangre de drago, Sangre de cristo

Jatropha cinerea (Ortega) Müll. Arg. *(Jatropha canescens, Mozinna canescens, M. cinerea)*
Ashy limberbush, Sangre de drago, Lomboy

Jatropha cuneata Wiggins & Rollins
Limberbush, Leatherplant, Sangre de drago

Jatropha macrorhiza Benth. *(Jatropha arizonica)*
Nettlespurge, Ragged nettlespurge

Description

Jatropha cardiophylla is a curious appearing plant, as are most others of the genus. This small bush has numerous, extremely flexible, wand–like stems arising from a central base. The stem bark is reddish–brown. Heart-shaped/triangular leaves form in groupings along the stem. They are shiny, wider than long, and have rounded teeth. The small, white–tubular flowers hang delicately from the upper stems. They are followed by small, rounded, and encased seeds.

Jatropha cinerea is a tall plant with yellowish–brown stem bark. When young, the undersides of the ovate leaves are felty. J. cuneata is also a stout, many–branched shrub, but unlike J. cardiophylla and J. cinerea, its leaves are wedge–shaped.

Jatropha macrorhiza, technically not a Limberbush–type, represents an entirely different growth morphology. The other Jatrophas profiled here are semi–woody perennials – J. macrorhiza is herbaceous. Yearly, the plant's above ground foliage dies back to the ground. From a large, thickened tap-root, several 1'–2' tall stems arise supporting large and palmately lobed dark–green leaves. A 3–celled fruit follows the small rose–pink flowers.

Quite possibly the most unique characteristic of many Jatrophas is their distinctive sap. When a branch is clipped close to the base, a deep reddish–brown thickened fluid (Jatropha macrorhiza has clear sap) weeps from the wound, looking surprisingly blood–like.

Distribution

Jatropha cardiophylla reaches its northern most limit just north of Tucson, Arizona. From 2,000'–3,000' look for the plant on rocky hillsides and foothills. In southern Arizona's Senita Basin, J. cinerea is found in isolated pockets. From this point, the plant is found south into Mexico. Collection is not recommended in the United States because of its limited distribution.

Jatropha cuneata is found along with the previously described species, but it is of larger distribution. Look for the plant among gravelly flats and slopes from southern Yuma to southwestern Pima County, Arizona. Look for J. macrorhiza from 3,500'–7,500' throughout southern Arizona, New Mexico, and Texas. Antelope horns is a common companion plant.

Chemistry

Condensed and hydrolyzable tannins.

Medicinal Uses

All varieties of Limberbush are extremely astringent. The roots by weight contain approximately 5% tannic acid. This dominant phenol group (hydrolyzable tannin) is the reason why these plants are able to tan hides. When in contact with cellular protein structures hydrolyzable tannins constrict, tighten, and alter these surfaces. Like Wild rhubarb, due to its drastic effect on cell surfaces, therapeutic use of Limberbush is somewhat limited.

Externally use the fresh sap or stem poultice to soothe and astringe burns, bites, and stings. Its use on weepy rashes and hive outbreaks is also of some value. Internally Limberbush tea is used to quell acute diarrhea; it is a purely symptomatic gastrointestinal astringent. The tea can also be gargled for mouth sores, spongy and bleeding gums, and a sore throat.

Jatropha macrorhiza has a similar array of tannins, but it also contains strongly purgative compounds. Liken its effect to very strong Rhubarb. Enough J. macrorhiza to provide a laxative effect will almost certainly elicit

rebound constipation. Consider recognizing this species for its visual beau-
ty and not as a medicine.

Indications

» Diarrhea
» Skin eruptions/Burns/Cuts/Stings (external)
» Mouth sores/Spongy and bleeding gums (gargle)

Collection

Clip several stems at the plant's base and apply the sap as needed or cut
them into small ½″ sections and dry.

Preparations/Dosage

» Stem decoction: 2–4 ounces 2–3 times daily
» Sap/Stem poultice: externally as needed

Cautions

Use Limberbush internally for several days at a time. If used longer the
plant may irritate the kidneys. Do not use during pregnancy due to the
plant's potential vasoconstrictive effect on uterine lining.

Other Uses

Like Wild rhubarb, it is a plant to know about if attempting to tan hides –
the old way.

Mallow

Malvaceae/Mallow Family

Malva neglecta Wallr. *(Malva rotundifolia)*
Common mallow, Cheeseweed

Malva parviflora L.
Little mallow

Description

Mallow is a clump–forming or spreading annual/short–lived perennial.
It has a thickened and short taproot. The plant increases in size quickly

even in the presence of just modest rainfall. The large 5–7 lobed leaves have heart–shaped bases, serrated margins, and long petioles. Typically, the 5–petaled flowers are inconspicuous, white to pale lavender or pink-ish, cleft, and ¼"–⅔" long. The fruit is a round, flattened, button–like, seed disk. Each disk separates into 10–12 sections or carpels. Throughout parts of the Southwest that have winter–spring influenced Pacific rains, Mallow is an initiatory plant that when at its peak literally can cover anything on the ground.

Distribution

This European native is commonly found throughout the United States. It is here to stay and is thriving in the West. Look for the plant anywhere the ground has been disturbed, but particularly around edges of building and structures, irrigated lands, yards, and roadsides.

Chemistry

Polysaccharides: arabinogalactans, β–d–glucan, l–arabinose, d–xylose, l–rhamnose, d–galactose, d–galacturonic acid, and d–glucuronic acid.

Medicinal Uses

Mallow has several distinct medicinal effects practically identical to Marsh-mallow, Hollyhock, and Globemallow. The tea is soothing to a dry and ir-ritating cough. Bronchial irritation present typically in the beginning or ending stages of a lung cold or bronchitis is equally soothed.

Mallow's polysaccharides are stimulating to innate immunity, and specifically leukocyte activities are enhanced. The plant's immunological effect is not necessarily strong, but it is helpful during the wintertime cold and flu season, or when immune depression is present.

Some of these Mallow family constituents are eliminated through the kidneys. The urine quality change that follows has a soothing and antiin-flammatory effect on the area. Lower urinary tract irritation is lessened, as is episodic kidney inflammation. Mallow has an age–old use as a kidney stone preventative. Drink a cup of tea daily if prone to lithic deposits. Its taste is pleasant enough to warrant long–term use without revulsion.

If suffering from gastritis Mallow is soothing to inflamed gastric mu-cosa. It is well combined with Artemisia douglasiana or A. filifolia in heal-ing peptic ulcers. Like Globemallow, the fresh or dried plant can be used as a drawing poultice. The tissue stimulating and softening effect provided by Mallow is of use in resolving boils, abscesses, and removing splinters. Combine it with other immune stimulating or circulation enhancing herbs for a more profound effect.

Indications
»   Bronchitis with an irritative cough
»   Cystitis/Urethritis
»   Kidney irritation
»   Urinary tract gravel, as a preventive
»   Gastritis
»   Boils/Abscesses/Splinters (internal and external)

Collection
The entire plant – leaves, stems and roots – are usable. In loose and moist soils, the taproots pull up easily. When split they are starchy and white.

Preparations/Dosage
»   Leaf infusion/Root decoction: 4–8 ounces 2–3 times daily

Cautions
There are no known cautions for Mallow with normal usage.

Manzanita
Ericaceae/Heath Family

Arctostaphylos spp. Adans.
Big bearberry, Manzanilla, Coralillo

Description
Manzanita is an evergreen bush or small tree reaching 3′–18′ in height. The outer red bark is thin and visually striking, on some varieties peeling freely and on others remaining smooth and intact. Forked branches form in tangles at branch ends making these plants practically impenetrable when growing in thickets. The leaves are usually ovoid, thickened, and often point skyward. The small, pink, and urn–shaped flowers form in clusters at branch ends and then transition into small 4–10 seeded tan fruit.

Distribution

Coastal mountainous regions of California have the densest populations of the plant. From this area, they radiate south and eastward to Texas. Typically, a mid–mountain plant throughout the Southwest, look for Manzanita with other Chaparral Scrub plants, such as Silk tassel and Scrub oak. It is found on exposed hillsides and rocky slopes.

Chemistry

Phenolic glucosides: arbutin, methylarbutin and hydroquinone; tannins: caffeic acid, gallic acid, catechol and ellagic acid; triterpenoids: uvaol, ursolic acid, lupeol, α–amyrin, β–amyrin, erythrodiol and oleanolic acid; anthocyanidins: delphinidin and cyanidin; quercitrin and quercetin.

Medicinal Uses

Manzanita inhibits lower urinary tract bacterial strains that thrive in alkaline urine. In the presence of alkaline urine, arbutin (a main constituent of Manzanita) is broken down into hydroquinone and is subsequently responsible for the plant's antibacterial qualities. Escherichia coli, a typical urinary tract pathogen, thrives in alkaline urine. In the presence of normal acidic urine (or Manzanita influenced urine), this bacterium finds attachment to cell walls difficult. Combining the use of Manzanita (or most other Heath family plants, such as Madrone or Cranberry) with diet changes that include more animal source proteins, along with limiting simple carbohydrates, often promptly resolves alkaline urinary tract infections.

Manzanita is also a urinary tract astringent. The plant's tannin complexes responsible for this tone lax urinary tract tissues by imparting a local tightening effect. Use it when there is dragging urinary pain in combination with dribbling of urine and mucus discharge.

As a postpartum sitz bath, Manzanita is useful in tonifying and soothing vaginal and cervical tissues. Since Manzanita is moderately inhibiting to Candida albicans it is well worth combining topical applications with internal use of Thuja, Cypress, or Garlic.

Indications

» Lower urinary tract infection with alkaline urine
» Vaginitis with or w/o Candida involvement
» As a postpartum sitz bath

Collection

Gather Manzanita leaves from late spring to summer after flowering when the ripe fruit is present. The arbutin content is most concentrated at this time, less so when the plant is in flower.

Preparations

Several things can be done to facilitate the breakdown of arbutin and methylarbutin into hydroquinone, therefore increasing the plant's effectiveness. Simply drying the leaf starts the conversion. Hydroquinone is also increased by rehydrating the leaves in a small amount of water for 3–4 hours. After this initial soak, decoct normally.

Dosage

» Leaf decoction: 4–6 ounces 2–3 times daily
» DPT (40% alcohol, 10% glycerin): 60–90 drops 2–3 times daily
» Fluidextract: 30–50 drops 2–3 times daily
» Sitz bath: as needed

Cautions

Manzanita may have a vasoconstricting effect on uterine lining, so it is contraindicated during pregnancy. The plant's tannins can have an irritating effect on gastric mucosa and the kidneys; limit consecutive use to two weeks. With the addition of Marshmallow and/or Corn silk, length of usage can be increased somewhat.

Other Uses

Although seed–filled and mealy, Manzanita's edible fruit are good for making jams and jellies. They taste apple–like[18].

---

18   Manzanita means little apple in Spanish.

Marsh Fleabane
Asteraceae/Sunflower Family

Pluchea camphorata (L.) DC. *(Erigeron camphoratus)*
Salt–marsh fleabane

Pluchea sericea (Nutt.) Coville *(Berthelotia sericea, Eremohylema sericea, Poly-*
pappus sericeus, Tessaria sericea)
Arrowweed, Cachanilla

Description

Pluchea camphorata is a tall and herbaceous annual. Its leaves are large, serrated, ovoid, and form alternately along stems. The mature flower clusters develop in large corymbs and are purplish–pink. The whole plant is somewhat sticky and has a strong camphor–like odor. When not in flower the plant may easily be confused with Camphorweed: Marsh fleabane has reddish stems, Camphorweed does not.

Pluchea sericea is a thicket–forming shrub. The plant's wand–like stems can reach 10′ in height, but usually they are less. The leaves are lanceolate, have prominent mid–veins, and alternate along the upper stems. Both the leaves and twigs on newer branch growth have a distinctive coating of hair. These appressed hairs cover the plant making its appearance somewhat silvery. The flower clusters are situated at the branch ends and are reddish–purple to lavender. Moreover, like others in the Sunflower family, the mature seeds are wind carried by their delicate tufts.

Distribution

Pluchea camphorata grows throughout most of the United States. In the West it is typically found at low–elevations in saline–alkaline moist soils. Look to the edges of slow moving rivers, around ponds, lakesides, and on moist alluvial fans.

Pluchea sericea is also found in low–lying moist soils, along drainages, streams, and on river and pond sides. It is well distributed throughout the low elevation Southwest. It ranges from southern California, east to southern Nevada, Utah, southern Colorado, south through much of Arizona, along the Rio Grande in New Mexico, and finally to the Trans–Pecos region of Texas. Both species are often found side by side.

Chemistry
Flavonoids, triterpenes, and sesquiterpenes.

Medicinal Uses
Although different plant parts are used, applications for both species generally overlap. Being the more stimulating of the two, Pluchea camphorata moves blood to surface tissues more so than P. sericea. The roots of P. sericea and the herb portion of P. camphorata made into various topical preparations are decidedly antiinflammatory and antioxidant to damaged tissues. Both plants are well applied to wounds. They facilitate healing and resolve tissue edema and swelling.

Internally both plants are sedating to gastrointestinal tract cramps associated with diarrhea. The tea, used longer–term, is diminishing to irritative–inflammatory conditions of the gastrointestinal tract walls, such as gastritis or colitis. If feverish, the hot tea of P. camphorata is diaphoretic and as a cold tea, it is diuretic. The plant may also stimulate menses as well as sedate period cramps.

Indications
» Wounds/Cuts/Abrasions (external)
» Cramps, gastrointestinal, with associated diarrhea
» Inflammation, gastrointestinal
» Fevers, dry

Collection
Gather the roots of Pluchea sericea and the herbage of P. camphorata, minus the flowers if allergic to Sunflower family pollen.

Preparations/Dosage
» FPT/DPT (60% alcohol): 30–60 drops 2–3 times daily
» Leaf/Root tea: 4–6 ounces 2–3 times daily
» External preparations: as needed

Cautions
Do not use during pregnancy.

Mesquite
Fabaceae/Pea Family

Prosopis velutina Wooton *(Neltuma velutina, Prosopis chilensis var. velutina, P. juliflora var. velutina)*
Velvet mesquite

Prosopis pubescens Benth. *(Prosopis emoryi, P. odorata, Strombocarpa odorata, S. pubescens)*
Screwbean mesquite, Tornillo

Prosopis glandulosa var. torreyana (Prosopis juliflora var. torreyana)
Western honey mesquite, Algarroba, Chachaca

Prosopis glandulosa (Prosopis juliflora var. glandulosa)
Honey mesquite

Description

Depending on soil and water conditions, Velvet mesquite grows to be a large shrub, or a small to moderate–sized tree. Older Velvet mesquites found along bottomlands and riversides have large, multi–branched trunks and can reach 50′–60′. The same tree growing in less hydrated soils, along secondary drainages or on hillsides, are 10′–20′ tall. The older bark is fissured and dark, and where the tree has sustained some injury from insects or branch damage a light brown to almost clear sap may weep from the wound. Composing each leaf is 1 or 2 sets of primary leaflets; each contains 9–30 sets of secondary leaflets. They are small and densely pubescent. Like most other Mesquites, this species has leaf–node–originating paired spines. The spines tend to be more abundant on young branches. The 2″–5″ long yellow flower spikes are cylindrical and composed of numerous small flowers. The seedpods are 4″–8″ long, narrow, and tend to gently curve in one direction or another. Like the leaves, the outer pod covering is pubescent. They are light tan in color when mature.

Screwbean mesquite is a large and spiny shrub or small tree. The older trunk bark is fibrous and stringy. The primary leaflets develop in sets of 1 or 2. Secondary leaflets number 5–9 sets and are small and covered with a dense coating of hair. The pale gray spines develop from leaf nodes. Cream flower spikes are 1½"–2" long. They are typical for the genus. The most characteristic part of the plant is its tightly spiraled, tan seedpods. These natural corkscrews are 1"–2½" long and encase small tan seeds.

Western honey mesquite, a large shrub or small tree, reaches 20' in height. Its pinnate leaves are composed of 1 set of primary leaflets and 8–20 sets of secondary leaflets. They are between ½"–1" in length and are typically hairless or have hair only along the margin. Large spines form in pairs at leaf nodes. The cream–yellow flower spikes are 2"–5" long. When mature the seedpods are tan and are 4"–10" long. Honey mesquite is similar in appearance to Western honey mesquite, although this species' larger leaves give it a weeping appearance. It is an attractive small tree.

Distribution
From 1,000'–4,500' Velvet mesquite is found just south of the Mogollon Rim in central Arizona and continues south through the bulk of the state. The tree is found along washes, drainages, rich bottomlands, and increasingly on drier slopes and mesas.

Look for Screwbean mesquite from sea level to 3,000' along major drainages throughout most of our southwestern deserts. In Arizona, the tree is found along the Colorado, Gila, Bill Williams, and Santa Cruz Rivers. In New Mexico look for it from the southern expanse of the Rio Grande to Texas until Devils River. In southern Utah, southern Nevada, and southern California the tree is also common along major drainages.

Western honey mesquite grows from sea level to 6,000' throughout much of southeastern California, southern Nevada, and in a small segment of Utah's Washington County. In Arizona look along practically the entire length of the Colorado and Gila Rivers, in isolated pockets in Cochise County, to southwestern New Mexico, particularly along the Rio Grande. It follows this course into Texas and reaches its eastward limit at Corpus Christi. Honey mesquite begins where Western honey mesquite leaves off. From southeastern New Mexico the tree covers much of Texas, southeastern Colorado, Kansas, Oklahoma, and finally to the Shreveport area of Louisiana. It is a tree of Desert Grasslands, plains, and prairies.

Chemistry
Condensed and hydrolyzable tannins.

Medicinal Uses

Like other Pea family plants, namely Acacia and Mimosa, Mesquite leaf powder is applied to cuts and scrapes to lessen superficial inflammation and astringe minor bleeding. The leaf tea is used to soothe sunburn, rashes, bites, and most other red and weepy conditions. The tea can also be gargled for sore throats and mouth sores.

The liquid or hardened sap, mixed with water and salt is soothing to conjunctivitis. The solution's antimicrobial activity will increase if mixed equally with Prickly poppy tea. Even though the sap has some inherent mucilage, over time the tannins can prove drying to the eyes. Therefore it is best to use it for several days at a time, then alternate to Prickly poppy or Desert anemone alone.

The hardened sap is one of the most reliable (and convenient) remedies for heartburn and gastritis. Simply suck on a grape–sized nodule like a piece of hard candy. Its mucilage–tannin mixture will soothe most gastric discomforts in 10–15 minutes.

Indications

» Cuts/Scrapes/Inflammations (external)
» Sore throats/Mouth sores (gargle)
» Conjunctivitis (eyewash)
» Gastritis/Heartburn

Collection

From late spring to early summer, gather the leaves when they are fully mature. During the spring and summer a pan can be set out under the tree's wounds in order to catch the weeping sap. Older nodules of hardened sap are also collected; they are found on older and younger trees alike. Gather Mesquite pods from mid to late summer, still on the tree when they are tan and brittle.

Preparations

The collected liquid sap is strained and diluted with 5 parts of distilled water. The hardened sap is slowly simmered in 32 parts of distilled water. After it has completely dissolved strain the solution well through a paper towel. Either solution is made isotonic by adding salt. See directions under eyewash. By applying low heat, the liquid sap can also be dehydrated for future use.

Store the pods in a refrigerator or freezer if not using them immediately, as every bean potentially contains a small insect. If there is a sudden occurrence of winged insects flying around indoors, look to the bucket of forgotten Mesquite pods in the corner – that is their source.

Dosage
»   Leaf infusion, topically or as a gargle: as needed
»   Eyewash: 2–3 times daily for 2–3 days, then rotate to a tannin free solution
»   Gum nodule: as needed

Cautions
There are no known cautions with normal usage.

Other Uses
½–1 pound of dried, mature pods are put into 2–3 gallons of water and slowly boiled. After several hours strain the Mesquite pod tea and continue to simmer. Reduce until a thickened consistency is reached. You now have a tasty and sweet syrup that can be used on pancakes, desserts, and other similar things.

Use an electric or hand grinder to make the meal or flour from the dried pods. All types of baked goods (cookies, breads, etc.) can be made with the meal–flour.

Mimosa
Fabaceae/Pea Family

Mimosa dysocarpa Benth. *(Mimosa wrightii)*
Velvet–pod mimosa, Gatuno

Mimosa aculeaticarpa Ortega *(Mimosa biuncifera)*
Wait–a–minute bush, Catclaw mimosa

Description
Mimosa dysocarpa is a 3′–6′ high perennial bush. The plant's thorns are spaced alternately along its branches. Smaller stems are distinctive in that they are 5–ridged. Mimosa's leaves are doubly compound and are

composed of 5–10 sets of primary leaflets and 6–12 sets of smaller second-ary leaflets. The pink to rose flowers form in cylinder–like spikes and are about an inch long. With age, the flowers become light in color giving them a distinctive 2–toned appearance. The 1″–2″ long seedpods contain numer-ous light brown seeds. The plant is called Velvet pod mimosa because the seedpods (and stems) are covered with fine appressed hair making them velvety to the touch.

Mimosa biuncifera is also between 3′–6′ tall but occasionally it be-comes larger, particularly when growing in moister soils. It is a many–branched shrub that forms in dense or open groupings. Unlike Catclaw acacia, which has alternating stem thorns, this species' branches have 2 re-curved thorns per node. The leaves are bipinnate. Its primary leaflets are composed of 4–7 sets and secondary leaflets have 6–13 sets. The small ball–like flower clusters are typically cream–colored, but occasionally they are pink or lavender. The reddish–brown pods have weak margin thorns. The seeds are smooth, dark brown, and almost a ¼″ long.

Distribution
Look for Mimosa dysocarpa between 4,000′–6,500′ in canyons and along hillsides and slopes from southern Arizona, east to New Mexico and west-ern Texas. M. dysocarpa prefers upper Desert Grasslands and Oak Wood-lands as its primary habitat. M. biuncifera is found between 3,000′–6,000′ throughout Arizona, New Mexico, and a large extent of Texas. Look for the plant in middle mountain drainages and along hillsides.

Chemistry
Hydrolyzed and condensed tannins.

Medicinal Uses
Use Mimosa like most other southwestern legume shrub–trees: as a tan-nin–based mild astringent. Topical preparations are soothing to abraded tissues and scraped skin. Compounding this effect with Mimosa's mild antimicrobial qualities makes the plant equally useful in diminishing the chances of superficial cuts becoming infected. A Mimosa leaf wash is well applied to sunburned skin. Most find it mildly soothing and cooling to in-flamed tissues. As a gargle, Mimosa is useful in astringing bleeding gums, canker sores, and sore throats.

Indications
»   Scrapes/Cuts/Skin abrasions/Burns (external)
»   Mouth sores/Sore throats (gargle)

Collection
When Mimosa's leaves are fully developed, usually after mid–spring, clip the branch ends from the plant. Dry these whole, then strip the leaves from the branch ends. Keep the leaves as medicine.

Preparations/Dosage
»   Leaf wash/Powder/Poultice: apply as needed
»   Leaf infusion: gargle as needed

Cautions
There are no known cautions with normal usage.

Other Uses
The dried beans can be cooked and eaten after one or two changes of water.

Mormon Tea
Ephedraceae/Joint–fir Family

Ephedra spp. L.
Mexican tea, Brigham tea, Joint fir, Popotillo, Tepopote, Canatillo

Description
Depending on species, Mormon tea varies in size. Some species are low–growing sub–shrubs; others like Ephedra trifurca can develop sizable trunks and attain heights of 6'–7'. Mormon tea's thin, wand–like branches are its most characteristic feature. They look to be large clumps of stiff–spiny grasses. Branch color varies depending on species and season. Some are bluish–green and then others are yellowish–green. At each branch node, small leaves, oppositely paired or in sets of 3, form virtually un–noticed. In the spring, small male and female cones develop on separate plants. They are clustered around branch nodes. After the female cone is successfully pollinated 1–3 small seeds are produced.

Distribution

At varying elevations, Mormon tea is common throughout our western deserts. Look for the plant in many different topographies. Flats, basins, rocky slopes, and hillsides are some typical habitats for the plant.

Chemistry

Flavonoids: lucenin 1, vicenin 2, and an array of tannins.

Medicinal Uses

Even though our native Mormon tea species supposedly contain no ephedrine and only traces of pseudoephedrine, the plant still is useful as a sinus passage decongestant, and in a limited capacity, as a bronchial dilator. Apparently, Mormon tea contains enough 'sub–ephedrates'[19] to make this effect noticeable. In addition, the plant's flavonoid content may contribute to these properties. Take the tea or tincture throughout allergy season for hayfever. Moreover, used before allergy season Mormon tea reduces allergic tendencies by strengthening mucus membranes.

Traditionally, Mormon tea has been used for urinary troubles. The tea tends to calm bladder and urethral irritation and can be useful in diminishing kidney irritability through its soothing diuretic properties. In addition, the tea is astringing to mouth, esophageal, and upper stomach irritations. This attribute is common in many plants with substantial flavonoid–tannin complexes. Surface membranes tend to be strengthened; inflammation is sedated through Mormon tea's interaction with cell walls.

Indications

» Rhinitis
» Irritation, urinary tract
» Irritation, gastric

Collection

Throughout mid to late spring when new branch growth is at its peak, snip the last foot of green growth. Chop these branch ends into smaller sections for tea or tincture preparations.

---

19 Not reflected in lab analysis most Mormon tea species do contain CNS stimulating agents. Cardiovascular stimulation is notable after taking these plants (diaphoresis/stronger pulse).

Preparations

Aside from the basic tea and tincture preparations, one efficient technique used for Mormon tea is as follows: cut the dried branches into 1" pieces. Put the pieces into a blender. Blend until most of the chlorophyll–laden cortical layers separate from the fibrous inner material, resulting in a green–yellow powder and small fibrous bundles. Sift the powder from the fiber with a mesh strainer. Encapsulate the powder; discard the fiber bunches. Take 1–2 capsules 2–3 times daily for head–centered allergy and hayfever reaction.

Dosage

»   Branch decoction: 4–6 ounces 1–3 times daily
»   DPT (50% alcohol): 30–60 drops 1–3 times daily
»   Capsules (00): 1–2, 1–3 times daily

Cautions

Use Mormon tea in moderation during pregnancy. Due to the plant's substantial tannin concentration, it has potential as a uterine wall vasoconstrictor. Like Chinese ephedra, do not take it if suffering from cardiovascular disease.

Mountain Marigold
Asteraceae/Sunflower Family

Tagetes lemmonii A. Gray
Lemmon's marigold

Description

Mountain marigold is an herbaceous perennial that freezes back to the ground during winter months. In mid–summer when at its peak it usually stands 3' tall by 3' wide with an array of suspended yellow daisy–like flowers. If the leaves are closely examined oil glands can be clearly seen. The volatiles contained within these glands are responsible for the mint–anise, slightly skunky odor that permeates the air if the plant is brushed against or crushed.

Distribution

Mountain marigold is a mid–mountain plant of southeastern Arizona and northern Mexico. It is found from 4,000'–8,000' among Oaks and Conifers in canyon bottoms where the soil is more apt to be nutrient rich and moist.

Chemistry

Acetylenic thiophenes, flavonoids, benzofurans, and carotenoids: lutein and zeaxanthin.

Medicinal Uses

Mountain marigold tea is soothing to stomach and upper small intestinal irritation. If the upper gastrointestinal tract is inflamed, this plant offers relief through its mild antiinflammatory and analgesic properties. Use it if suffering from gastritis, pre–ulcer conditions, and gas pains.

The plant has an interesting effect on the nervous system and corresponding emotional outlook. Shortly after the fresh plant tincture is taken, a calming quality can be felt along with a lightness of mind, sometimes to the extent of giddiness. I have seen the effects of this plant useful in times of fixated emotional morbidity.

If feverish, the hot tea is a reliable way to initiate sweating. Mountain marigold is predictably vasodialating. The plant's aromatics shift blood flow to the surface of the body, dilating the pores of the skin, therefore facilitating diaphoresis. An oil or salve can be made from the dried flowers and applied to poorly healing skin, cuts, and scrapes. It is nutritive to tissues and will expedite healing.

Indications

» Gastric irritation/Gas pains
» Fevers, dry
» Poorly healing tissues/Scrapes (external)

Collection

From late spring to late summer collect the upper foliage with or without the flowers (the flowers are rich in carotenoids and flavonoids).

Preparations

Tincture fresh, or dry the leaves and flowers for tea or topical use.

Dosage
» FPT: 30–60 drops 3–4 times daily
» Leaf infusion: 4–8 ounces 3–4 times daily
» Oil/Salve made from the flowers: topically as needed

Cautions
There are no known cautions with normal usage.

Night Blooming Cereus
Cactaceae/Cactus Family

Selenicereus grandiflorus (L.) Britton & Rose *(Cereus grandiflorus, Cactus grandiflorus)*
Sweet scented cactus, Queen of the night

Peniocereus greggii (Engelm.) Britton & Rose *(Cereus greggii)*
Queen of the night, Reina de la noche

Description
Selenicereus grandiflorus is a thin–stemmed cactus that creeps along the ground and climbs into surrounding vegetation. The fleshy stems have 5–6 ridges that extend along its length and are lined with small groupings of spines. The white–cream flowers are large, showy, and fragrant. They are 8"–10" wide with thin and linear sepals surrounding the larger petals. They open in the evening and close with the morning sun. The small fruit are orange–red and contain numerous small seeds.

Peniocereus greggii is a weak–stemmed and thin cactus growing up through other bushes for support. Typical support–protection plants are Creosote bush, Catclaw, and other desert shrubs. The weakly spined branches are usually 4–5 ribbed, grayish–green, and somewhat branched. They are easily mistaken for dead sticks so a trained eye is often needed to find the plant when not in flower. The above ground stems occasionally die back each year only to grow anew from a large tuber. The flowers, similar to Selenicereus grandiflorus', are very large, fragrant, and open for one night only in the spring to early summer. A group of plants in a local vicinity has the uncanny ability of flowering during the same night. The fruit are small and ovoid and similar in most respects to S. grandiflorus'.

Distribution

Selenicereus grandiflorus is indigenous to the West Indies but is widely cultivated as an ornamental and occasionally can be found in nurseries in warmer parts of the country. It grows well as an indoor potted cactus. Peniocereus greggii is found throughout lower elevations in western Texas, southern New Mexico, and Arizona. Look to Creosote bush mesas and hillsides. It is never an easy plant to locate in the wild but once it is found there are usually others in close proximity.

Chemistry

Selenicereus grandiflorus: hordenine; roots of Peniocereus greggii: peniocerol, desoxyviperidone, viperidone, viperidinone, and β–sitosterol.

Medicinal Uses

The therapeutic applications for Selenicereus grandiflorus and Peniocereus greggii generally overlap, although P. greggii is considered the weaker of the two. S. grandiflorus has a well–documented western tradition, which spans more than 150 years. First used by Homeopathic practitioners, then by the Eclectic Doctors, and finally by some non–conformist, standard–practice doctors, all agreed, Cactus (as S. grandiflorus was formerly called) was a useful cardiovascular medicine. Traditional Mexican use of P. greggii appears to be similar, although specific differences are not known. Both species will be referred to as Night blooming cereus.

Use Night blooming cereus to slow and strengthen a rapid, thready, and excitable pulse. Individuals who tend to be of a nervous temperament and who are prone to palpitations, shortness of breath, and weakness, all resulting from over work or emotional upset will benefit from Night blooming cereus. Similar to Hawthorn, a gloomy and dark outlook accompanying the above symptom set also indicates Night blooming cereus. Older individuals should use it as a heart tonic for mild to moderate heart enlargement or weakness from tobacco use.

Just how Night blooming cereus enlivens the heart is still under debate, but it appears that it may augment adrenergic–sympathetic responses affecting the organ. The plant combines well with thyroid sedating herbs such as Lycopus or Leonurus in diminishing hyperthyroidal heart palpitations. Fluid retention tends to lessen around the extremities, particularly around the ankles if dependent upon cardiac weakness. Unlike Digitalis, Night blooming cereus does not have a cumulative effect, so there is no danger of build–up toxicity. The plant best suits functional disturbances and is of only moderate value in organic valvular irregularities such as mitral and aortic regurgitations.

Indications
» Cardiac irregularities dependent upon weakness
» Tachycardia/Arrhythmia/Palpitations

Collection/Preparations
Unless island hopping in the Caribbean, collecting Selenicereus grandiflorus will probably be from nursery stock. Clip several stems and/or flowers from the plant. Cut these into small ¼"–½" pieces and tincture fresh. If a group of Peniocereus greggii is found in the desert, be light–handed about collection. Clipping several branches from a plant will not have a detrimental effect due to its massive storage root. However, if in flower, leave it to set seed. Do not collect the root in the wild, as the plant is endemic and isolated in the United States. Occasionally P. greggii can be found propagated at native plant nurseries throughout the Southwest, if so using the root is permissible. Process and tincture the stems and/or roots the same as S. grandiflorus. Drying either plant will diminish its medicinal strength.

Dosage
» FPT of Selenicereus grandiflorus: 5–15 drops 1–4 times daily
» FPT of Peniocereus greggii: 10–25 drops 1–4 times daily

Cautions
Do not use Night blooming cereus if there is a strong and bounding pulse, typically exhibited in robust individuals with strong constitutions. In these individuals, Night blooming cereus may raise blood pressure. Inversely in asthenic types, the plant typically lowers blood pressure or will have no effect on the matter. Do not use while pregnant or nursing.

Ocotillo
Fouquieriaceae/Ocotillo Family

Fouquieria splendens Engelm.
Coachwhip, Candlewood, Jacob's staff

Description

Like many plants of the southwestern deserts, Ocotillo is semi–succulent and appears bizarre compared to temperate–zone plant life. This multi-stemmed, long lived perennial often lives to be 150 or 200 years old. A mature, well–nourished plant can produce upwards of 100 spiny vertical stems. The stem bark is distinctly patterned and is comprised of living material, which is yellowish and waxy, and non–living material, which is grayish and serves a protective function. The oval green leaves are waxy as well. Depending on rainfall, Ocotillo abundantly produces leaves and correspondingly loses them in drier times. This cycle can occur numerous times a year. At the branch ends conical red flower spikes are followed by valved seed capsules.

Distribution

Ocotillo is typically found from 6,000' and lower throughout the Sonoran, Mojave, and Chihuahuan Deserts. Look for the plant on mesa tops, rocky slopes, and plains.

Chemistry

Dammarenediol and its triterpenes derivatives; iridoid glucosides: gali-oside, splendoside, asperocotillin, adoxoside, adoxosidic acid, and loganin; kaempferol, quercetin, isoquercetin, rutin, cinnamic acids, caffeic acids, scopoletin, leucocyanidin, and ellagic acid.

Medicinal Uses

Ocotillo tends to be a mild expectorant. It increases bronchial secretion somewhat, making thickened phlegm easier to dislodge. The plant is also sedating to a dry and spasmodic cough. Both of these activities make Oco-tillo useful in wintertime lung afflictions.

Ocotillo has a general decongesting effect on lymphatic and venous circulation of the pelvic area. This use is well applied to hemorrhoids, pel-vic lymph enlargements, and prostatitis. It is speculated that Ocotillo is ef-fective here by its clarification of lipid–lymph uptake via the portal circula-tion. Overall, this influence enhances extracellular fluid movement of the area, lessening trunk–pelvic congestion. Traditional use of Ocotillo among Hispanic New Mexicans has been for sore throats, tonsillitis, and to simu-late menses.

Known locally by Mexican vaqueros as a wound healer on horses and other stock animals, the root seems to have a powerful topical effect on tissue cuts, gouges, tears, etc. For both people and animals, keep the poultice, salve, or other preparations applied until tissue mending is complete.

Indications
» Dry cough with thickened phlegm
» Hemorrhoids
» Lymph enlargements, pelvic
» Prostatitis
» Wounds (external)

Collection
After finding a many–branched and healthy Ocotillo, select a thick limb close to its outside circumference. With a hand–held saw make a clean lateral cut removing the stem from the base of the plant. As opposed to snapping the branch from the base by pulling downward, using a saw will ensure there is minimal surrounding damage. With a knife, strip the spiny bark from the core wood. The leaves can be collected with the bark as well.

Ocotillo root can be used equally, and is slightly more potent than the bark. I recommend collecting the root only if the plant has already been disturbed – possibly through subdivision development/blading, etc. Killing a mature plant – often 100–150 years old – for root material, when a stem can be similarly applied, is a short–sighted activity[20].

Preparations
Because of Ocotillo's nonpolar constituents, the plant is extracted well with alcohol. Although a vita–mix blender is (eventually) effective, the dried bark can be difficult to powder. The fresh plant tincture tends to be the most efficacious preparation.

Dosage
» FPT/DPT (70% alcohol): 30–60 drops 2–3 times daily
» Bark decoction: 4–6 ounces 2–3 times daily
» External preparations: as needed

20   In a number of states Ocotillo is labeled as a protected plant. This designation seems to be more of a revenue–generating procedure (pay $ for a collection permit) rather than a preservation tactic. Although regionally abundant, keep the legalities in mind when harvesting the plant.

Cautions
Do not use Ocotillo during pregnancy.

Other Uses
Living Ocotillo fences can be made by burying the cut stems (just below a joint is optimal) an inch or two in the ground. Secured and watered they root easily.

Dry the mature flowers for a beverage tea. A combination of Ocotillo flowers and Sumac fruit is a superb mixture – healthy and tasty.

Passionflower
Passifloraceae/Passionflower Family

Passiflora mexicana Juss. (*Cieca mexicana, Monactineirma mexicana, Passiflora contrayerva*)
Mexican passionflower

Passiflora foetida L. (*Dysosmia foetida, D. hircina, Passiflora baraquiniana*)
Corona de cristo

Passiflora incarnata L. (*Passiflora edulis var. kerii*)
Maypop, Purple passionflower

Description
All Passionflowers are vining plants that trail on the ground or climb into supporting vegetation. Anchoring tendrils are opposite deeply lobed leaves, which alternate along the stem. The flowers form on axillary peduncles of varying length and depending on species, they are generally a showy affair of different color. Normally there is a base of 5 or 10 tepals. Resting on top of this arrangement is a fringed corona, comprised of numerous filaments. Above this are 5 stamens and 3 styles in a whorled pattern. The fruit are many seeded and depending on species can be sweet and aromatic.

Passiflora mexicana's leaves are deeply 2–lobed, appearing much like a pair of pants. The mid–vein area traversing each lobe often has a whitish coloration. The corona is purplish–pink. P. foetida has 3–5 lobed leaves. They are grayish–green and felty. Its corona is lilac–colored. P. incarnata has 3–lobed leaves with pale blue–violet filaments.

Distribution

Look for Passiflora mexicana throughout southeastern Arizona between 2,500'–5,000'. The plant is commonly found growing up among Mesquites along streams and gullies that run with seasonal water. P. foetida ranges from southern Arizona and southern New Mexico to Texas. It is considered a weed throughout much of the tropical world. P. incarnate grows in warmer temperate regions. It is found throughout the southeast and as far west as Texas. Other species are planted as ornamentals throughout warmer parts of the west. The bulk of over 300 species exist throughout Tropical America.

Chemistry

For Passiflora incarnata: indole alkaloids: harman, harmine, harmalin, harmol, and harmalol; flavonoids: orientin, isoorientin, vitexin, and isovitexin; cyanogenic glycosides.

Medicinal Uses

Passionflower is a multi–faceted sedative. It is applicable to several different stress patterns and if used properly can take the place of herbal regimens that comprise a number of herbs. Firstly, use Passionflower to ease anxiousness and tension. Stronger doses of 1–2 teaspoons of tincture taken before bed can be quite effective in alleviating insomnia.

If timed well Passionflower diminishes mild seizure activity. Take the herb before an episode fully manifests. The plant is also indicated in diminishing tics and muscle spasms from fright, anger, or other vicissitudes of life.

Passionflower tends to be one of the most reliable herbs in curbing cravings and anxiety in substance withdrawal. Make Passionflower a primary herb if quitting Cannabis, opiates, alcohol, or nicotine habits. It is calming to the nerves and soothing to the mind when the body is craving to be re–intoxicated. It is of particular use in the tremors of alcohol withdrawal.

The plant fits individuals with excessive cardiac force that have a strong pulse, hypertension, and noticeable surface vasodilation – blood movement – around the upper chest and neck. Use Passionflower to lower blood pressure and slow the heart rate. It is one of the best remedies in aborting tachycardia.

The plant is underrated in its application to bronchial complaints when there is an irritative, spastic cough that is difficult to stop. Its spasmolytic effect is also serviceable in bronchial constriction and shortness of breath when nervousness is exacerbating the episode. The plant is calming to griping and spasmodic diarrhea from food reactions or the catch all – irritable bowel syndrome.

Indications

» Anxiety/Tension
» Spasm, muscle
» Mild seizure activity/Tics
» Insomnia
» Substance withdrawal
» Tachycardia with hypertension and forceful pulse
» Cough, spasmodic/bronchial constriction
» Diarrhea, spasmodic

Collection

Passiflora mexicana and P. foetida are summer bloomers and are collected from late summer to early fall when in full flower. Ideally, prune the whole vine with leaf, flowers, and immature fruit. Also, collect the cultivated varieties in bloom. Passionflowers that are medicinally potent stink when in flower or when their foliage is crushed. Let their rank smell be an indicator to different species' potency.

Preparations/Dosage

» FPT/DPT (50% alcohol): 60–90 drops 2–3 times daily or 1 teaspoon in acute situations
» Fluidextract: 20–40 drops 2–3 times daily
» Herb infusion: 4–8 ounces 2–3 times daily

Cautions

Do not use Passionflower during pregnancy due to its weak contractile inhibition of uterine smooth muscle. Although the plant has use in replacing anti–anxiety or sedative pharmaceuticals, full doses of both simultaneously will prove synergistic and will leave the recipient overly sedated.

Other Uses
Passiflora edulis is primarily cultivated in warmer parts of the world for its edible fruit. As a medicine, the plant is inferior. Inversely the other varieties, principally the southwestern natives, will have semi–edible fruit with medicinal/sedative overtones.

Penstemon
Scrophulariaceae/Figwort Family

Penstemon spp. Schmidel
Beardtongue

Description
Depending on species, Penstemon generally takes on three varying morphologies. It is either small, delicate and ground hugging, upright and herbaceous, or robust and shrub–like. Whatever the type, these perennials have opposite leaves. Upper leaves are sessile and tend to clasp the stem. Lower leaves are petioled. Often they are thickened, lance or ovoid shaped, and smooth and glaucous. The flowers form in racemes and are found in a wide array of colors: red, pink, and purple are common. The tubular flowers have 5 united petals and are often 2–lipped. The oval seed capsules contain many small brownish seeds.

Distribution
With over 200 species worldwide, most occur in the American West. Penstemon frequents varying elevations: from the low elevation arid desert, to the high mountains with Conifers and Aspen, some variety of Penstemon will probably be close. Look to the edges of draws, gullies, rocky hillsides, meadows, and along trail and roadsides. It is a common plant.

Chemistry
Iridoid glycosides, phenolic acids, and anthocyanines.

Medicinal Uses
Although Penstemon remains largely under–utilized as a plant medicine, in terms of strength it appears to be on–par with Figwort (Scrophularia spp.), another Figwort family plant. That is to say both are mild medicines

that exhibit minor antiinflammatory qualities.

Use Penstemon topically as a mild therapy for stings, bites, rashes, and poorly healing tissues. Its structure–enhancing anthocyanines, mainly responsible for the flower's coloration, are very useful in augmenting skin repair, so the most effective preparation should include both leaf and flower material. These qualities also make the plant applicable to cut and wound healing. Combining Penstemon's structure enhancing compounds with its soothing and cooling attributes makes it a worthy application for many conditions.

Indications
» Rashes/Bites/Stings (external)
» Wounds/Cuts (external)

Collection
When in flower clip the upper herbage and use it either fresh or dry. Emphasis on tissue repair can be increased by collecting more flowering racemes.

Preparations/Dosage
» Oil/Salve/Poultice: as needed

Cautions
There are no known cautions with normal usage.

Periwinkle
Apocynaceae/Dogbane Family

Vinca major L.
Big leaf periwinkle

Description
Periwinkle is a trailing perennial with dark green and ovate–pointed leaves. They are 2"–3" long, opposite, waxy, and have wavy margins. The non–flowering stems grow close to the ground and root profusely at the nodes. The showy and solitary purple flowers form from leaf axils. The corollas are 5–lobed and base–fused. Like many other Dogbane family plants,

when a leaf or stem is broken a milky latex exudes from the wound. The plant in the West reproduces not sexually, but by spreading rhizomes.

Distribution
Periwinkle is originally native to southern Europe and northern Africa. In warmer areas throughout the United States, it is found as an ornamental escapee. From pockets in the northwest part of the country, it is found in horseshoe pattern: down the west coast through most of California, then throughout the Southwest and Southeast, finally to the mid–eastern states. Temperature extremes, sun exposure, and lack of moisture limit the plant's expanse. Look to shaded streamsides and around old farms and homesteads.

Chemistry
Alkaloids: majvinine, reserpinine, vincamajoreine, vincawajine, majoridine, methoxyvellosimine, and lochvinerine.

Medicinal Uses
Like caffeine, through Periwinkle's vasoconstricting effect on peripheral blood vessels, it can be useful in diminishing the pain and sensitivity of an acute stage migraine headache. Systemically as well, the plant lessens passive hemorrhaging. Use it to quell mild bleeding from hemorrhoids, nosebleeds, and urinary tract injury. Profuse menstruation, as well as mid–cycle bleeding, also diminishes under Periwinkle use.

Indications
»   Migraines, acute pain
»   Hemorrhoids, bleeding
»   Nosebleeds
»   Hemorrhaging, passive, urinary tract
»   Menorrhagia/Mid cycle–bleeding

Collection
Gather the leafing vine with or without the flowers. Tincture the plant fresh, or dry for other preparations.

Preparations/Dosage
»   FPT/DPT (50% alcohol): 20–40 drops 1–3 times daily

Cautions

Do not use during pregnancy or while nursing. Periwinkle may slightly lower blood pressure, so it is not recommended if taking cardiovascular medications.

Pipevine
Aristolochiaceae/Pipevine Family

Aristolochia watsonii Wooton & Standl. *(Aristolochia porphyrophylla)*
Watson's birthwort, Watson's dutchman's pipe, Desert pipevine, Arizona snakeroot, Yerba del indio, Raíz del indio

Description

Aristolochia watsonii carpets the ground or surrounding rocks in small patches. Occasionally a foot or two of vine growth can be found growing up into supportive bushes. Its leaves are green, reddish–green, or even purple. They are alternate, triangular–hastate, and have pronounced light-er mid–veins. The pipe–shaped tubular flowers are green/purple with in-ner purple spots and a purple lined mouth. The fruit is a greenish–purple winged/valved capsule.

Most species (350 or so) of Aristolochia are known as carrion flow-ers. They emit musky/rank/rotting odors in order to attract their particu-lar pollinators. This species is pollinated by sand flies, better known as 'no–see–ums'.

Distribution

Aristolochia watsonii is found throughout much of Arizona, southern New Mexico, and possibly to western Texas (listed in some of the older keys). Within its range it is fairly common, but often missed due to being very inconspicuous. It primarily is found next to dry stream beds, seasonal drainages, wash sides, and occasionally on lesser traveled dirt roads. Using coverage plants, it is often associated with Acacia, Mesquite, or Palo verde, and is mostly found between 2000'–4500'.

Chemistry

Aristolochia general: aristolochic acid derivatives with various carbon skel-etons, aporphines, benzylisoquinolines, isoquinolines, protoberberines, protopines, amides, chlorophylls, mono–, sesqui–, and diterpenoids, lignans, biphenyl ethers, flavonoids, tetralones, benzenoids, and steroids.

Medicinal Uses

Most Aristolochia species throughout the world have significant medicinal histories. From internal to external use, they are effective medicines for an array of issues other plants simply don't address (or a complex combination of plant medicines are needed to duplicate Aristolochia's influences).

Unfortunately though, over the past two decades a particular toxicity issue has become apparent with the regular ingestion of a number of Asian species: notably Aristolochia fangchi and A. manshuriensis. Chinese–Herbs Nephropathy (CHN) has been coined describing a situation of rapidly progressive interstitial nephropathy. In extreme cases continued ingestion has resulted in renal cancer and/or deterioration resulting in transplant, or even death linked to untreated renal failure.

Aristolochic acids (especially AA1 and AA2), a group of compounds found in varying quantities in likely all Aristolochia species, are at the toxicities' center. A large number of these species contain high levels of offending AAs. Chinese species are not the only plants to have been implicated. Renal disease has also been correlated with a number of Japanese, European, and Indian species. American varieties potentially have the same issues.

Aristolochia watsonii, at least according to one chemical analysis, contains low amounts of toxic AA1 and AA2, but higher amounts of low–toxicity AA3. This may seem like good news, but the problem that occurs with relying upon just one analysis is the same problem that is encountered when just one study or one sample is relied upon: the chance of one stand–alone observation being inaccurate is much greater than a number of independent, yet similar in conclusion, observations being inaccurate. So until more research is available on A. watsonii's chemistry, I suggest using Aristolochia watsonii, and indeed all other species of Aristolochia, only externally[21].

The external application of Pipevine is not outside the realm of

21   It indeed pains me to reclassify this plant as potentially more toxic than therapeutic (internally). Adverse reaction documentation has passed the speculative threshold. Unlike the opaque and biased 'the sky is falling' viewpoints on Comfrey, Ephedra, and Kava, it is clear that Aristolochia should not be used internally even in small amounts.

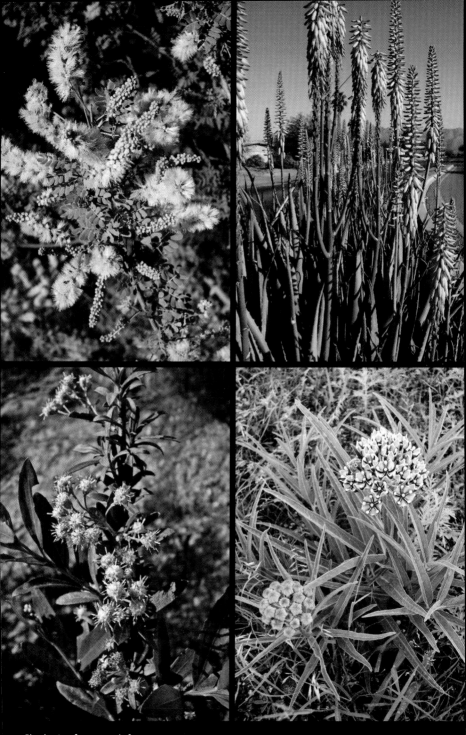

Clockwise from top left:
1. Acacia (*Acacia greggii*); 2. Aloe (*Aloe vera*); 3. Antelope horns (*Asclepias asperula*); 4. Baccharis (*Baccharis salicifolia*).

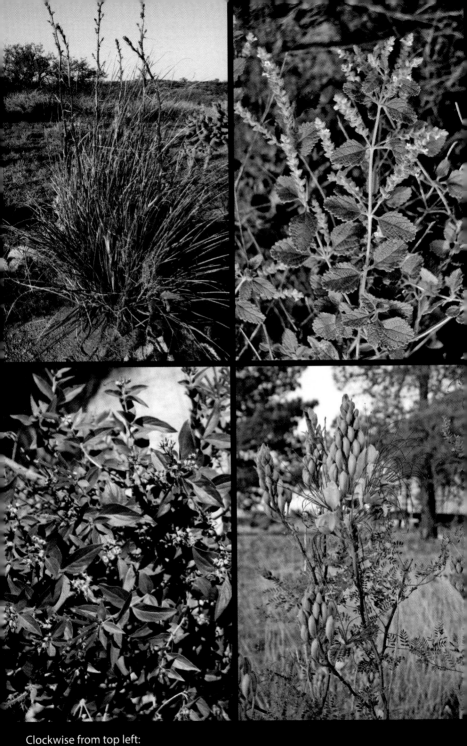

Clockwise from top left:
5. Beargrass (*Nolina microcarpa*); 6. Beebrush (*Aloysia wrightii*); 7. Bird of paradise
(*Caesalpinia gilliesii*); 8. Bouvardia (*Bouvardia ternifolia*).

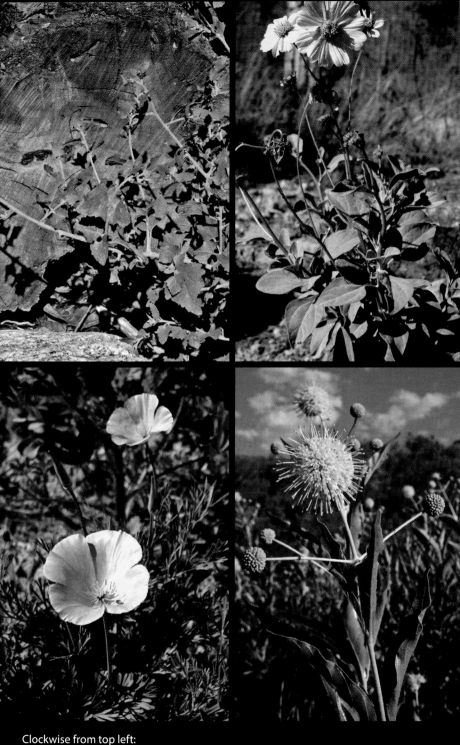

Clockwise from top left:
9. Bricklebush (*Brickellia californica*); 10. Brittlebush (*Encelia farinosa*); 11. Buttonbush (*Cephalanthus occidentalis*); 12. California poppy (*Eschscholzia californica subsp. mexicana*).

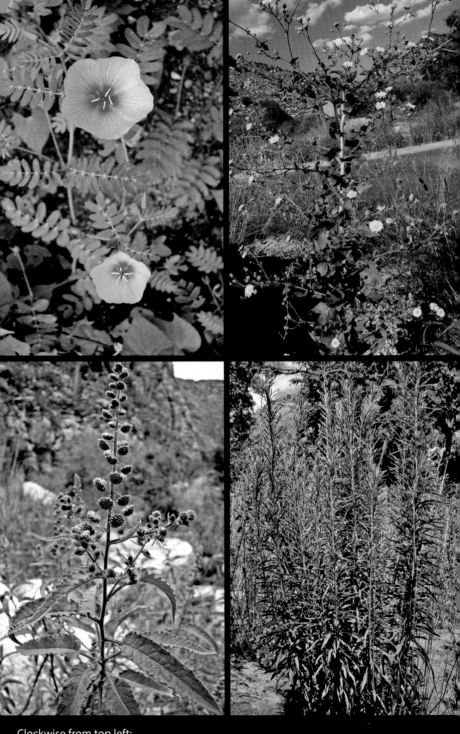

Clockwise from top left:

13. Caltrop (*Kallstroemia grandiflora*); 14. Camphorweed (*Heterotheca subaxillaris*); 15.
Canadian fleabane (*Conyza canadensis*); 16. Canyon bursage (*Ambrosia ambrosioides*).

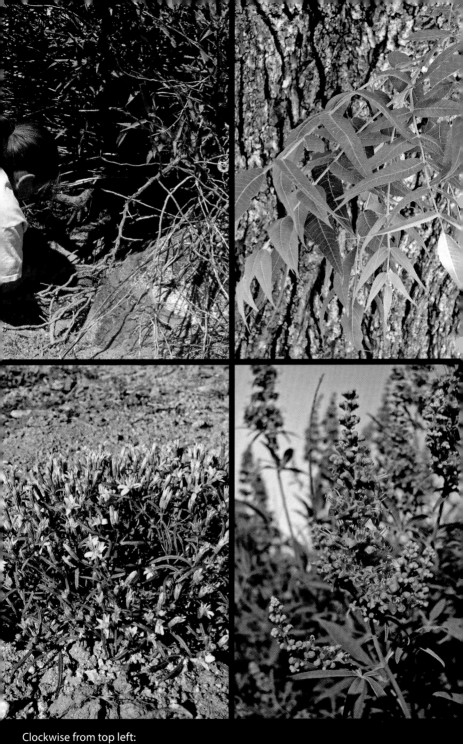

Clockwise from top left:

17. Canyon bursage (*Ambrosia ambrosioides*); 18. Canyon walnut (*Juglans major*); 19. Chaste tree (*Vitex castus, anaus*); 20. Chinchweed (*Pectis papposa*)

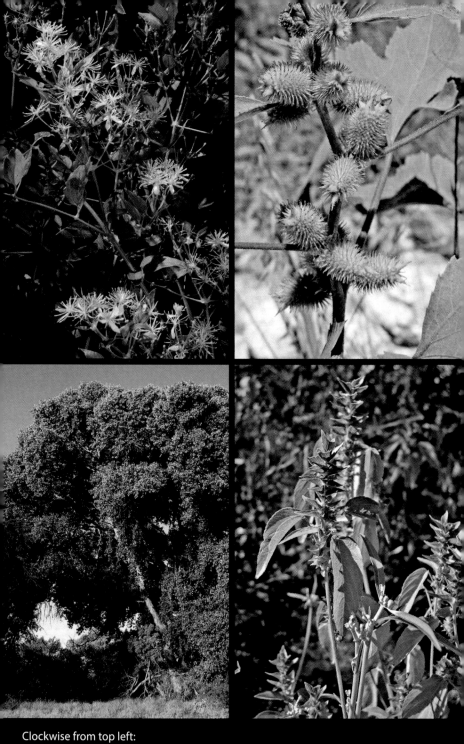

Clockwise from top left:
21. Clematis (*Clematis ligusticifolia*); 22. Cocklebur (*Xanthium strumarium*); 23. Copperleaf
(*Acalypha neomexicana*); 24. Cottonwood (*Populus fremontii*)

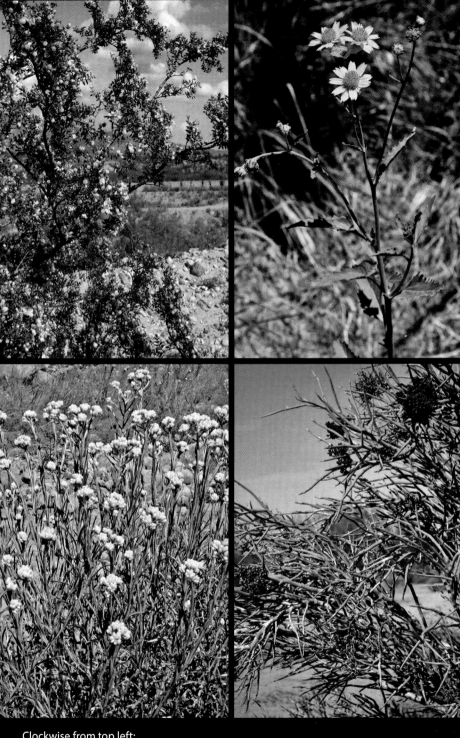

Clockwise from top left:
25. Creosote bush (*Larrea tridentata*); 26. Crownbeard (*Verbesina encelioides*); 27. Crucifixion thorn (*Castela emoryi*); 28. Cudweed (*Pseudognaphalium leucocephalum*).

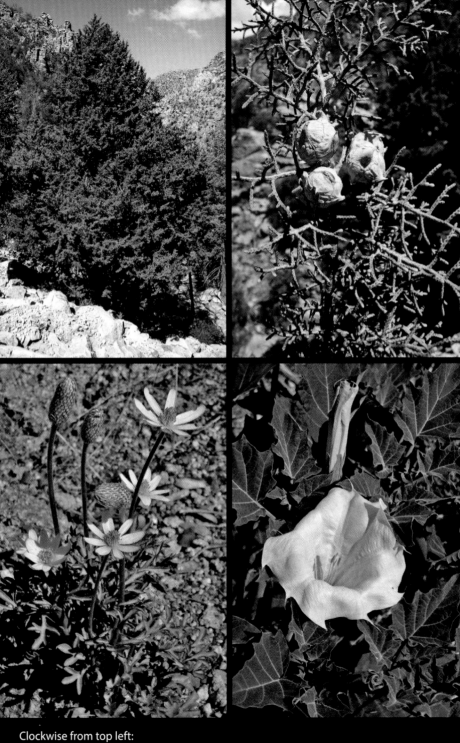

Clockwise from top left:
29. Cypress (*Cupressus arizonica*); 30. Cypress (*Cupressus arizonica*); 31. Datura (*Datura wrightii*); 32. Desert anemone (*Anemone tuberosa*).

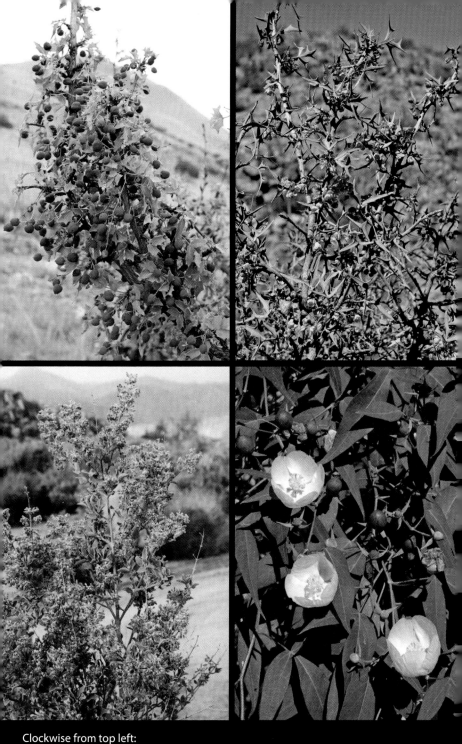

Clockwise from top left:

33. Desert barberry (*Berberis fremontii*); 34. Desert barberry (*Berberis trifoliolata*); 35.
Desert cotton (*Gossypium thurberi*); 36. Desert lavender (*Hyptis emoryi*)

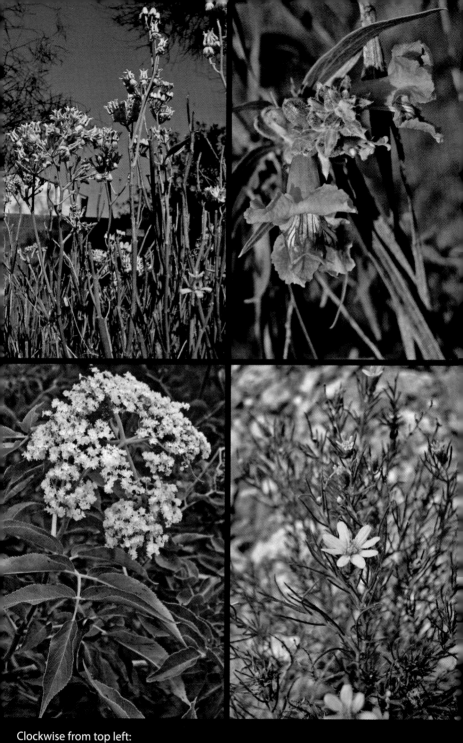

Clockwise from top left:
37. Desert milkweed (*Asclepias subulata*); 38. Desert willow (*Chilopsis linearis*); 39. Dogweed (*Dyssodia acerosa*); 40. Elder (*Sambucus nigra subsp. cerulea*)

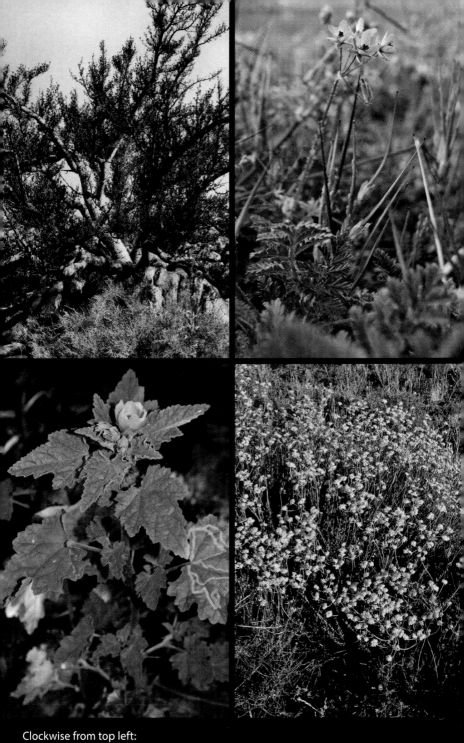

Clockwise from top left:
41. Elephant tree (*Bursera microphylla*); 42. Filaree (*Erodium cicutarium*) 43. Flat–top–
buckwheat (*Eriogonum fasciculatum*); 44. Globemallow (*Sphaeralcea coulteri*)

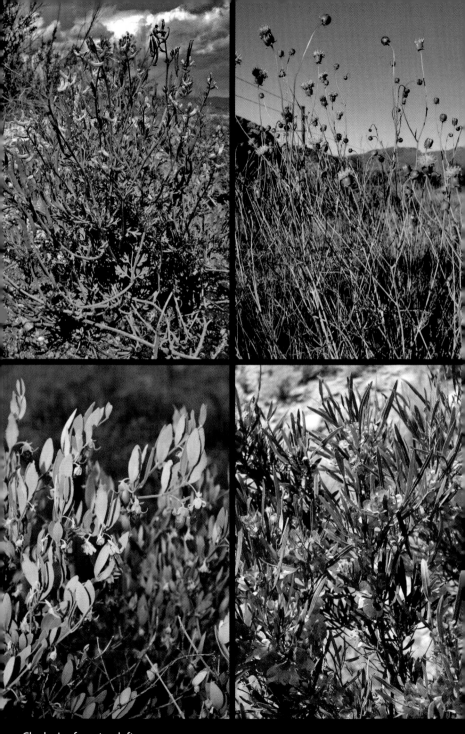

Clockwise from top left:

45. Golden smoke (*Corydalis aurea*); 46. Greenthread (*Thelesperma megapotamicum*); 47.

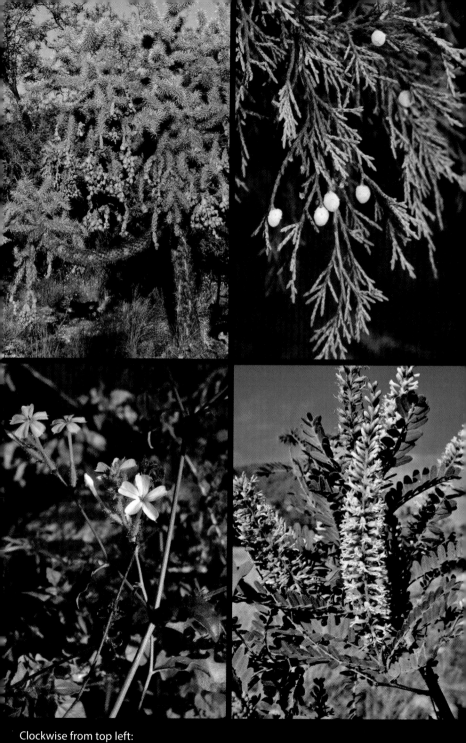

Clockwise from top left:

49. Jumping cholla (*Cylindropuntia fulgida*); 50. Juniper (*Juniperus scopulorum*); 51.
Kidneywood (*Eysenhardtia orthocarpa*); 52. Leadwort (*Plumbago zeylanica*)

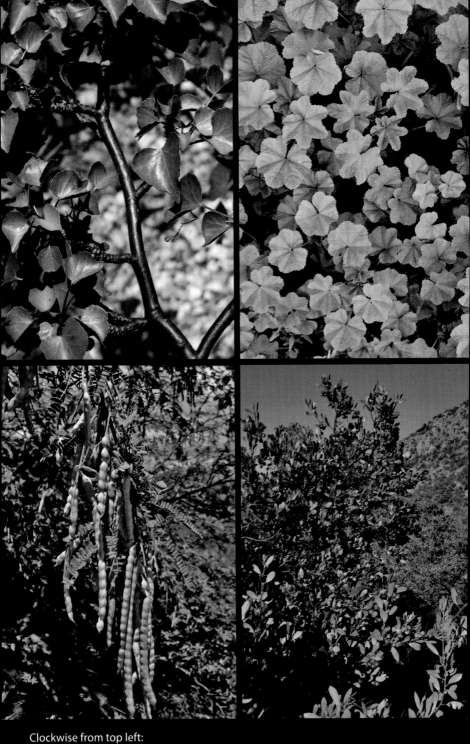

Clockwise from top left:
53. Limberbush (*Jatropha cardiophylla*); 54. Mallow (*Malva parviflora*); 55. Manzanita
(*Arctostaphylos pungens*); 56. Mesquite (*Prosopis velutina*).

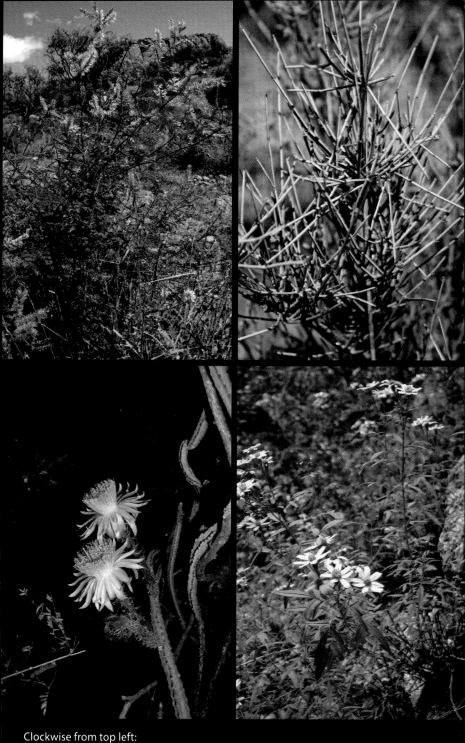

Clockwise from top left:
57. Mimosa (*Mimosa dysocarpa*); 58. Mormon tea (*Ephedra aspera*); 59. Mountain marigold (*Tagetes lemmonii*); 60. Night blooming cereus (*Peniocereus greggii*).

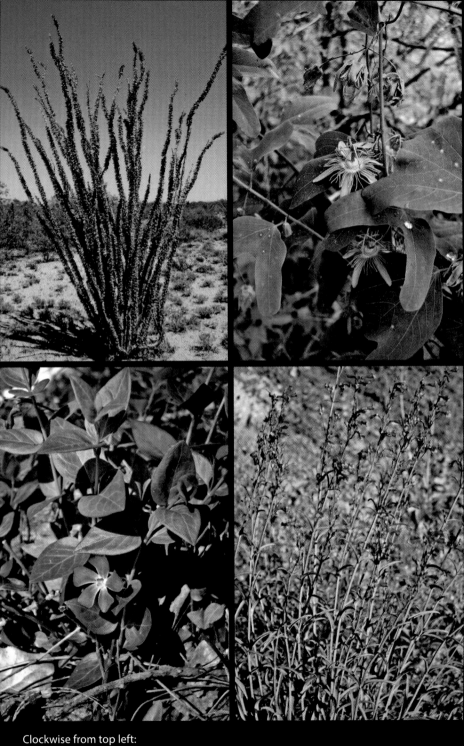

Clockwise from top left:
61. Ocotillo (*Fouquieria splendens*); 62. Passionflower (*Passiflora mexicana*); 63. Penstemon (*Penstemon parryi*); 64. Periwinkle (*Vinca major*).

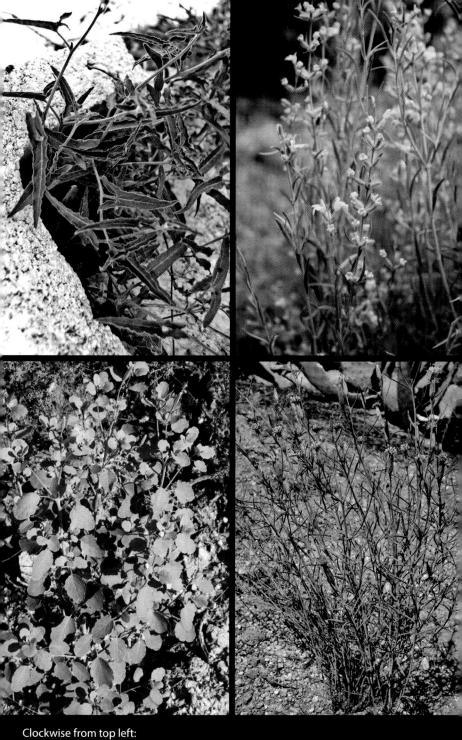

Clockwise from top left:
65. Pipevine (*Aristolochia watsonii*); 66. Poliomintha (*Poliomintha incana*); 67. Poreleaf
(*Porophyllum gracile*); 68. Poreleaf (*Porophyllum ruderale* subsp. *macrocephalum*)

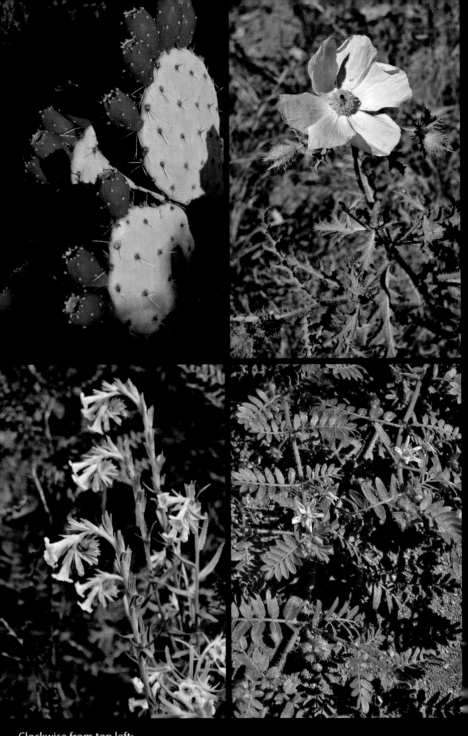

Clockwise from top left:
69. Prickly pear (*Opuntia engelmannii*); 70. Prickly poppy (*Argemone pleiacantha*); 71. Puncturevine (*Tribulus terrestris*); 72. Purple gromwell (*Lithospermum multiflorum*).

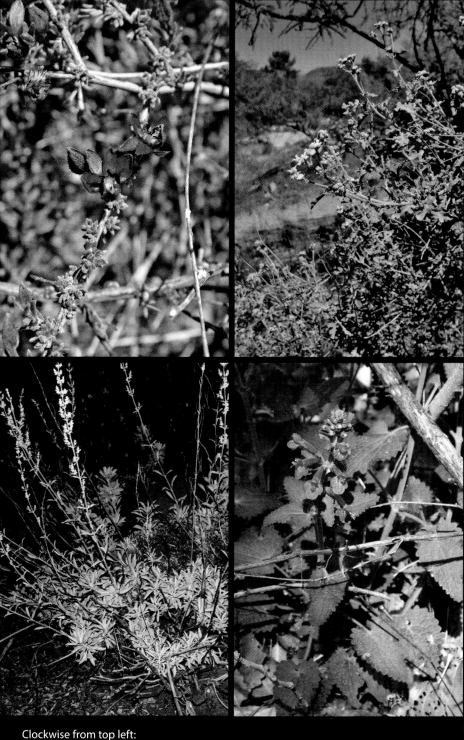

Clockwise from top left:
73. Ratany (*Krameria erecta*); 74. Rayweed (*Parthenium incanum*); 75. Red betony (*Stachys coccinea*); 76. Sage (*Salvia apiana*).

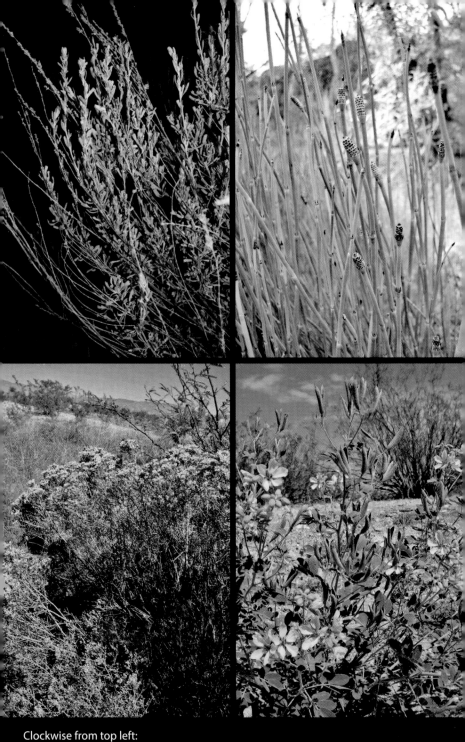

Clockwise from top left:
77. Sagebrush (*Artemisia tridentata*); 78. Scouring rush (*Equisetum hyemale*); 79. Senna
(*Senna covesii*); 80. Snakeweed (*Gutierrezia microcephala*)

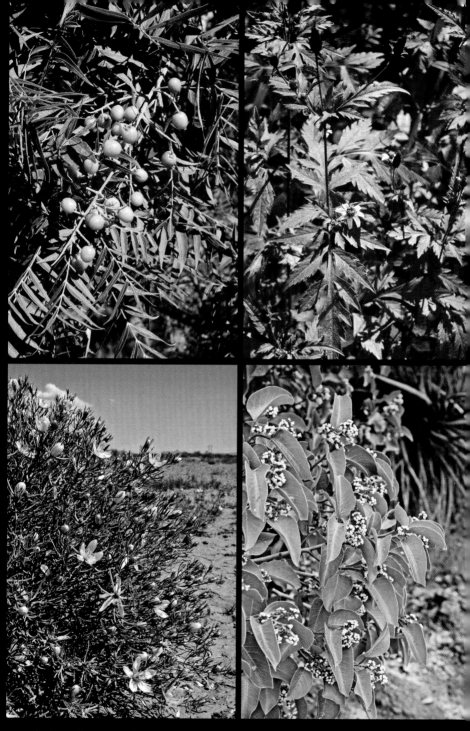

Clockwise from top left:
81. Soapberry (*Sapindus saponaria var. drummondii*); 82. Spanish needles (*Bidens pilosa*);
83. Sumac (*Rhus ovata*); 84. Syrian rue (*Peganum harmala*).

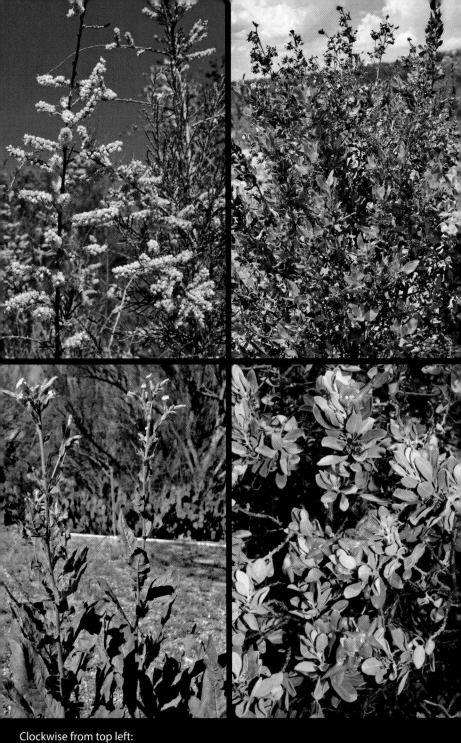

Clockwise from top left:

85. Tamarisk (*Tamarix chinensis*); 86. Tarbush (*Flourensia cernua*); 87. Texas ranger (*Leucophyllum frutescens*); 88. Tobacco (*Nicotiana obtusifolia*)

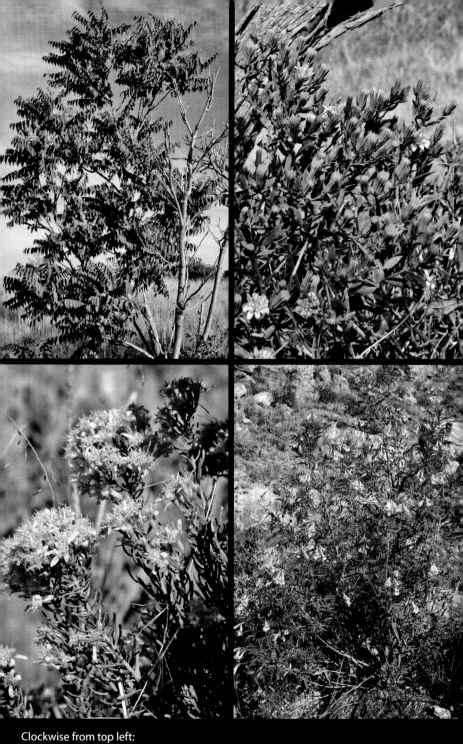

Clockwise from top left:
89. Tree of heaven (*Ailanthus altissima*); 90. Trixis (*Trixis californica*); 91. Trumpet flower
(*Tecoma stans*); 92. Turpentine bush (*Ericameria laricifolia*)

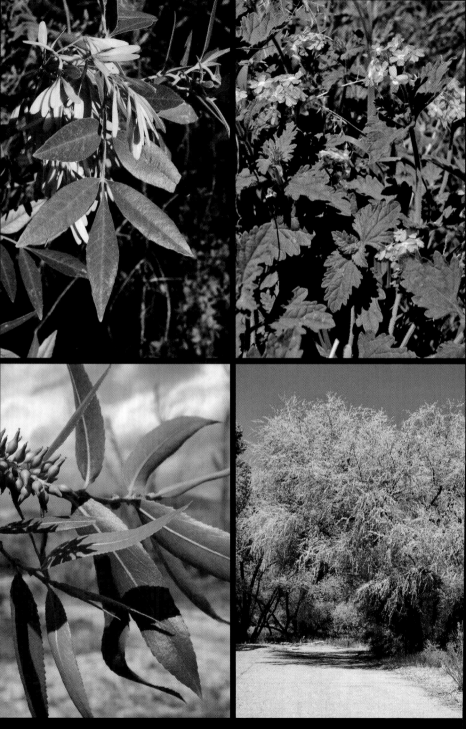

Clockwise from top left:
93. Velvet ash (*Fraxinus velutina*); 94. Verbena (*Glandularia gooddingii*); 95. Western black willow (*Salix gooddingii*); 96. Western black willow (*Salix gooddingii*).

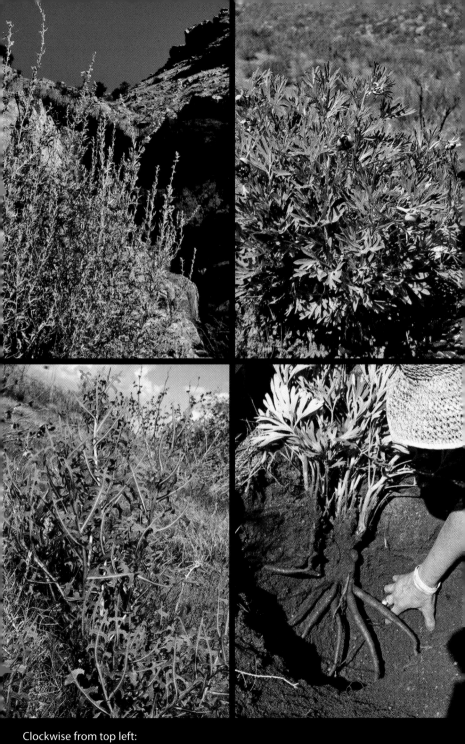

Clockwise from top left:
97. Western mugwort (*Artemisia ludoviciana*); 98. Western peony (*Paeonia californica*);

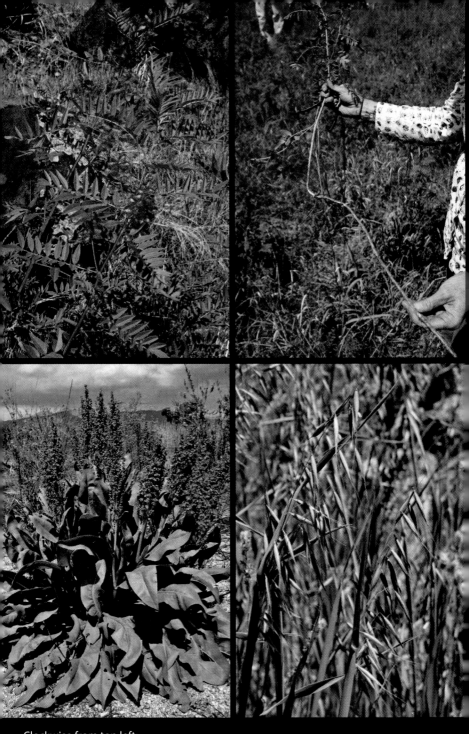

Clockwise from top left:
101. Wild licorice (*Glycyrrhiza lepidota*); 102. Wild licorice (*Glycyrrhiza lepidota*); 103. Wild oats (*Avena fatua*); 104. Wild rhubarb (*Rumex hymenosepalus*).

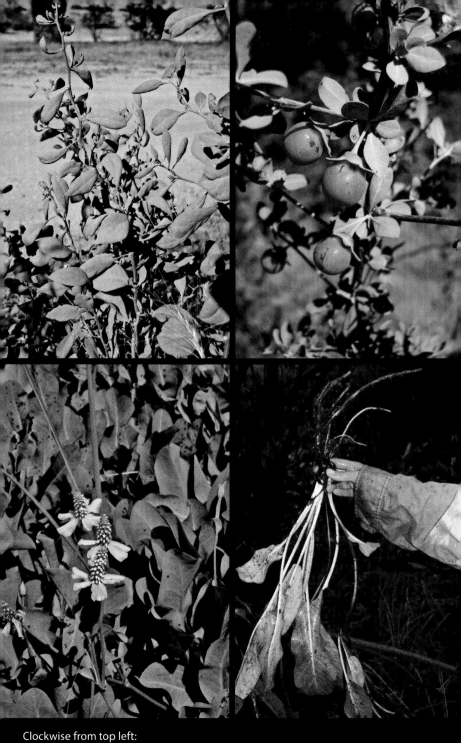

Clockwise from top left:
105. Wolfberry (*Lycium pallidum*); 106. Wolfberry (*Lycium pallidum*); 107. Yerba mansa
(*Anemopsis californica*); 108. Yerba mansa (*Anemopsis californica*)

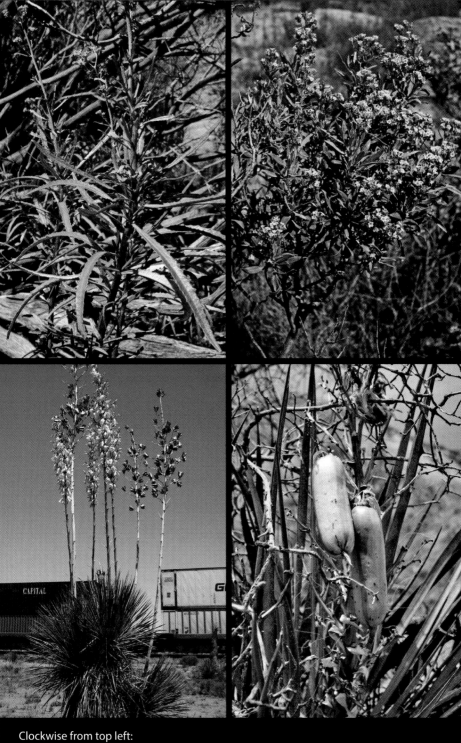

Clockwise from top left:
109. Yerba santa (*Eriodictyon angustifolium*); 110. Yerba santa (*Eriodictyon trichocalyx var. lanatum*); 111. Yucca (*Yucca baccata*); 112. Yucca (*Yucca elata*).

intelligent use. Most Aristolochia's are known as topical snakebite medicines – our species is no different. Aristolochic acids have powerful neutralizing effects on venoms of most poisonous snakes. If springtime rattlesnake encounters are common, keep the salve or ointment made with 1–part Pipevine root and 1–part Echinacea handy. In conjunction with standard anti–venom therapies (and internal Echinacea), keep the bite covered with this mixture. Other venomous bites and stings (scorpion, cone–nose insects, brown recluse, and black widow) will also respond well to this combination.

Indications
» Snakebite, venomous (external)
» Insect/Spider bites, venomous (external)

Collection
As a root medicine start digging about 6"–8" to one side of the plant where the stems emerge from the ground. Depending on soil conditions, reaching depths of 1'–2' may mean the use of a hand trowel...or a pic–axe. When collecting Aristolochia watsonii I prefer locating plants under shrubs next to drainages. These soils tend to be less compacted and slightly more aerated with decomposing leaf litter. Once a hole is started slowly dig towards the plant and locate the forked tap–root. Keep tracing down next to the root until the very last of it is located. Gently pry it loose – sometimes these roots will have to be re–traced on the opposite side to include wayward forks. Be sure to get the entire root – any 4"–6" inch piece that is left in the ground will not re–sprout. The foliage is of no medicinal consequence – though if the plant is in seed be sure to spread around the capsules.

Preparations/Dosage
» External preparations: salve, ointment, oil, all as needed

Cautions
For external use covering a limited surface area, there is little to no caution for the plant.

Poliomintha
Lamiaceae/Mint Family

Poliomintha incana (Torr.) A. Gray *(Hedeoma incana)*
Frosted mint, Bush mint

Description
Typically a small–sized shrub (3′ x 3′ is about average), Poliomintha is distinct due to its dense coating of felt–like leaf and stem hair. Light and snowy in appearance the plant's narrow leaves are ½″–1″ long an oppositely arranged. The flowers are pale blue–purple and organized in axillary clusters. Poliomintha's seeds (nutlets) are smooth and oblong. A pleasant–scented Mint family bush, it is easily identifiable due to its coloration (very light) and scent.

Distribution
Poliomintha is found from south–central Utah along the Green and Colorado River drainages, to central–west/southwest Colorado. Specifically it occupies a large expanse of the Colorado Plateau in Arizona to several isolated groups in central/southern New Mexico and western Texas. Another grouping is found on the north face of the San Bernardino Mountains in California. A plant of sandy soils of the Painted and Chihuahuan Deserts, look for it between 4000′–7000′.

Chemistry
Essential volatiles: pulegone, 1,8–cineole, linalool, isopulegone, α–terpineol, and 8–hydroxy–4– p–menthen–3–one.

Medicinal Uses
Use Poliomintha like Pennyroyal (Mentha pulegium) and Western pennyroyal (Hedeoma spp.). Whole plant preparations have predictable effects on a number of systems. Through Poliomintha's carminative influence, taken with or after meals, it diminishes stomach distension and related gas and bloating. Like others in its class it tends to dilate stomach vasculature, delivering more blood to the area, therefore diminishing stasis and inactivity. Although not as reliable as Peppermint, the plant will be found settling to nausea.

If feverish, the hot tea will stimulate sweating, helping to reduce core temperate via surface heat dissipation. It is best used when the skin is hot and dry.

As a simple stimulatory emmenagogue, Poliomintha will trigger menstruation, suppressed from causes such as stress, sickness, or climate–temperature changes. It is especially valuable when the whole pelvic area feels cold and contracted.

Indications
» Gas/Bloating/Nausea
» Fever, dry skin
» Menstruation, suppressed

Collection
Gather the herb portion, in flower or not. Remove the flowers and leaves from the stems; discard the stems. Tincture the flowers and leaves fresh, or dry them for tea.

Preparations/Dosage
» FPT: 20–40 drops 1–3 times daily
» Infusion: 4–6 ounces 1–3 times daily

Cautions
Do not use while pregnant or nursing.

Other Uses
The essential oil makes an effective (pleasant–scented) insect repellent. Add 10 drops per ounce of alcohol and apply as a spray.

Poreleaf
Asteraceae/Sunflower Family

Porophyllum gracile Bernh. *(Porophyllum caesium, P. cedrense, P. confertum, P. junciforme, P. leucospermum, P. nodosum, P. ochroleucum, P. pinifolium, P. vaseyi)*
Slender poreleaf, Odora, Yerba del venado, Deerweed

Porophyllum ruderale (Jacq.) Cass. *(Cacalia porophyllum, C. ruderalis, Kleinia porophyllum, K. ruderalis, Porophyllum ellipticum, P. latifolium, P. macrocephalum, P. porophyllum, Tagetes integrifolia)*
Papalo

Description
Porophyllum gracile is a small, many–branched perennial, not more than 2′ tall by the same wide. Except for a few linear leaves, the slender branches are practically leafless. In the spring P. gracile's bluish–green coloration distinguishes it from surrounding plants. The inconspicuous flowers are purplish–white. They are supported on ½″–¾″ long involucres. New stem growth, leaves, and flowers are strongly aromatic.

Porophyllum ruderale is a 1′–2′ tall annual with ovoid, mostly opposite, and thickened leaves. Like P. gracile, the involucres are also thickened, and on them rest inconspicuous and purplish–white flower heads. When crushed the whole plant is aromatic. The odor is pungent and not at all unpleasant.

Distribution
Porophyllum gracile populates hillsides and basins of the Chihuahuan, Mojave, and Sonoran Deserts. From 4,000′ and below, P. gracile is found throughout southern Nevada, southern California, and Arizona. P. ruderale is essentially a southern Arizona plant. South from the Peloncillo and Baboquivari Mountains it is found between 3,500′–5,000′ on rocky slopes, hillsides, and canyons.

Chemistry
Acetylenic thiophenes; monoterpenes: α–pinene, sabinene, and myrcene; sesquiterpene: β–cubebene; fatty acid derivatives: 7–tetradecene,

cis–4–decenal, pentadecanal, and heptadecanal.

Medicinal Uses

Use Poreleaf when in need of a simple gastric carminative. If the stomach feels full and distended from improper dietary choices, several sprigs of the fresh plant or a little of the fresh plant tincture will be found relieving. Eating several leaves or flowers has the uncanny ability of making anyone with trapped stomach air, burp. For colicky babies it can be thought of as an equivalent to Catnip, working well to relieve trapped gas and spasm.

Indications

» Dyspepsia with bloating
» Nausea
» Colic

Collection

In the spring or summer when new growth is apparent, collect the top several inches of fresh branches from the plant. Leave older, woody sections as they have little value, which is evidenced by their lack of pungency.

Preparations

Individuals whom live close to Poreleaf will benefit most from the plant, as eating a small handful of the fresh herb is by far the most efficacious way of receiving its benefits. The fresh plant tincture is second in serviceability. After drying the plant, the pungency diminishes. The herb infusion is less effective than the fresh plant or the fresh plant tincture.

Dosage

» Fresh leaves and flowers: eaten as needed
» FPT: 30–60 drops 2–3 times daily
» Leaf infusion: 4–8 ounces 2–3 times daily

Cautions

There are no known cautions with normal usage.

Other Uses

Porophyllum ruderale's or Papalo's use as a carminative spice (like Cilantro) predates Columbus' arrival in the Americas. It's best used fresh, like cilantro.

Prickly Pear
Cactaceae/Cactus Family

Opuntia engelmannii Salm–Dyck ex Engelm.
Nopal, Nopalitos, Tunas

Description
At maturity this succulent cactus stands 4'–6' tall by 8'–10' wide. The bulk
of the plant is composed of connected pad–like stems that arise from a
thickened base. The green, pancake–like and elliptical pads are uniformly
covered by thorn clusters. Smaller thorns, called glochids are intermingled
with larger thorns. They are particularly abundant on the circumference of
the pad. New flower bud and pad growth commences in mid–spring. The
bright yellow flowers bloom in late spring to early summer. Each flower
only lasts one day. They open early in the morning and close at midday
when it is the hottest. Early to mid–summer the burgundy pear–shaped
fruit develop.

Distribution
From south–central California, Prickly pear is found eastward to central
Texas. It grows as far north as South Dakota and south through Colorado,
Arizona, and New Mexico. The plant thrives in numerous ecosystems in-
cluding dry deserts, grasslands, and Juniper–Oak Woodlands. Look for
Prickly pear on hillsides, canyon bottoms, and lower desert basins. From
coast to coast, there are dozens of Prickly pear species, but this is primarily
a plant of the arid West.

Chemistry
Carbohydrate–containing polymers, consisting of a mixture of mucilage
and pectin; betalains: betaxanthin, betanin, vulgaxanthin, miraxanthin,
and portulaxanthin; rhamnose, galactose, galacturonic acid; calcium
oxalate.

Medicinal Uses
Prickly pear is a versatile, safe, and exceedingly common plant medicine.

With supplemental food uses and a common themed usage history, the cacti is well–worth knowing. Additionally, most species of Prickly pear (collectively called Platyopuntia) can be used like this one.

Taken before meals, the cactus reduces blood sugar concentrations by 15–20% in individuals with NIDDM (non–insulin dependent diabetes mellitus). This effect is mainly achieved through the plant's soluble fiber content, which slows down dietary sugar uptake. The plant's soluble fiber also binds with cholesterol–containing bile acids, limiting their re–uptake by the portal circulation. This effect limits the liver's overproduction of 'bad' cholesterol, ultimately lowering plasma LDLs (low density lipoprotein).

Several ounces of pulp mixed with a small amount of water has a cooling effect on esophageal and stomach irritations, be they from acid reflux or gastritis. This antiinflammatory effect soothes irritated gastric membranes. Not only does Prickly pear mucilage serve as a protectant to damaged stomach lining, it also has the ability of augmenting the quality of gastric mucus making it useful as a stomach ulcer healer.

Slices of Prickly pear pad applied to acute injuries, such as contusions and sprains, will reduce tissue inflammation and edema. Additionally, swelling and discoloration will resolve more quickly. It is a simple remedy that works. Moreover, when applied to burns and inflammations, the pulp makes an excellent healing poultice. Consider it a good equivalent to Aloe vera.

The flowers of Prickly pear (and most other Opuntias) are high in flavonoids. Be it the flower infusion taken internally or other preparations applied topically, they are good for fortifying tissues that are slow to heal. In addition, flower preparations strengthen fragile capillaries and minimize varicosity development. The flower tea also tends to be diuretic and stimulates the kidney's excretion of uric acid. As a preventive therapy, use it to lessen uric acid kidney stones and gout–oriented conditions.

Indications

Pad:

» Diabetes mellitus, non–insulin dependent
» LDL, elevated
» Acid reflux/Gastritis
» Ulcer, gastric
» Burns (external)
» Swellings/Contusions (external)

Flowers:
»   Poorly healing tissues (internal and external)
»   Fragile capillaries/Varicosities (internal and external)
»   Water retention
»   Uric acid kidney stones/Gout

Collection/Preparations

When harvesting Prickly pear be aware of the very small thorns or glochids – they may not be seen but they are certainly felt. Find a sizable plant, one that looks healthy and has no signs of environmental stress or insect damage. Locate one pad in the bunch that is oriented away from the others. Take two good–sized rocks that fit well into your hands and scrape the larger thorns from the pad. After this is complete, cut along the outer circumference of the pad, removing the thorns that were missed. Holding the pad with a gloved hand, cut it from the plant. Now cut the pad down the middle as if you are cutting open a bagel. Scrape the pulp from the pad's center into a bowl. This will keep in a refrigerator for 2–3 weeks. Repeat this process as needed when stores get low.

For internal use, start by mixing several ounces of Prickly pear pulp with several ounces of water. Blend if needed, then drink this mixture. Store–bought Prickly pear slices are not as effective as our freshly made preparations. Indian–fig or Mission prickly pear (Opuntia ficus–indica), which has soluble fiber content but is also high in glucose, is not as helpful for hyperglycemics. In addition, Prickly pear fruit juice, which can be bought at many health food stores, is lower in soluble fiber and higher in simple–sugar content than whole pad preparations.

Dosage

»   Pulp slurry/Cooked pad: 1–2 ounces before meals
»   External pulp/Flower infusion/Salve: apply as needed
»   Internal flower infusion: 4–8 ounces 2–3 times daily

Cautions

Do not use in IDDM (insulin dependent diabetes mellitus). Eating excessive amounts of the raw pad or fruit has been known to cause 'Cactus fever', a feverish state with accompanying chills. It is self–resolving but has been known to give people a scare who are attempting to exist solely from the plant in survival situations.

Other Uses

The young pads can be eaten raw or cooked after the thorns have been removed by boiling, brushing, or roasting. The tart taste is from calcium oxalate accumulation. For a tasty treat, a ripe fruit is split down the middle and the inner pulp is eaten, with or without the seeds. Prickly pear fruit serves as a popular juice, jelly, and wine base.

Prickly pear is a host plant for Cochineal (Dactylopius coccus), a small, cottony–web forming insect. Although not popular today because of displacement by synthetic dyes, years ago the British used the pigment derived from the insect to dye their army's coats red, hence 'Red coats'. Crushed and applied to cuts and scrapes Cochineal is significantly antimicrobial.

Prickly Poppy
Papaveraceae/Poppy Family

Argemone spp. L.
Cowboys' fried egg, Chicaolte, Cardo santo

Description

Prickly poppy stands about 2' tall with alternately spaced clasping bluish–green leaves. The 2"–3" diameter flowers develop from spring through summer. Large, white, and paper–thin petals surround a core of orange stamens, which seem to be always alive with insects of various types. The oblong and spiky seedpods start to appear in mid–summer. After beginning to dry, these capsules open and release miniscule dark black–brown seeds. When young Prickly poppy can be mistaken for Wild lettuce. The similarities end when a leaf or stem is broken. A yellow–orange sap weeps from the wound, very unlike the milky sap that exudes from Wild lettuce.

Distribution

Prickly poppy is found throughout the West. It frequents disturbed soils such as roadsides, dry riverbeds, and overgrazed land.

Chemistry

Major alkaloids: dihydosanguinarine, sanguinarine, berberine, protopine, chelerythrine, and coptisine.

Medicinal Uses

Prickly poppy is a multi–faceted plant. It contains compounds that are both medicinal and if consumed in larger quantities, toxic. With the plant's array of compounds in mind, it can be likened to a combination of Bloodroot, Desert barberry, and California poppy.

As a sedative, Prickly poppy works best when there is pain from acute injury making sleep difficult. Its quieting effect on afferent pain signals gives some relief if the situation is dependent upon muscular rigidity. Prickly poppy is also useful in sedating smooth muscle constriction of bronchial and intestinal tissues. The herb fits when there is a hectic and spasmodic cough with bronchial heat and hyperactivity. Likewise, the herb has value if there is intestinal cramping with associated bouts of diarrhea.

Externally the oil or salve made from the seeds is an excellent burn dressing. It is soothing and pain relieving to inflamed and abraded tissues. The externally applied tea is antimicrobial, assisting cuts and broken skin in staying free of pathogens. An isotonic tea of the herb, strained for very small leaf and stem hair, makes a soothing eyewash. It reduces conjunctiva inflammation. Styes also diminish with its use.

Indications

» Pain, muscular
» Insomnia/Restlessness
» Cough, spasmodic
» Cramps, intestinal
» Infection, bacterial (external)
» Burns/Abrasions (external)
» Conjunctivitis (eyewash)

Collection

Collect Prickly poppy throughout the spring and summer. With pruners snip the upper half of the plant, including the leaves, flowers, and seedpods. Be sure to wear gloves while collecting the plant: the fine hairs are sharp and course.

Preparations

After drying the uncut herb, garble everything from the stems. Chop them into ¼"–½" pieces. Use both parts for medicine.

Dosage

» Herb infusion: 2–4 ounces 2–3 times daily
» DPT (50% alcohol): 20–40 drops 2–3 times daily
» Eyewash: 3–4 times daily

Cautions

Even in moderate quantities, problems can potentially develop when the seeds or particularly the refined seed oil is ingested regularly. In northern India Mustard seed oil, unknowingly adulterated with Prickly poppy seed oil (Argemone mexicana) has been the cause of numerous deaths. Individuals succumb as a result of massive interstitial fluid disorganization, vascular deterioration, and subsequent edema. It is important to note that ingesting a refined seed oil, which by nature is a highly potentiated substance, is very different from ingesting the crude seed–herb preparations used here.

Although seed preparations of Prickly poppy have been used as a mildly stimulating laxative, it is best to err on the side of caution and not use these preparations internally, or at least not by themselves. If seed preparations are used, keep their use short term: 2–3 days at a time. The internally used whole herb is less toxic. Short–term use of 2–3 weeks at any one time is relatively safe. Individuals taking this plant should be healthy and not involved in any major pharmaceutical regimens. Pregnant and lactating women and children should not use Prickly poppy internally.

Puncturevine

Zygophyllaceae/Caltrop Family

Tribulus terrestris L.
Goathead, Sandbur, Bullhead

Description

Puncturevine grows mat–like and can cover expansive stretches. The entire plant is hairy. The leaves are composed of 4–7 small compound leaflets. They develop on long horizontal stems that sometimes reach 7′–8′ in length, though normally they are only 2′–3′ long. In the summer, the small and 5–petaled, bright yellow flowers open in the morning and close soon after when confronted by the hot sun. The seed capsules are 5–sectioned and break apart at maturity; each section is double–spined and contains several seeds. They are viable for at least five years, making eradication next to impossible. The seed capsules or goatheads as they are *affectionately* called are legendary for the discomfort they cause to bare feet.

Distribution
A non–native from southern Europe, Puncturevine now is distributed widely throughout the West. Look for the plant in disturbed areas such as roadsides, vacant lots, and along fields and pastures.

Chemistry
Sapogenins: terrestrosin, ruscogenin, and hecogenin; harmine and nor–harmine; flavonoids: quercetin and rutin.

Medicinal Uses
Although terminology and descriptions of effects differ, western, Chinese, and Ayurveda perspectives coincide on Puncturevine use. In relation to the cardiovascular system, the plant fits individuals with moderately elevated blood pressure whom suffer from angina pectoris. The coronary artery, which supplies blood to the heart, is dilated through Puncturevine's influence. This effect quenches the organ's literal cry for oxygen, thus diminishing heart constriction and pain. Puncturevine's mild blood pressure lowering effect is additionally useful for hypertensive individuals with a sedentary lifestyle.

Puncturevine is useful in diminishing the formation of both uric acid and oxalate based kidney stones, be it from injury, dehydration, or metabolic excess. Its diuretic tendency, combined with the plant's soothing effect on urinary tract mucus membranes, makes the plant's application to urinary irritability well suited.

Puncturevine is known to alter/augment circulating androgens, particularly DHEA (dehydroepiandrosterone) and testosterone within the body. Although the mechanism of action is still unclear, its effects are noticeable: libido is increased, and in men, erectile response is heightened, as is the quantity and quality of sperm. Nocturnal emissions or spermatorrhea lessens under its use. Many men using the plant (it combines well with Ginseng) often notice a related sense of increased physical strength and will – a good tonic for older men and the metrosexual alike. Women too may notice an increase in libido.

Traditionally Puncturevine is used for skin outbreaks that exhibit redness and heat. Since the plant is significantly antiinflammatory and hence somewhat mediating to allergic reactivity, topical and internal use of Puncturevine is of value in treating eczema and psoriasis. Of interest also is the plant's stimulatory effect on melanocyte proliferation, making external seed preparations of use in treating vitiligo.

Indications
» Hypertension with fluid retention
» Angina pectoris
» Kidney stones, as a preventative, both uric acid and oxalate types
» Decreased libido/Low sperm count and poor quality
» Skin allergies/Eczema/Psoriasis (internal and external)
» Vitiligo

Collection
Collect Puncturevine from mid to late summer after responding to seasonal rains. It is easily pulled up, roots and all. Be mindful of the seed capsules or goatheads – they can gouge hands easily if aggressively handled. Collect the seed capsules in the late summer to early fall.

Preparations
Although the whole plant is somewhat active, the mature and dried capsules with seeds are the strongest parts. Puncturevine lends itself to most preparations.

Dosage
» Herb/Seed infusion: 2–4 ounces 2–3 times daily
» FPT/DPT (60% alcohol): 30–40 drops 2–3 times daily
» Topical preparations: as needed

Cautions
There have been reports of toxicity reactions when the plant is too enthusiastically eaten by stock animals. Cases of liver and kidney problems and sun–sensitivity do arise in these circumstances. With this in mind, prudence suggests if the herb is to be used as a simple, keep the duration to short term (several weeks). In formula, longer term use is acceptable. Do not use during pregnancy, while nursing, or with liver or kidney disease.

Purple Gromwell
Boraginaceae/Borage Family

Lithospermum multiflorum Torr. ex A. Gray
Stoneseed, Puccoon

Description
Purple gromwell is a small and herbaceous perennial. Vertical stems, reaching 1'–2' in height, arise from the root crown. The leaves and stems are verdant and somewhat hairy. The leaves form alternately along stems and are narrow and elongated. Each leaf has a prominent mid–vein. The yellow flowers form in terminal clusters and are scorpioid shaped. Each tubular flower has 5 small petaled lobes. The small seeds are white and very hard, hence the name Litho–spermum (stone–seed). The plant's taproot is long and slender. Purplish splotches are evident on the root's crown.

Distribution
From Wyoming, the plant grows south to Arizona and New Mexico. Throughout the Southwest, it can be found from 6,000'–9,500'. Look to Pine and Juniper Woodlands. The plant is fond of flats and slopes.

Chemistry
Naphthoquinone, hydroxycinnamic acid ester: rosmarinic acid; γ–linolenic acid; pyrrolizidine alkaloids, chlorogenic acid, succinic acid, and lithospermic acid.

Medicinal Uses
The medicinal potency of Purple gromwell is largely due to the purplish–red pigments contained in the roots. These pigments, mainly composed of naphthoquinone, are also pronounced in Lithospermum erythrorhizon, a much–researched Chinese species. In addition, many species not profiled here are also medicinally potent.

Topically the plant has use in wound healing, mainly through its antiinflammatory–antioxidant properties. Furthering this effect is Purple gromwell's moderate antibacterial quality. Purple gromwell is also inhibiting to various fungal strains, so its application is warranted in topical skin and nail fungi. There is also promise in the plant sedating the excesses of psoriasis and eczema.

Although lately lab research has shown Lithospermum ruderale to be broadly sedating to gonadotropic and thyroid stimulating hormone activity, due to the presence of pyrrolizidine alkaloids, internal use of the plant should be avoided. Incidentally, this hormonal altering activity coincides with the Shoshone's sterility inducing/contraceptive use of the plant. The roots and seeds of L. virginianum were once used by the Eclectic physicians and lay practitioners alike as a soothing diuretic. The tea was also indicated in dissolving urinary tract gravel.

Indications
» Wounds/Cuts/Scrapes (external)
» Infection, bacterial/fungal (external)
» Psoriasis/Eczema (external)

Collection
Gather the plant in the spring or summer using the foliage or flowers as an indicator. The roots are usually small but older plants can produce sizable woody taproots. After digging the roots, discard the foliage as it is non-medicinal.

Preparations/Dosage
» Root decoction: topically as needed
» DPT (50% alcohol): topically as needed
» Oil/Salve/Poultice: as needed

Cautions
Purple gromwell contains liver-toxic pyrrolizidine alkaloids, as do many other Borage family plants (particularly the Amsinckia and Cryptantha genera) in the Southwest. Internal use is to be avoided.

Other Uses
Purple Gromwell has potential as a dye plant. The Chinese variety, Lithospermum erythrorhizon, was used in silk staining.

Ratany
Krameriaceae/Ratany Family

Krameria grayi Rose & Painter *(Krameria bicolor, K. canescens, K. sonorae)*
White ratany, Chacate

Krameria erecta Willd. ex Schult. *(Krameria glandulosa, K. parvifolia, K. imparata, K. interior, K. navae)*
Range ratany, Chacate

Krameria secundiflora DC. *(Krameria diffusa, K. lanceolata, K. prostrata)*
Three fans, Prairie bur

Description
These low–growing shrubs form into mound–like clumps. They are densely branched and can be somewhat spiny. The herbage is grayish–green and hairy. The small linear leaves, particularly on younger branches, are stem hugging. The crimson–purple flowers are composed of 3–5 petals and can appear strangely beak–like. The seedpods, the size of a cultivated cherry, appear as oddly inflated globes surrounded by small barbed spines. Krameria is a reputed partial root parasite. Creosote bush and Triangle–leaf bursage are typical hosts.

Distribution
The three species profiled here generally overlap in habitat. Both Krameria grayi and K. erecta are found from 5,000′ and below through much of Arizona, southeastern California, and southern Nevada, to western Texas. They are common to desert mesas, foothills, and alluvial fans where soils are rocky. K. secundiflora, found from 4,000′–7,000′, ranges from southeastern Arizona east to Florida.

Chemistry
Catechin and epicatechin; proanthocyanidin derivatives: procyanidin and propelargonidin; neolignans and norneolignans: ratanhiaphenol 1 and 2.

Medicinal Uses
Many species of Ratany, some not profiled here, have a rich western

medicinal history. Up until the early 20th century these plants were widely used in Western Europe and later here in the United States.

Virtually all of Ratany's medicinal benefits derive from its astringency. The tea used as a mouthwash is tonifying to gums and can be used with Ginger or Prickly ash for added tissue stimulation. It is of use in periodontitis and spongy and receding gums, and is also relieving to aphthous stomatitis (canker sores).

Ratany diminishes diarrhea through its astringent effect on the gastrointestinal tract and its contents. Moreover, passive hemorrhaging, be it bronchial, uterine, urinary, or gastrointestinal tract centered, is diminished. Menorrhagia, or excessive menstruation dependent upon perimenopause or subnormal levels of reproductive hormones, is often reduced by Ratany, albeit symptomatically. The plant serves as a tissue and capillary bed constrictor and does not affect circulating hormone levels. If there is no underling infection, colliquative sweating is often lessened with Ratany. The addition of Sage often augments its effectiveness.

When applied topically to weepy sores, cuts, rashes, and stings, Ratany astringes, lessens inflammation, and facilitates healing. The salve is used to shrink hemorrhoids and diminish associated bleeding. Rectal suppositories made with Ratany oil are used to encourage healing of anal fissures. It combines well with Yerba mansa for these purposes.

Indications
» Periodontitis/Spongy and bleeding gums/Canker sores (mouthwash)
» Diarrhea
» Menorrhagia
» Hemorrhaging, passive
» Sweating, colliquative
» Hemorrhoids/Anal fissures (external)

Collection/Preparations
The rootbark of thick roots and the flexible secondary roots are the articles of choice. If either part has an inner reddish layer it will make for a strong preparation. Although not quite as strong, herb preparations can be used as well – a dosage increase will compensate for potency differences.

Dosage
» FPT/DPT of rootbark (50% alcohol, 10% glycerin): 15–30 drops 2–3 times

daily
» Cold infusion: 2–4 ounces 2–3 times daily, topically as needed
» Suppositories: 1–2 daily (one being used before bed)

Cautions
Like most tannin plants internal use should be limited to short term: 2–3 weeks concurrently, or else gastric and/or renal irritation may result. Ratany is not recommended during pregnancy due to its vasoconstricting effect on uterine lining.

Rayweed
Asteraceae/Sunflower Family

Parthenium incanum Kunth
Mariola, Crowded rayweed

Description
Rayweed is a small, woody–based perennial shrub 2'–3' in height. The plant is densely branched and may even droop due to abundant leaf mass. The leaves are grayish–green, lobed, and are alternately arranged along the stems. Above the foliage small cream flowers form in flattop panicle groupings.

Distribution
From 2,500'–5,000' Rayweed is found from the Grand Canyon area in northern Arizona to Pima and Cochise Counties in southern Arizona, east to central New Mexico, and finally to the Edwards Plateau and Rio Grande Plain in Texas. Usual locations for it are along rocky hillsides and on the edges of gullies. It prefers alkaline, calcrete–laden soils and is most abundantly found throughout the Chihuahuan Desert.

Chemistry
Sesquiterpene lactones: tetraneurin, fruticosin; triterpenoids; flavonoids: quercetin, penduletin, quercetagetin, polycladin, and artemetin.

Medicinal Uses
A ½–cup of Rayweed tea before meals is a stimulating bitter. Digestive

secretions are amplified, augmenting protein and fat digestion. It, like other bitters, can be used before meals to restore appetite and proper digestive response to food. In time, this will provide better assimilation of nutrients. The plant is also a bile stimulant, as are most plant bitters. Some individuals may find Rayweed mildly laxative, making it indicated in constipation dependent upon stress, poor eating habits, and a suppressed urge to defecate.

Indications
» Indigestion
» Congestion, liver/gallbladder
» Constipation, mild

Collection
Before flowering, from early to mid–summer, gather the leaves of Rayweed.

Preparations/Dosage
» Leaf infusion: 2–4 ounces 2–3 times daily

Cautions
Do not use during pregnancy or while nursing.

Other Uses
The related Mexican plant, Guayule (Parthenium argentatum), was briefly cultivated in the US during WWI and WWII for its rubber content. Rayweed too has a notable, yet smaller, rubber content.

Red Betony
Lamiaceae/Mint Family

Stachys coccinea Ortega
Scarlet betony, Texas betony, Scarlet hedgenettle

Description
Herbaceous, perennial, and rhizomatous, Red betony displays opposite leaves. They are generally triangular, slightly cordate, petioled, and have

serrated margins. The basal leaf growth is more significant than the stem leaf growth. The spikes are interrupted and comprised of red–scarlet, tubular, and two–lipped (lightly mottled larger lower lip) flowers. After going to seed the calyx tips are spiky to the touch. The entire plant has a subtle Catnip–like scent.

Distribution

Red betony's main area in the United States (it's also common in Mexico) is southeastern Arizona. From the Mogollon Rim north of Phoenix, south to the Santa Ritas, then east to the Chiricahuas and Peloncillos, it is encountered along lower to mid–elevation foothill and mountainous draws, streamsides, and canyons, almost always in moist soils with full to semi–shade. It's also found in similar habitats, however sporadically, throughout southern New Mexico to West Texas (at least it was found at one time in Texas – recent vouchers are scarce). Although it's most common between 3000'–6000', its minimum to maximum elevation is listed as 1500'–8000'. The plant is easy to cultivate. Its ornamental use is common.

Chemistry

Stachys general: Iridoids, flavonoids, phenolic acids, and diterpenoids.

Medicinal Uses

A mild plant medicine, Red betony belongs to a lesser–used segment of the Mint family. As opposed to the highly aromatic members that are commonly used (Peppermint, Monarda, Sage, etc.) Red Betony's influence tends to be more subtle.

Less stimulating but more sedating, in many respects Red betony is close in application to Wood betony (Stachys/Betonica officinalis). Drink a strong cup of tea (best preparation) if suffering from a stress–oriented headache, especially if neck tension and mental agitation are contributing factors. Try it before bed, particularity if there is an underlying state of inflammation that makes sleep difficult to achieve (not necessarily pain, but restlessness from allergy or an auto–immune situation for instance). The tea also makes a decent free–radical quencher in reducing the liver excitability of a hangover – red–irritated eyes, headache, and sluggishness.

Indications

»   Headache, stress–type

» Agitation/Insomnia, with underlying inflammation

Collection
To collect the leaves simply pinch and remove them from the central stems. The flower spikes are equally utilizable and are clipped from the plant with pruners. Mix the flower spikes and leaves in equal portions or use the leaves solo if not in flower. Later in the season (early fall), the plant is leggy and comprised of mostly stem growth. If this is the case, simply clip the upper ⅔, stem and all, and dry for tea. Once dry garble the herb (with gloves – the calyxes are spiky).

Preparations/Dosage
» Infusion: 4–8 oz. 2–3 times daily
» Fresh juice: 1–2 oz. 2–3 times daily
» FPT/DPT (50% alcohol): 30–60 drops 2–3 times daily

Cautions
There are no cautions with normal usage.

Sage
Lamiaceae/Mint Family

Salvia apiana Jeps.
White sage

Salvia carnosa Dougl. ex Benth *(Salvia dorrii)*
Purple sage, Desert sage

Salvia mohavensis Greene
Mojave sage

Salvia clevelandii (A. Gray) Greene
Cleveland sage, Chaparral sage

Description
All Salvias have square stems, opposite leaves, and to varying degrees are aromatic. Tubular flowers form in whorls around upper stems and most

develop interrupted spikes. Each calyx and corolla are 2–lipped.

Salvia apiana is a 3′–5′ foot tall perennial. The petioled leaves are ob-lanceolate and 1″–3½″ long. Leaves and upper stems are made silvery-white by a covering of appressed hair. Whorled flower clusters develop on the upper stem sections. They are white or speckled with lavender.

Salvia carnosa is a highly variable species with many varieties exhibit-ing leaf and flower differences. This small shrub is less than 3′ high. Leaves are spatula shaped, linear, or obovate. They are covered with a fine layer of appressed hair making their appearance silvery. Whorled flowers form on upper branch stems and are blue.

Salvia mohavensis is a small, many–branched shrub generally 3′ tall. Leaf blades are oblanceolate or deltoid, green, and covered with short leaf hair. The whorled flowers are pale blue or lavender. S. clevelandii is also about 3′ in height. Its leaves are ½″–1½″ long, oblong, and coated with a grayish pubescence. The flowers are blue–lavender. The whole plant is ex-tremely fragrant.

Distribution

Salvia apiana is found in California from the coastal ranges of Santa Bar-bara and San Diego Counties, east to the desert's edge, and south. Look to dry slopes in Chaparral Scrub areas. Its range is small, yet where it occurs, it is abundant.

From Washington to Arizona, S. carnosa is extensively distributed throughout the Desert West. Look to Juniper–Pinyon Woodlands and Sage-brush Deserts. Salvia mohavensis is found from 1,000′–5,000′ in desert re-gions of southern Nevada, southeast California, and western Arizona. Look to dry rocky slopes and canyon walls. S. clevelandii is found on dry slopes, below 3,000′ in Chaparral Scrub areas and in the coastal mountains of southern California.

Chemistry

Volatile oil content for Salvia general: α–pinene, camphene, β–pinene, myrcene, α–phellandrene and β–phellandrene, 3–carene, p–cymene, 1,8–cineole, limonene, cis–ocimene, trans–ocimene, γ–terpinene, terpi-nolene, linalol, camphor, borneol, 4–terpineol, α–terpineol, bornyl–acetate, β–caryophyllene, γ–cadinene, α–cadinene, and farnesol; diterpenes: car-nosic acid, carnosol, rosmanol, epirosmanol, isorosmanol, salvicanol, and rosmadial.

Medicinal Uses

Salvia's medicinal potency is essentially indicated by its strong aromatic smell. Like most other Mint family plants, the stronger the smell, the stronger the medicine.

If there is a dry fever and a strong determination of blood, a hot cup of Sage tea will be diaphoretic. Inversely, the room temperature tea or tincture curbs colliquative sweating, particularly when body temperature is normal, the skin is soft and relaxed, and the extremities are cool.

Sage is decidedly carminative. It is useful taken as a spasmolytic for gas pains and flatulence. Its dilatory nature moves blood, hence activity to the stomach walls.

Several different varieties of Sage have been used in English herbal medicine for memory loss, forgetfulness, and to 'strengthen the brain'. Lately it has been discovered that the essential oil of several varieties of Sage, namely Salvia officinalis and S. lavandulaefolia, inhibit AChE (acetylcholinesterase) in cholinergic neuronal synapses of the brain. This has promise in diminishing the dementia and cognition loss of Alzheimer's disease. Even in non–Alzheimer's study subjects, improved attention and recall has been observed. Apparently, Sage blocks AChE from breaking down acetylcholine into inactive choline and acetate. This activity keeps AChE in the synapse longer, thus improving brain nerve transmission[22].

The plant's monoterpene content, which is largely responsible for this effect acts strongest as a whole complex. The plant's aromatics are much less potent taken out of context and used in an isolated fashion, even if recombined to mimic the plant's natural essential oil ratios. This is not a new phenomenon. Most plants work best as whole herbal medicines, not standardized extracts.

Applied externally Sage is strongly antiinflammatory and antioxidant. It is efficacious in relieving the pain and redness from burns and other injuries. Its use rivals Lavender in these conditions.

Inhale the steam from a cup or pot of hot tea for pharyngitis, tonsillitis, and strep throat. This process concentrates Sage's antimicrobial aromatics to the back of the throat where the majority of the bacterial colonization occurs. This done for five minutes three times a day, along with internal immune stimulating herbs such as Wild indigo, Echinacea, or Myrrh, combined with rest, is a useful plan. Of course the traditional

22   AChE inhibition through pharmaceuticals is the primary conventional treatment for Alzheimer's disease.

gargle with the hot tea is also useful – it will need to be done every couple of hours to assist in recovery.

Lastly, Sage tea is an age–old remedy that mother's use to halt breast milk production after their young have been weaned. 1–2 cups a day is the standard amount. Even though the exact mechanism is unknown, the plant's effect on lactation is the same as on excessive sweating...that is to diminish.

Indications
» Fever, dry, moderate temperature
» Sweating, colliquative
» Gas/Spasm, gastrointestinal
» Memory loss
» Cognition, poor
» Alzheimer's disease
» To lessen breast milk
» Burns (external)
» Pharyngitis/Tonsillitis/Strep throat

Collection
Due to the plant's characteristic smell, gathering Sage is always a pleasant experience. Collect the leaves and flowering parts only, as these have the greatest concentration of aromatics.

Preparations/Dosage
» Herb infusion: 4–8 ounces 2–3 times daily
» FPT/DPT (50% alcohol): 30–60 drops 2–3 times daily
» Spirit: 20–30 drops 2–3 times daily
» Essential oil: topically as needed
» Ointment/Oil/Salve: as needed
» Steam inhalation: 2–3 times daily

Cautions
Do not use the essential oil during pregnancy or while nursing.

Other Uses
Sage's use as a seasoning needs little mention, though that it is also a car-minative is of no coincidence. Southwestern Sages, particularly Salvia

apiana, are used ceremonially as a 'smudge'. Known as White sage, it tends to be more fragrant and less irritating than Sagebrush, which is also used ceremonially in a similar fashion.

Sagebrush
Asteraceae/Sunflower Family

Artemisia tridentata Nutt. *(Seriphidium tridentatum)*
Big sagebrush, Mountain sagebrush

Description
This evergreen bush varies in size depending on rainfall and soil conditions. In ideal circumstances where the winters are cold and there is adequate precipitation, the plant reaches 9'–10' in height, but 3'–4' is more common with average soil, rainfall, and warmer temperatures.

The trunk of Sagebrush is woody, thickened, and on older plants, is covered by grayish–brown stringy bark. The leaves are wedge–shaped and typically have 3 blunt teeth. However, they sometimes have 4–9 teeth, and occasionally are completely lacking teeth and are entire. The leaves' silvery–blue appearance results from the plant's dense coating of leaf hair. When the aromatic leaves are crushed, a distinctive sage–like smell is apparent; the plant's pungency is also evident when it is well hydrated and daytime temperatures are high. In the fall, the small yellow flowers form in panicles at branch ends. Throughout most of its range, Sagebrush is a prolific seeder, demonstrated by various removal programs designed to clear western grazing lands of the plant.

Distribution
Sagebrush is a dominant plant common to western rangelands. It is found from British Columbia and South Dakota south to the Rocky Mountains, New Mexico, central Arizona, and California.

Chemistry
Artemeseole, camphor, carvacrol, 1–8–cineol, α–pinene, β–pinene, thujol, and thujone, among other constituents.

Medicinal Uses

Sagebrush is a strong and multi–faceted medicinal plant, capable of affecting a number of organ systems more profoundly than the best Mugwort, a closely related herb. As a cold tea, Sagebrush is an aromatic bitter.
It is stimulating to hydrochloric acid, pepsinogen, and other gut secretions
(as are most Artemisias). This compounded with its carminative and bile
stimulating effects increases the body's digestive prowess. With Sagebrush
protein and fat are digested and assimilated more efficiently. Less gas and
cramping associated with gastrointestinal tract weakness will be observed.

The cold tea is diuretic. The hot tea is strongly diaphoretic, particularly when the skin is hot and dry, the pulse is strong, and there is a general
feeling of contained body heat. The plant can break the most stubborn of
fevers.

Sagebrush is broadly antimicrobial and anti–parasitic. Long hailed as
a treatment for some food and water borne illnesses, it inhibits Salmonella
spp. and Escherichia coli, among other pathogenic organisms responsible
for food poisoning. Modern findings and traditional use also support the
plant being used in amebic infections, i.e. montezuma's revenge–traveler's
diarrhea, and as a broad–spectrum vermifuge. Pinworms and roundworms
are the surest parasites Sagebrush will eliminate.

The plant is stimulating to menses mainly through its essential oil
(and thujone) content. The hot tea or tincture put in hot water, is particularly useful in dilating uterine capillary beds, thus delivering more blood
and activity to the area. This usually is enough to stimulate menses if slow
to start from a recent viral infection or even from moving to a colder locale.

When applied topically, Sagebrush is significantly antimicrobial and
antifungal. Various external preparations are all useful in inhibiting numerous Staphylococcus, Streptococcus, and fungal varieties. From ringworm and athlete's foot to wounds and ulcers that need some infection
fighting help, the plant is powerful. Compounding this influence is Sagebrush's analgesic effect. Acute pain from contusions, sprains, and blows
along with chronic pain from rheumatoid arthritis or bothersome old sport
injuries, are all quieted.

A warm poultice or fomentation is decidedly sedative to menstrual,
intestinal, and stomach cramps. Moreover, the plant makes a strong antimicrobial respiratory tract medicine. Inhaling the volatile oil filled steam
of the tea is useful for bronchitis, especially when lung mucus is thickened and difficult to expectorate. The inhaled steam rivals White sage and

Eucalyptus in treating strep throat and sinusitis.

Indications

- » Indigestion
- » Cramps/Flatulence, gastrointestinal
- » Congestion, liver/gallbladder
- » Fever, dry skin
- » Food poisoning
- » Diarrhea, amebic
- » Pinworm/Roundworm infestation
- » Amenorrhea with water retention and feelings of coldness
- » Infection, fungal/bacterial (external)
- » Contusions/Sprains (external)
- » Cramps, menstrual (external)
- » Cramps, gastrointestinal (external)
- » Bronchitis (inhaled steam)

Collection/Preparations

In the spring, before flowering, snip the last 8"–10" of new growth from the branch ends. These clippings can either be wrapped in small bundles or chopped into smaller manageable pieces for drying.

Dosage

- » Leaf infusion (cold or standard): 2–4 ounces 1–2 times daily
- » FPT/DPT (60% alcohol): 10–30 drops 1–2 times daily
- » Inhaled steam: 2–3 times daily
- » External preparations: as needed

Cautions

Due to Sagebrush's thujone and related essential oil content, do not use it during pregnancy or while nursing. Additionally, its use should be discontinued if there are sensations of dizziness, nausea, or headache. Internally use Sagebrush consecutively for 1–2 weeks or less.

Other Uses

Although the smoke is harsh on the eyes and respiratory tissues, Sagebrush smudge has a rich historical and present day ceremonial use. It is known as the 'other' Sage.

Scouring Rush
Equisetaceae/Horsetail Family

Equisetum laevigatum A. Braun *(Equisetum funstonii, E. kansanum)*
Smooth scouring rush, Cola de caballo

Equisetum hyemale L. *(Equisetum praealtum, E. robustum var. affine, Hippochaete hyemalis)*
Scouring rush, Cola de caballo, Canutillo de llano, Caballo

Description
Similar in appearance, Equisetum laevigatum and E. hyemale are perennials that arise from spreading rhizomes. Their wand–like stems are hollow and jointed. Fertile stems are distinct in appearance: they have small cylinder–like cone terminations. Given its prominent silica formed ridges, E. hyemale's stems are the rougher of the two species profiled.

Distribution
Both Equisetum species discussed here are found throughout most of the United States and much of Canada. They are commonly encountered along stream sides and the moist soils of springs and seeps throughout an array of elevations in the Southwest.

Chemistry
Flavonoids: chlorogenic acid, kaempferol, dihydrokaempferol, hydroxycinnamic acid, equisetumpyrone, quercetin, protogenkwanin, gossypetin, luteolin, apigenin, protoapigenin, genkwanin, and naringenin; silicic acid, silica, calcium, potassium, and phosphorus.

Medicinal Uses
Souring rush is essentially a Horsetail analog and can be treated as a substitute or a replacement for this better known plant. Mainly a urinary tract medicine, most find Scouring rush to be soothing to the bladder, kidneys, and related areas. It specifically is of use in diminishing urinary tract irritability and painful urination. Internal preparations are also mildly diuretic and will assist in the elimination of fluid accumulation (non–organic causes) around the ankles, wrists, and mid–sections of the body. Moreover,

when taken as a daily tea, kidney stone formation is reduced through the plant's ability of increasing urine volume.

Although its mechanism of action as a hemostatic is not clearly understood, the plant lessens passive hemorrhaging. Use it if there is blood in the urine from physical injury or gastrointestinal bleeding from ulceration or other non–malignant inflammatory processes. Internal preparations may even be useful if there is blood–tinged sputum from a severe cough.

Topically and internally the plant facilitates wound healing and tissue repair. This is mainly due to Scouring rush's flavonoid, silica, and silicic acid content. The plant is also used to strengthen the hair, nails, and skin. Connective tissues throughout the body are augmented. The plant makes a good tea for fortifying bones damaged by injury, or weakened from osteoporosis.

Indications
» Urination, painful/irritated
» Fluid retention
» Kidney stones, as a preventative
» Hemorrhaging, passive
» Ulceration, gastrointestinal
» Hair, nails, skin, bones, and connective tissues, weakened
» Wounds (external and internal)

Collection
Equisetum arvense (Horsetail) has the highest quercetin content in its new spring growth – approximately 50% of its total flavonoid content (Scouring rush species are potentially similar). Therefore it is best to gather any Equisetum species during this time. As spring changes to summer, the plant's quercetin content quickly diminishes.

Fertile and infertile stems alike can be collected of Scouring rushes. Clip the stems at their bases. Use them fresh or dry. After drying, the stems are easily separated into 1"–2" sections for storage.

Preparations/Dosage
» Fresh juice: 1 ounce 2–3 times daily
» Herb infusion: 2–4 ounces 2–3 times daily
» Poultice: as needed

Cautions

It is possible that Scouring rush, exposed to common agricultural run–off, produces several toxic compounds. Therefore do not collect and use the plant around contaminated areas. In addition, excessive quantities of the tea or juice may irritate the kidneys.

Other Uses

The abrasive qualities of Scouring rush are practically legendary, but surely are exaggerated. It has been said that the plant was once used to sharpen knives and clean and polish pots and metals – an herbal equivalent to steel wool.

Senna

Fabaceae/Pea Family

Senna hirsuta var. glaberrima (M.E. Jones) H.S. Irwin & Barneby *(Cassia gooddingii, C. leptocarpa var. glaberrima, Ditremexa glaberrima)*
Slimpod senna, Woolly senna

Senna armata (S. Watson) H.S. Irwin & Barneby *(Cassia armata, Xerocassia armata)*
Spiny senna

Senna covesii (A. Gray) H.S. Irwin & Barneby *(Cassia covesii, Earleocassia covesii)*
Desert senna

Description

Senna hirsuta var. glaberrima is a 2′–3′ tall, herbaceous bush. When fully leafed–out and in flower the plant's sub–tropical appearance is distinctive. The leaves are deeply green and usually between 4″–7″ long. They are pinnately divided into 4–8 sets of long triangular leaflets. The leaves alternate along the branched stems and progressively diminish in size as they terminate inter–spaced with the flowers. Towards the outer reaches of the plant, the large, deep yellow–orange flowers have 5 petals and are quite noticeable in the summer. The brown pods are thin, usually 6″–10″ in length, and form in clusters of 2–3. The encased and small brownish seeds are tightly packed together in one long row.

Senna armata is a low–growing and deciduous bush usually 1′–2′ in height. Much of the year it is leafless, only to break the trend and form leaves in response to winter rains. The leaf axles terminate pointedly as spines. Bright yellow flowers are followed by tan and inflated seedpods.

Salvia covesii is a small and semi–herbaceous bush. In drier winters, the spring–formed leaves are very compact and hairy, giving the plant a greenish–sliver coloration. As with other Sennas, this plant also has characteristic yellow flowers followed by elongated small pods.

Distribution

Look for Senna leptocarpa var. glaberrima along wash embankments, roadsides, and drainage areas. From southeastern Arizona, this plant is found east to New Mexico and south through Mexico, Central America, to South America. Look for S. armata in the western desert of southern California, the extreme southern tip of Nevada, and along parts of the Colorado River Drainage in western Arizona. Typically, it can be found along washes and drainages in sandy soils. From 1,000′–4,000′ look for S. covesii along gravely wash sides, hillsides, and roadsides throughout southeastern California, southwestern Arizona, southern Nevada, and southern New Mexico.

Chemistry

Hydroxyanthracene glycosides: sennosides; naphthalene glycosides; flavonoids; mucilage (galactose, arabinose, rhamnose, and galacturonic acid).

Medicinal Uses

Senna is a straightforward stimulant laxative. Similar to Aloe, Senna's anthraquinones affect the small and large intestines. The plant increases transit time and peristalsis while decreasing intestinal fluid absorption.

Mixing the plant with a carminative herb such as Ginger or Peppermint will limit its griping (gastrointestinal cramping) potential. Taken before bed and dosed properly, Senna will soften the stool and stimulate a bowel movement for the next morning[23]. Some of the plant's glycosides are

23   It is also important to address dietary and constitutional factors for long–term relief. Fiber and water intake, upper gastrointestinal and hepatic response to food, and psychosomatic factors are all important issues to address when resolving chronic constipation.

broken down in the colon by bacterial activity. The resulting metabolites, particularly rheinanthrone, are responsible for much of the plant's effect.

Because the pods contain polysaccharide–starches the rate at which Senna delivers its stimulant–anthraquinones is somewhat slowed, making them gentler in effect. The leaves lack these substances, which is the main reason why they tend to be harsher in activity.

Indications
» Constipation, general

Collection
The leaves, flowering racemes, seedpods, and immature seeds are all active. The leaves have the largest quantities of anthraquinones. The fully mature seedpods have small amounts and the mature seeds are nearly devoid of these compounds. Dry all parts after collection.

Preparations
A cold infusion made with the pods is the choice preparation. Although the leaves can also be used, consider them harsher in activity.

Dosage
» Cold infusion: 1–2 grams of whole pods to 1 cup of water, taken before bed
» Fluidextract (40% alcohol): 5–20 drops before bed

Cautions
Due to the plant's potential sympathetic stimulation of uterine contractions, do not use it during pregnancy. Senna will have a laxative effect in nursing infants through mothers drinking the tea. Senna is not recommended in constipation from dehydration, as the plant's effect on intestinal electrolyte absorption will exacerbate the situation. Also muscular tetany has been observed with excessive consumption – electrolyte balance, particularly of potassium, is disorganized by Senna. Excess consumption of the tea or over–the–counter preparations will cause habituation and dependence. Senna is best used for 1–2 weeks at a time, or longer in combination with supporting herbs.

Snakeweed
Asteraceae/Sunflower Family

Gutierrezia microcephala (DC.) A. Gray *(Brachyris microcephala, Gutierrezia sarothrae var. microcephala)*
Sticky snakeweed, Thread–leaf snakeweed, Matchweed, Resinweed, Escoba de la víbora, Yerba de la víbora, Collálle

Gutierrezia sarothrae (Pursh) Britton & Rusby *(Brachyris divaricata, Galinsoga linearifolia)*
Broom snakeweed, Snakebroom, Matchweed, Escoba de la víbora, Yerba de la víbora, Collálle

Description
Snakeweed is a clump–forming perennial bush. The small, linear–green leaves are apparent from mid–spring though early to mid–fall when the plant flowers. The leaves are semi–resinous and when crushed they are sticky and aromatic. When in flower the small yellow blooms cover the upper portion of the plant giving it a frosted appearance.

The two most abundant species in the West are Gutierrezia microcephala and G. sarothrae. They differ mainly in floral characteristics. G. microcephala's flowers are cylindrical and have 1 or 2 ray and disk flowers per head. G. sarothrae's flower heads are shaped more or less like a slender top, each flower having 3–8 ray and disk flowers.

Distribution
Snakeweed is a common plant widely distributed throughout the West. It is found nearly from sea level to almost 10,000' and in great abundance on over–grazed rangelands. Gutierrezia microcephala is found from southern Colorado west to the White Mountains of California, east through much of Arizona, New Mexico, and southwestern Texas. From 2,000'–6,000' the plant inhabits several different vegetation zones: Oak–Juniper Woodlands, Desert Grasslands, and the Mojave Desert. Look for the plant on slopes, flats, and hillsides. G. sarothrae has the widest range of the two. Throughout the western interior, the plant is found from 3,000'–6,000' on flats and plains.

Chemistry
Terpenes: geraniol, γ–humulene, trans–verbenol, verbenone, α–pinene, β–pinene, limonene, nopinone, myrentol, polyalthic acid, and daniellic acid; flavonoids: sarothrin, calycopterin, jaceidin, and sudachitin.

Medicinal Uses
Snakeweed is mainly used externally to reduce joint soreness, particularly from rheumatoid arthritis. Being broadly antiinflammatory and especially sedative to muscular–skeletal pain, it will be found particularly helpful to sufferers of 'fibromyalgia'. Not only is soaking in a bath of Snakeweed tea before bed the preferred method of application, it is also generally relaxing and therefore will assist deeper sleep states, making it doubly beneficial for some people. Additionally, a small amount of the tea can be sipped while soaking for added benefit. The liniment, oil, or salve can be applied for similar relief of isolated painful areas. Like its close relative Turpentine bush, Snakeweed is antimicrobial. Applied to cuts and scrapes it will facilitate healing by its retarding effect on bacterial growth.

Indications
» Arthritis, rheumatoid/osteoarthritis (internal and external)
» Pain, chronic, muscular (internal and external)
» Cuts/Scrapes (external)

Collection
Collect Snakeweed from late summer to early fall in bloom or not, though allergy sufferers may prefer to gather the plant without flowers. Prune the upper new growth. This can either be bundled with rubber bands or string, or collected loosely and then dried.

Preparations
Use several ounces of the dried material to make a gallon of tea. This then is added to bath water. It is best to infuse the herb due to its volatile oil content.

Dosage
» Leaf infusion: add to bath water; internally, 1 cup daily
» Oil/Salve/Liniment: as needed

Cautions

Do not use during pregnancy due to the plant's potential uterine stimulant effect. Large amounts internally may irritate the liver.

Soapberry
Sapindaceae/Soapberry Family

Sapindus saponaria var. drummondii (Hook. & Arn.) L.D. Benson
Western soapberry, Jaboncillo, Palo blanco

Description

Soapberry is a large bush or small tree capable of reaching 30' in height, but typically, it stands 10'–15' tall. With age the tree's bark becomes gray and fissured. At first glance Soapberry looks to be some sort of stunted Walnut but upon closer examination the deciduous and pinnate leaves are smaller than and not serrated like Walnut's. Soapberry has between 13–19 leaflets that are 2"–4" long by ½"–1" wide. At branch ends, the small and whitish flowers develop into pyramidal shaped panicles. Upon maturation, the fruit are yellowish–green. After drying they become translucent: the outer amber portion of the fruit is partially see–through, enabling the viewer to peer through its crinkled outer coating to the seed inside. In sandy soils, in canyons and small drainages, Soapberry tends to grow in thickets where the tree sprouts from laterally growing roots.

Distribution

From 2,500'–6,000' Soapberry is found along canyon sides and drainages particularly where soils are sandy. Look for the plant from central Arizona, east to the Gila River and Rio Grande Drainages in New Mexico, to Texas, and east to Louisiana.

Chemistry

Triterpenes: α–amyrin, β–amyrin, and hederagenin; flavonoids: luteolin and rutin; various saponins; lipids, mostly found within the seed: arachidic, linoleic, oleic, palmitic, and stearic acids.

Medicinal Uses

Much like Yucca, Soapberry's medicinal effect is derived from its saponin content interacting with the gastrointestinal tract's walls and contents. Use Soapberry when arthritic conditions are dependent upon poor intestinal health, particularly when poor dietary habits and constipation are factors. The plant's saponins form complexes with harmful colonic flora by–products and inhibit their systemic absorption, therefore proving systemically antiinflammatory.

Soapberry is also directly antimicrobial. But unfortunately, the plant does not discriminate between good and bad enteric microbes. When using the plant, internal supplementation with Lactobacillus acidophilus may be necessary to keep functional levels of these good microorganisms intact. Soapberry is broadly anti–protozoal. Its use is warranted in traveler's diarrhea and other similar conditions.

Indications

» Arthritis, dependent upon constipation and poor intestinal health
» Diarrhea from protozoal infection

Collection

Gather the leaves from late spring through mid–summer. The fruit should be gathered from early to mid–fall.

Preparations/Dosage

» Leaf infusion: 2–4 ounces 1–3 times daily
» Fruit decoction: 1–2 ounces 1–3 times daily
» Capsule (00), powdered leaf: 2–4, 1–3 times daily
» Capsule (00), powdered fruit: 1–2, 1–3 times daily

Cautions

Traditionally Soapberry has been used to stupefy fish. In various studies, the plant has been shown to kill snails and mollusks, and even has spermicidal properties, so the plant is not completely benign. Dosed properly, like any plant, its use is therapeutic. That said, do not use Soapberry during pregnancy, while nursing, or with children. In addition, diarrhea can result with over use. It is best to use Soapberry for two consecutive weeks or less, and then rotate to another non–saponin plant.

Other Uses

A soapy wash can be made with the crushed and dried fruit.

Spanish Needles
Asteraceae/Sunflower Family

Bidens pilosa L. *(Bidens adhaerescens, B. alba, B. leucantha, Centipeda minuta, Coreopsis leucantha, Kerneria pilosa)*
Bur marigold, Pitchforks, Stick tight, Beggar's ticks

Description
Spanish needles is a 3'–4' tall herbaceous annual. The pinnate leaves are composed of 3–5 leaflets and are oppositely arranged. These large leaflets are lance to oval shaped and have toothed margins. The flowers form at branch ends and arise from leaf axils on long petioles. They are composed of mostly yellow disk flowers. Less uniform in appearance are the slightly larger white ray flowers. The seeds are linear, 4–sided and have 2–4 awns terminating one end. They stick to clothes and animal fur easily, and are typically transported this way – a rather successful method, considering the extent of Spanish needles' range.

Distribution
This species is originally native to South America, but now is found throughout the tropical and subtropical world. In the United States, it ranges from southern California to southern Arizona and east to Florida. Look to disturbed lowlands, moist riverbanks, fields, and vacant lots.

Chemistry
Coumarins: aesculetin; triterpenes: β–amyrin, friedelan, lupeol, and lupeol acetate; flavonoids: quercetin and others; monoterpenes: borneol and limonene; sesquiterpenes: β–caryophyllene, germacrene d and t–muurolol; phenylpropanoids; steroid: daucosterol; benzenoid: phenylheptatriyne; alkenynes; diterpene: phytylheptanoate.

Medicinal Uses
Spanish needles tea augments the quantity and quality of gastric mucus. It does this by activating prostaglandin activity within the epithelial lining of the gut wall. This effect increases tissue vascularity and glycoprotein content of gastric mucus[24]. All of these activities make Spanish nee-

24   Proper viscosity and quantity of gut mucus are important in maintaining

dles of use in any ulcer healing approach. The plant also has application in pre–ulcerous gastritis.

Traditionally the plant is used in treating a variety of cardiac ailments by healers in Central America. Research has confirmed that Spanish needles' blood pressure lowering effect mainly comes from the plant's ability to diminish influxes of extracellular calcium within aortic smooth muscle. This subsequently reduces tonicity of those muscle fibers, thus lowering blood pressure. Although Spanish needles has little effect on sodium excretion, it has been shown to diminish both essential and sodium induced hypertension.

In its effect on the large and small intestines, Spanish needles is similar to Canadian fleabane. Both have flavonoid contents that are sedating to inflammatory processes, particularly if they are autoimmune mediated. It specifically diminishes excessive lymphocyte proliferation, making it of value in ulcerative colitis or crone's disease. Moreover, the plant tends to lessen diarrhea through its mild astringency.

Spanish needles is used as a treatment in some areas of the tropical world where malaria is problematic. This plant (and other species, such as Bidens frondosa, B. bipinnata, and B. ferulaefolia) has been found to retard the growth of Plasmodium falciparum, one of the main parasites responsible for malaria. Spanish needles is used advantageously as a co–therapy with pharmaceuticals where drug resistance is an issue. Although no research to my knowledge has been conducted, there is potential in Spanish needles being of similar use in retarding Babesia growth. The organism is responsible for babesiosis, or various 'tick fevers', particularly of concern throughout the northeast and northwest parts of the country. Both Plasmodium falciparum and Babesia reproduce within red blood cells.

Topically applied, Spanish needles is somewhat antimicrobial and is useful in retarding bacterial growth responsible for infections. The tea as a wash, or the oil or salve, tends to be soothing to redness and irritation. Likewise, an eyewash made of the herb is cooling to inflamed conjunctiva. As a urinary tract medicine the plant is mild but worthy of note. Although not a urinary tract disinfectant, the plant is soothing to bladder and urethra irritability, and lessening to hematuria.

stomach health and in healing gastric and duodenal ulcers. Incidentally, continual emotional anxiety and tension have a diminishing effect on the gut's protective mucus layer, thereby exposing the stomach's sensitive mucosal layer to the causticness of innate hydrochloric acid. This greatly increases the chances of ulcer formation.

Indications

» Ulcers, gastric/duodenal
» Gastritis
» Colitis, ulcerative
» Hypertension, essential and sodium induced
» Malaria, as a co–therapy with conventional medications
» Wounds/Cuts (external)
» Conjunctivitis (eyewash)
» Urinary tract irritability, with passive hemorrhaging

Collection

From late spring through summer, collect the herbaceous portions of the plant.

Preparations/Dosage

» Herb infusion: 4–8 ounces 2–3 times daily
» FPT/DPT (50% alcohol): 30–60 drops 2–3 times daily
» Wash/Oil/Salve: as needed

Cautions

There are no known cautions with normal usage.

Sumac

Anacardiaceae/Cashew Family

Rhus microphylla Engelm.
Little leaf sumac, Desert sumac

Rhus trilobata Nutt.
Squaw bush, Lemonade berry, Skunk bush

Rhus ovata S. Watson
Sugar bush, Sugar sumac

Description

As a moderately sized, deciduous shrub, Rhus microphylla grows to be 6' high by 6' wide. Its branches are weakly spiny and form in dense tangles.

Comprising each leaf are 5–9 small pinnate leaflets. The white and very small 5–petaled flowers appear before the leaves in the early spring. The leaves and then the fruit develop shortly after. The small and hair–covered red fruit are sticky, edible, and form in clusters at the branch ends. If particularly abundant they can cause the branches to droop.

Rhus trilobata is a slightly larger shrub. The leaves are comprised of 3 leaflets. They are lobed and non–leathery. The plant also develops edible–tart fruit. R. ovata is a large evergreen shrub occasionally reaching 12' in height. The oval leaves are leathery, entire, and are slightly longer than wide. Dense fruit clusters follow small cream flowers. The plant is adapted to brush fires, particularly in the Chaparral Scrub of southern California where seeds germinate more successfully and root crowns sprout prolifically after burns.

Numerous species of Rhus not discussed here can also be used medicinally. It is also important to be aware of the differences between Western poison oak (Toxicodendron diversilobum) and Western poison ivy (Toxicodendron rydbergii) and non–toxic Rhuses. Poison oak's form is variable and can be shrub to vine–like. The leaves are divided into 3 leaflets, are usually shiny, and can be entire or present small serrations or lobes. Western poison ivy is typically a shrub with non–aerial roots. The fruit at maturity, for both plants, are white as opposed to the red–sticky fruit of non–toxic Rhuses. When a stem or leaf is broken, a white, milky, and urushiol–containing sap is noticeable. This does not occur in non–toxic Rhuses.

Distribution

Rhus microphylla is found on rocky slopes and mesas from 3,500'–6,000'. In Arizona from the Rincon and Santa Rita Mountains, the plant is found east to New Mexico and Texas along the Rio Grande and Pecos River Drainages. From Oklahoma, it ranges south. It is a typical Chihuahuan Desert plant.

R. trilobata, an extremely variable species, is found at numerous elevations and can grow as high as 7,000'. It is extensively found throughout the West. R. ovata frequents Chaparral Scrub areas of southern California. In central Arizona the plant is found below the Mogollon Rim, although it does not reach into lower elevations where water scarcity and higher temperatures are limiting factors.

Chemistry
Condensed and hydrolyzable tannins.

Medicinal Uses
Sumac leaves are astringent due to their array of tannins. Use a fresh leaf poultice or the externally applied tea for stings, bites, rashes, and sunburn. The plant is decidedly soothing to skin irritations and superficial inflammations. The leaf powder applied topically will quickly astringe mild bleeding from cuts and scrapes. As a gargle for sore throats, mouth sores, and receding and bleeding gums, it is useful. A strong cup of tea will also prove lessening to episodic diarrhea.

Indications
- » Burns/Cuts/Scrapes (external)
- » Sore throats/Bleeding gums (gargle)
- » Diarrhea

Collection
Clip the leaves from the upper portion of the plant. Use fresh or dry normally.

Preparations/Dosage
- » Leaf infusion: 2–4 ounces 2–3 times daily
- » External preparations: as needed

Cautions
Keep consecutive, internal use of the leaf to short term (2–3 weeks). Longer–term use, as with most other tannin containing plants, may inhibit gastric function, irritate the kidneys, and be mildly vasoconstricting to uterine lining. It is not recommended during pregnancy.

Other Uses
The red sticky fruit of Sumac makes a refreshing, lemon–like beverage. Add 4 ounces of fresh fruit to 1 gallon of water. Let this stand for 24 hours, strain, and sweeten to taste. The fruit can also be dried for later use.

Syrian Rue

Zygophyllaceae/Caltrop Family

Peganum harmala L.
Harmal, Wild rue

Description
As a small perennial bush, Syrian rue typically stands 2′ tall by about the same wide. The plant is herbaceous but dense due to its many–branched stems and finely divided leaves. They form alternately along stems, are smooth, green, semi–succulent, and linear. Flowers form at branch ends and are white with 5 petals. Syrian rue's capsules are 2–4 celled and contain many seeds.

Distribution
Syrian rue has a wide native Central Asian and Middle Eastern distribution. In this country, it is an escapee, and is most concentrated around the southern–most part of the border between Arizona and New Mexico. From there it is found along primary and secondary roadsides to the El Paso area. An isolated grouping now exists in central Nevada.

Chemistry
Indole alkaloids: harmol, harmalol, harmine, harmaline, harmalidine, and isoharmine; a non–indole alkaloid: vasicine; anthraquinones.

Medicinal Uses
Syrian rue is a broadly acting medicinal plant with significant pharmacological activity. This is due to its indole group of alkaloids, which have been extensively researched. Seed preparations are the choice article and tend to be mildly mood elevating and sedative. This is generally thought to be due to the plant's monoamine oxidase inhibition (and other neurotransmitter influences) which reduces serotonin re–uptake in neuronal synapses.

Although Syrian rue's immediate mood–altering effects are more pronounced than St. Johns wort's, after time its influence tends to diminish. Syrian rue is better used in formula with other mood–elevating herbs, as alone (especially in excess) it may impede coherent thought process, and cause gastrointestinal upset.

Coincident with Syrian rue's traditional use as an antipyretic, research also suggests the plant's indole alkaloid group reduces body temperature slightly. This is due to the plant's effect on the hypothalamus and other cerebral centers responsible for body temperature regulation. This activity suggests the plant is of use in lowering a high fever. Being inhibiting to various bacterial and fungal strains, the tincture or seed poultice applied topically is broadly antimicrobial. Use it on bacterial and fungal skin infections.

Indications
» Depression, mild
» Fever
» Infection, bacterial/fungal (external)

Collection
Just before the seedpods split and open, clip them from the plant. Place them loosely in a paper bag and dry. Crush the papery seedpods with your hands in the bag. Discard the seedpods. Keep the seeds for medicine.

Preparations
The seed tincture is the most efficacious internal preparation. Additionally, the seed tincture's dark red–burgundy color is striking.

Dosage
» DPT (60% alcohol): 30–60 drops 2–3 times daily
» Seed poultice/Powder/Oil/Salve: topically as needed

Cautions
Do not use Syrian rue with other psychoactive pharmaceuticals, particularly MAO inhibitors. The plant should not be used during pregnancy (or nursing) due to its potential emmenagogue activity. Toxic central nervous system and gastrointestinal effects will be seen if taken in excess.

Other Uses
A dye from the seeds, called Turkish red, was used in textile coloring and in dying Turkish rugs.

Tamarisk
Tamaricaceae/Tamarisk Family

Tamarix aphylla (L.) H. Karst.
Athel

Tamarix chinensis Lour. *(Tamarix juniperina, T. pentandra, T. ramosissima)*
Salt cedar

Description
Tamarix aphylla is a large, pyramidal, 30'–50' tall tree, with thin but dense foliage. The tree's overall appearance is delicate yet robust. The trunk bark is reddish–brown to gray. The scale–like leaves make the tree's appearance deceivingly Cypress–like, which did cause some botanical confusion at the end of the 19th century when botanists were trying to classify the tree. The leaves are grayish blue or green and glaucous. The branches are numerous and thin. The small white to pink, 5–petaled flowers form in spike–like panicles on branch ends.

Tamarix chinensis appears nearly identical to T. aphylla, with one notable exception: T. chinensis is a large bush or small tree. It never approaches the size of T. aphylla. In addition, as described below, how and where this plant grows is another useful distinguishing characteristic.

Distribution
Tamarix aphylla is non–native and is originally from Eurasia. In this country it was originally planted as a windbreak, shade, or ornamental tree. The majority of these trees throughout the Southwest originate from approximately a ½–dozen Algerian cuttings. Chances are, all clones here are from 1 or 2 trees abroad. Look for the tree throughout the hot and dry Southwest. Old farms, homesteads, and ranches are good places to look. Rarely does the tree escape cultivation.

Tamarix chinensis, indigenous to the same regions, is found along streams, wash sides, and irrigation ditches throughout the California deserts, east through Arizona, New Mexico, and to Texas. Up to nearly 6,000' and along waterways the plant can grow so densely it is known to choke out many native species. The plant is considered a noxious weed due to its aggressive nature. Its range expands yearly.

Chemistry

Polyphenols: tamaridone, tamadone, gardenins, nevadensin, apigenin, tamarixellagic acid, dehydrotrigallic acid, isoferulic acid, gallic acid, isoquercitrin, and tamarixin.

Medicinal Uses

Use Tamarisk externally on weepy rashes, bites, stings, and other problems that either Mesquite or Acacia remedy. Tamarisk is astringent from an array of bark and leaf tannins. Due to these compounds, it is moderately antibacterial and antifungal. There are stronger medicinal plants for either type of infection but if it is the only plant available Tamarisk will come in handy.

Indications

» Scrapes/Cuts/Abrasions/Burns (external)
» Mouth sores/Sore throats (gargle)

Collection

Gather the leaves and/or bark. The bark has a higher tannin yield and is subsequently the stronger part.

Preparations/Dosage

» External preparations: as needed

Cautions

There are no known cautions for external use.

Tarbush

Asteraceae/Sunflower Family

Flourensia cernua DC. *(Helianthus cernuus)*
Varnishbush, Blackbrush, Hojase, Hojansen, Ojasé

Description

Tarbush is a 3'–4' high, semi–deciduous, long–lived shrub. Leaves are 1" long and ½" wide, green, oval, and covered with a sticky–shiny resin. Older branches are dark gray. New stem growth is much lighter. The bell shaped inflorescences lack ray flowers. They are nodding and situated in axillary and terminal groupings.

Distribution
Serving as an indicator plant, Tarbush is a typical Chihuahuan Desert resident. It is found from 3,500'–5,000' throughout valleys, slopes, and mesas. It ranges from southeastern Arizona through New Mexico's Rio Grande and Pecos River Basins to western Texas.

Chemistry
Mono and sesquiterpenoids: camphene, β–myrcene, 3–carene, limonene, 1,8–cineole, borneol, cisjasmone, β–caryophyllene, caryophyllene oxide, and globulol; lactones: tetracosan, pentacosan, hexacosan, heptacosan, octacosan, nonacosan, and triacontan; flavonoids: kaempferol, quercetagetin, kumatakenin, cirsimaritin, and hispidulin.

Medicinal Uses
Traditional Mexican usage is relied upon here in describing how Tarbush is best used. Few herbs surpass Tarbush's bitterness, therefore internally it is a stimulating bitter tonic, similar in use to Bricklebush. Tarbush enhances upper digestive process by stimulating an array of gastric secretions. This enables food to be more adequately digested. Use the tea before meals if chronic indigestion, gas, and stasis are common, particularly with protein-rich and fatty foods. Tarbush is also stimulating to bile production and release, thereby assisting in small intestinal fat digestion. Topically the plant is antifungal and antimicrobial, so apply external preparations to related complaints. Incidentally, these latter activities are common for resinous plants that must develop complex defense mechanisms for predator and elemental protection.

Indications
- » Indigestion/Digestive stasis
- » Congestion, liver
- » Wounds/Cuts/Scrapes (external)
- » Infection, bacterial/fungal (external)

Collection
Tarbush's leaves are most hydrated throughout the spring and summer.

Collect the upper herbage at this time.

Dosage
» Leaf infusion: 2–4 ounces before meals
» Oil/Salve/Wash: as needed

Cautions
Large doses of Tarbush can be nauseating and laxative. Do not use during pregnancy or while nursing. Additionally the plant should be avoided if there is a biliary blockage.

Texas Ranger
Scrophulariaceae/Figwort Family

Leucophyllum frutescens (Berl.) I.M. Johnston
Purple sage, Barometer bush, Rain sage, Cenizo

Description
A medium–sized semi–evergreen shrub, Texas ranger is comprised of ½"–1" long greenish–silver leaves. Ideally the plant's foliage is somewhat dense in growth, however during dry or cold periods it tends to be sparse. The tubular pink–purple flowers have a two–lipped five–lobed opening (very similar to Penstemon). Capable of multiple bloom times, Texas ranger's flowering frequency is dependent upon season and soil moisture. It's a showy bush that is commonly utilized throughout the Southwest for its ornamental appeal.

Distribution
Mainly a Texas plant, Texas ranger is indigenous to the Edwards Plateau, south through the Rio Grande Plain, and on to Mexico. To the west it inhabits the southern portion of the Trans–Pecos. It's almost always found in alkaline soil, particularly in rocky caliche/calcrete areas. As a planted ornamental, Texas ranger is common throughout New Mexico and Arizona (southern portions) and West Texas.

Chemistry
Betaines: glycinebetaine, trigonelline; iridoid glycosides; lignans.

Medicinal Uses

As a traditional tea plant, Texas ranger was once employed by southern Texans and Mexicans as a cold and flu sipping tea, particularly if the lungs were the main area of involvement (cough, bronchitis, etc.). It's mild tasting enough to be well–tolerated, by children too, even without sweetener. I suggest other herbs for a more robust cold–flu approach, however if in need of a mild tea that's just a bit of a sudorific, Texas ranger should be the one. The tea also makes a useful base for relevant tinctures – Ginger, Echinacea, Elephant tree, Yerba santa, etc. It combines well with equal portions of Mormon tea (as a decongestant) or one of the Mints as a stronger diaphoretic.

Due to Texas ranger being so mild, like Greenthread, Feather plume, Blue curls, or Mallow, it's fine to drink solely as a beverage.

Indications

»   As a cold/flu sipping tea

Collection

Prune a number of branches with ample leaf (and flowers, if possible) growth. Set these aside in a large cardboard box until dry. Garble the leaves and flowers from the branches. Discard the branches.

Preparations/Dosage

»   Herb infusion: 4–8 ounces 2–3 times daily

Cautions

There are no cautions for Texas ranger.

Tobacco
Solanaceae/Nightshade Family

Nicotiana glauca Graham *(Nicotidendron glauca, Siphaulax glabra)*
Tree tobacco, Punche

Nicotiana trigonophylla Dunal
Desert tobacco, Tobaco loco

Nicotiana attenuata Steud.
Coyote tobacco

Description

Nicotiana glauca is a short–lived bush or small tree. Distinctive in appearance, the plant has evergreen, ovate, and large bluish–green leaves. They are prominently veined, smooth, and glaucous. They alternate along the stems on long petioles. Clusters of long and yellow–tubular flowers develop on leafless branch ends. The flower tubes are 5–lobed and close during the evening. They are followed by an oval seed capsule containing numerous small brown seeds.

Nicotiana trigonophylla is an annual, biannual, or sometimes a short–lived perennial. It stands 1′–3′ in height. Large specimens have numerous multi–branched stems arising from their bases. The large leaves are oblong, green, and clasp the stem. They become smaller as they near the end of the branches' flowering top. The small, tubular, and cream to greenish white flowers form at branch ends. Like N. trigonophylla, the capsules contain many small brown seeds. The entire plant is sticky and covered with small hairs. It is common for it to be dust and debris covered.

Nicotiana attenuata is a 2′–3′ tall annual. Like N. trigonophylla, the whole plant is hairy and sticky. The leaves alternate along the stem, are lanceolate, and are 2″–6″ long. Lower leaves are petioled, whereas upper leaves are small and sometimes sessile. The tubular and white flowers form in racemes. They are followed by ovoid seed capsules which hold minuscule brown seeds.

Distribution

Nicotiana glauca is a native of Argentina and Chile. Since its accidental introduction from a California botanical garden approximately 100 years ago, it has become quite prolific in some areas. From 5,000' and below look for this plant in disturbed soils and along roadsides, streams, and wash sides.

The plant has colonized numerous waterways throughout the Southwest. The Salt and Gila Rivers in Arizona have dense stands of the plant. From the Rio Grande Plain in Texas, Nicotiana glauca is found east through parts of New Mexico, Arizona, to central California.

From 6,900' and below, Nicotiana trigonophylla is found from western Texas to Nevada and Utah. It ends its westward expansion in the Creosote bush and Joshua tree country of southern California. It is commonly found in Arizona and parts of New Mexico. Look for this native plant in disturbed soils, vacant lots, trail and roadsides, flood plains, and along washes and drainages.

Nicotiana attenuata has the largest range of the Tobaccos profiled here. From Montana and British Columbia, the plant is found south to Arizona, New Mexico, and California. From 1,000'–7,500' look to disturbed areas similar to where N. trigonophylla is found. On occasion, they are found side by side.

Chemistry
Major alkaloid for Nicotiana glauca: anabasine; N. trigonophylla: nornicotine; N. attenuata: nicotine.

Medicinal Uses
Tobacco's primary use is as a topical analgesic. External preparations are useful in relieving pain and sensitivity from contusions, sprains, and other sport–accident type injuries. Soaking in a bath made with Tobacco tea is limiting to joint soreness, aches, and pains from a hard day's work. Topical preparations are also well applied to muscular spasm be it from overwork or injury. All three species profiled either have substantial amounts of nicotine (N. attenuata), nornicotine (N. trigonophylla), or anabasine (N. glauca). Tobacco's alkaloid content has a well–documented inhibitory activity on body–brain pain transmission.

Alone, the oil or leaf bolus is soothing to hemorrhoids. With internal Ocotillo use, the combination will offer substantial relief. Additionally, I have found the fresh leaf poultice or warm fomentation one of the best topical analgesics for spider and insect bites.

Indications
» Pain, acute (external)
» Hemorrhoids (external)
» Insect bites and stings (external)

Collection
Gather Nicotiana glauca's large leaves and dry them using a dehydrator – otherwise leaf browning is common. Collect and dry the leaves of the other two species using no special technique.

Preparations/Dosage
» Fresh plant liniment/Poultice/Salve/Oil/Bath: topically as needed

Cautions
Do not use topical applications, particularly full body baths, with an existing heart irregularity, hypertension, or if pregnant. Even healthy individuals may feel some chest tightness with extended bath application. Tobacco is for external use only.

Other Uses
Tree tobacco's anabasine content makes the tea a useful insecticide, particularly against aphids.

Tree of Heaven
Simaroubaceae/Quassia Family

Ailanthus altissima (Mill.) Swingle
Chinese sumac, Ailanto

Description
Tree of heaven is a small to moderately sized tree occasionally reaching 80' in height. If not regularly pruned the tree is colony–forming. If manicured it resembles a small walnut tree. Its dark green leaves are composed of 6–12 pinnately arranged and pointed leaflets. Although some flowers are perfect, male and female flowers generally occur on separate trees with the male flowers having the strongest smell. The seeds are encased in oblong samaras.

Distribution

Tree of heaven's range is sporadic owing to the fact that it once was planted as an ornamental throughout the Southwest and potentially wider. It is extensively naturalized in old mining towns throughout California, Arizona, and New Mexico.

Chemistry

Quassinoids: ailantinol, ailanthone, shinjulactone, shinjudilactone, amaloride, and others; triterpenoids and tannins.

Medicinal Uses

It is said that Tree of heaven's early presence here in the Southwest is due to Chinese immigrants of the mid–19th century. The tree served these transplants as a transportable medicine: it was easily grown and remedied illnesses of travel. Tree of heaven contains a group of compounds called quassinoids, which are also found in Quassia and in a lesser–known southwestern shrub, namely Castela emoryi[25].

Tree of heaven is best suited to quell diarrhea and dysentery caused from protozoal infections. Like most Quassia family plants, Tree of heaven is active against an array of gastrointestinal tract pathogens, particularly Entamoeba histolytica, the cause of traveler's diarrhea, and Giardia. Tree of heaven is doubly beneficial because the plant is also tonic and rebuilding to weakened or damaged intestinal wall mucosa (which can easily result from these types of intestinal infections). Use Tree of heaven when diarrhea has become chronic and has caused a general state of weakness.

The quassinoids found in Tree of heaven have modest anti–malarial activity. This means bark preparations may prove useful in drug–resistant/ tenacious strains when used in combination with conventional medications for malaria.

In times of emotional stress when the nervous system has become hypersensitive (small insults are interpreted as greater dangers), Tree of

25   For most purposes Tree of heaven can be substituted for Castela. Medicinal uses for each significantly overlap. It only makes sense to collect Tree of Heaven in lieu of Castela. The former is a successful weed–tree and is extremely prolific and fast growing. Inversely, Castela is a very slow growing, long–lived, relic of older times. Considered a waning genus with a very low seed germination rate, it is estimated that only 'thousands' and not 'tens of thousands' of these bushes exist in the U.S. This makes Castela vulnerable to over harvesting by unknowing collectors.

heaven can prove soothing. The plant quiets extraneous muscular contractions and is useful in reducing mild seizure activity, tremors and shakiness, particularly from shock and trauma.

Indications

» Diarrhea and dysentery with accompanying blood and intestinal wall injury
» Amebic, protozoal infections
» Nervous system excitability/Tremors/Mild seizure activity

Collection/Preparations

Gather the trunk and branch bark in the spring, but it can be collected year round if necessary. Tree of heaven lends itself well to most preparations. A cold infusion extracts both quassinoids and tannins. If the tea is found nauseating, use alcoholic preparations as they are more easily tolerated by the stomach.

Dosage

» Cold infusion/Decoction: 2–4 ounces 2–3 times daily
» FPT/DPT (50% alcohol): 20–30 drops 2–3 times daily
» Fluidextract: 10–20 drops 2–3 times daily

Cautions

Too much Tree of heaven, particularly the tea, can cause nausea, weakness, and a cold–sweaty parasympathetic–like state. Do not use during pregnancy.

Trixis

Asteraceae/Sunflower Family

Trixis californica Kellogg
Cachano

Description

Trixis is a small, roundish, and mound–like shrub with fragile, grayish–white, and many–branched stems. With adequate rainfall, Trixis's foliage is dense and uniform. In drought conditions it tends to form unevenly on branch tips. The bright green leaves are lanceolate and typically are 1"–2" long. The margins are toothed or entire and occasionally curl slightly under the leaf body. The leaves are deciduous in response to lack of rain and cold temperatures. Trixis can flower throughout the year in response to adequate rain, but normally it is a spring to summer bloomer. The yellow flowers appear in dense and flat clusters. After flowering, the dried involucral tubes remain and are notable.

Distribution
From 2,000'–4,000', Trixis is found from scattered locations around the Grand Canyon and west to southern California. Throughout much of southern Arizona the plant extends east to New Mexico, particularly along the Rio Grande Drainage, and finally to southwestern Texas. Normally Trixis is found under shrubs and trees (such as Palo verde and Mesquite), in rocky crevasses, or in canyons that provide some protection from constant sun exposure.

Chemistry
Trixis general: flavonoids, sesquiterpene lactones, and trixanolides.

Medicinal Uses
Like many of the plants presented in this book, Trixis is not widely used north of the border. It is put forth here as a medicine deserving more experimentation. The plant is traditionally used externally on wounds, ulcers, and inflammations to expedite healing.

Indications
»   Wounds/Ulcers (external)

Collection
Clip the hydrated herbage with or without the flowers. Dry the herbage normally.

Preparations/Dosage
»   External preparations: topically as needed

Cautions
There are no known cautions with normal usage.

Trumpet Flower
Bignoniaceae/Bignonia Family

Tecoma stans (L.) Juss. ex Kunth
Tronadora, Palo amarillo, Retana

Description
As a tropical holdout in the Southwest, Trumpet flower stands out from late spring through summer with its verdant foliage and large and tubular–yellow flowers. It is a deciduous shrub usually reaching 4′–6′ in height. Its leaves are oppositely arranged along the branches. Leaflets are pinnately formed with 1 terminal leaflet ending the group. Like Desert willow, the seedpod is elongated. The seeds are surrounded by a winged membrane making wind disbursement likely.

Distribution
It is found from the Sonoran and Chihuahuan Desert regions of southern Arizona, New Mexico, and Texas to Florida, Mexico, and South America. The northern most reaches of Trumpet flower are determined by low temperatures. Look for the plant on foothills, rocky slopes, and among boulders where some cold protection can be gained against low nighttime temperatures.

Chemistry
Monoterpenes, triterpenes, benzenoids, phenylpropanoids, and flavonoids.

Medicinal Uses
The tea or tincture of Trumpet flower is taken internally before meals to stimulate appetite and digestive secretion. It is specific in treating atonic stomach conditions. Use the plant if after eating or drinking there is fullness, distention, and gastric burning. It also has a reputation for treating gastritis caused from long–term alcohol abuse.

Trumpet flower modestly reduces blood sugar levels. It is most useful for individuals with NIDDM (non–insulin dependent diabetes mellitus) who are *almost* able to control blood sugar elevations with exercise and diet therapies. Taken with meals Trumpet flower will give an extra push to blood sugar normalcy. Research suggests the plant is best for postprandial hyperglycemia as it is an intestinal glucose absorption inhibitor.

Like most other Bignonia family plants, Trumpet flower is inhibiting to Candida albicans. If a round of steroids or antibiotics has led to a Candida flare–up, Trumpet flower is of value both topically and internally. For vaginal Candida infections, soaking in a sitz bath made with the tea along with internal usage is an efficacious plan. Campsis radicans or Trumpet creeper, a plant native to the southeastern part of the country, is cultivated in warmer parts of the West and can be used similarly.

Indications
»   Indigestion
»   Gastritis from alcohol abuse
»   Diabetes mellitus, non–insulin dependent
»   Infection, Candida, localized and systemic (internal and external)

Collection
During the spring and summer, collect the branch ends with the leaves and/or flowers.

Preparations/Dosage
»   Herb infusion: 4–8 ounces 2–3 times daily
»   Sitz bath: 2–3 times daily

Cautions
Do not use in IDDM (insulin dependent diabetes mellitus).

Turpentine Bush
Asteraceae/Sunflower Family

Ericameria laricifolia (A. Gray) Shinners (*Bigelowia nelsonii, Ericameria nelsonii, Haplopappus laricifolius*)
Cancerweed, Yerba del pasmo

Description
Turpentine bush is a small rounded shrub typically reaching 2'–3' in height and width. In full sun locations, the plant is distinctly mound–like. However, among other shrubbery or trees it reaches upwards becoming less

uniform. Its small linear leaves are compact and form at the upper terminal branch ends often appressed and cloaking the stems. In the fall, yellow flower clusters appear at branch ends and with the leaves give the plant a leveled, flattop appearance. The leaves are very resinous and are sticky when crushed. They emit an oily and turpentine–like scent.

In stature and overall appearance, Burroweed (Isocoma tenuisectus) closely resembles Turpentine bush. The most prominent differences between the two plants are: Burroweed is slightly smaller and its leaves are pinnatifid. Turpentine bush's leaves are entire.

Distribution
From 3,000'–6,000', Turpentine bush can be found on rocky slopes and hillsides, usually among Scrub oak, Mesquite, and Palo verde. From eastern stretches of the Mojave Desert in California, Turpentine bush stretches across to south–central New Mexico.

Chemistry
Flavonoids: apigenin, jaranol, isokaempferide, kaempferol, luteolin, nepetin, quercetin, isorhamnetin, and rhamnocitrin; diterpene: grindelic acid.

Medicinal Uses
Topically use Turpentine bush to resolve slow to heal ulcers, wounds, bedsores, and other similar conditions. Turpentine bush is also broadly antimicrobial. A topical powder, salve, or poultice is useful in clearing infected cuts and other superficial skin injuries. A warm poultice or the salve facilitates the process of boils, abscesses, and pimples in coming to a head. Consider the essential oil of Turpentine bush to be a much stronger representation of the plant, at least regarding its antibacterial uses. I've seen very good results from applying the diluted essential oil to cuts, scrapes, and the like. I also believe its potential as a more potent internal medicine (versus the whole plant) is likely.

Turpentine bush has a sedating effect on smooth musculature and to some degree on the central nervous system. Traditionally, the plant has been used in treating convulsions and spasms, particularly if initiated from moving from a hot environment to a cooler one in a short time period. A warm poultice can be applied to local pain and spasm, such as over the abdomen for menstrual, intestinal, or stomach cramps. Internally the plant is decidedly stimulating to menses.

Indications
» Wounds, to speed healing (external)
» Spasm and central nervous system excitability (internal and external)
» Amenorrhea with uterine cramps (internal and external)

Collection
Before flowering when new stem and leaf growth is apparent, snip the upper 6″–8″ of growth. The herb can be dried normally or bundled much like
Snakeweed. When collecting have rubber bands or twine on hand for bun-
dling the upper herbage.

Preparations/Dosage
» Leaf infusion: 4–6 ounces 2–3 times daily
» DPT (50% alcohol): 30–60 drops 2–3 times daily
» Oil/Salve/Poultice/Powder: as needed
» Essential oil: 2–3 drops 1–2 times daily

Cautions
Do not use Turpentine bush during pregnancy or while nursing.

Velvet Ash
Oleaceae/Olive Family

Fraxinus velutina Torr. *(F. pennsylvanica subsp. velutina)*
Fresno

Description
Velvet ash is a tree of substantial size particularly when growing in moistened soils. Older trees can reach 30′–40′ in height, but usually they are less.
The tree's crown is dense, rounded, and somewhat symmetrical. The bark
is gray, fissured, and relatively soft. The deciduous leaves are 4″–6″ long
and are composed of 3–9 leaflets. Their characteristics can be highly variable: toothed to entire, hairy to glabrous, and leathery to thin. Male and
female flowers are borne on separate trees. Male flowers form in dense
clusters on branch ends and appear like strange gall formations. After being pollinated the female flowers form into 'keys' or seeds surrounded by a
single wing.

Distribution
Velvet ash can be found from western Texas, New Mexico along the Rio Grande and Gila River Drainages, throughout southeast and central Arizona to southwestern Utah, southern Nevada, and finally to southeastern California. Between 1,000'–6,000', the tree is encountered along streamsides, canyon bottoms, wash sides, and gullies.

Chemistry
Coumarins, secoiridoid glucosides, phenylethanoid glycosides, lignans, flavonoids, and tannins.

Medicinal Uses
With little modern update, the therapeutic use of Velvet ash comes to us largely from a time of the past. The bark tea is considered a digestive tonic. Use it before meals to stimulate digestive secretion and appetite. The plant is also used in corresponding liver sluggishness and biliary congestion. Larger doses are laxative.

Topical preparations of the bark are used for many types of slowly healing cutaneous conditions. Velvet ash's flavonoid content is mostly responsible for its therapeutic action on the skin and related tissues.

Indications
» Indigestion with liver/gall bladder sluggishness and mild constipation
» Skin conditions, poorly healing (external)

Collection
Gather the unfissured bark from the younger branches. Lay out in strips to dry.

Preparations/Dosage
» Bark decoction: 4–6 ounces 2–3 times daily
» Poultice/Oil/Salve: externally as needed

Cautions
Do not take large amounts during pregnancy due to the plant's laxative properties, which are remotely capable of sympathetically stimulating contractions. Moreover do not use it if there is a hepatic/biliary blockage.

Verbena
Verbenaceae/Vervain Family

Verbena bracteata Lag. & Rodr.
Prostrate verbena, Bigbract verbena

Verbena macdougalii A. Heller
New Mexican verbena, MacDougal verbena

Glandularia gooddingii (Briq.) Solbrig *(Verbena arizonica, V. gooddingii, V. verna)*
Desert verbena, Mock vervain, Southwestern mock vervain

Description

Verbena bracteata is a small, low–growing, and spreading annual or short–lived perennial. The leaves of this plant are deeply lobed and form oppositely along ridged stems. The entire plant is hairy. The flower spikes are long and composed mostly of leaf–like bracts. The flowers are small and pinkish–purple.

Verbena macdougalii is a 2–4 foot tall perennial. It is a stately plant compared to others of the genus. Oblong–ovate shaped leaves are serrated, hairy, and arranged oppositely on the plant's ridged stems. The small and purplish flowers are arranged in upright spikes on upper stem ends.

Glandularia gooddingii, a Verbena by relation and use, is a low–growing, clump–forming, and short–lived perennial. The leaves are arranged oppositely along conspicuously angled stems. They are triangular and deeply lobed or serrated. The stems and leaves are hairy. The light–purple flower clusters form at branch ends. Each flower, as with other Verbenas, is 5–lobed, 2–lipped, tubular, and held within a tubular 5–toothed calyx.

Distribution

At varying elevations, Verbena bracteata is widely distributed nearly throughout the entire country. Look to disturbed and moist soils, around cattle tanks, sumps, and bottomlands. V. macdougalii is found from Wyoming to western Texas, Arizona, and New Mexico. Throughout the arid Southwest, the plant is found at higher elevations (5,000'–8,500'). In more northerly locals look to lower elevation areas. Ponderosa pine forests and grassy meadows are common spots.

Glandularia gooddingii is found from nearly sea level to 6,000'. It is common in disturbed land, along drainages, mesas and on rocky slopes. The plant ranges from California, to Nevada and Utah, south and east to Arizona, New Mexico, and southern Texas.

Chemistry
Anthocyanines; flavonoids: naringenin and eriodictyol; triterpenoids.

Medicinal Uses
Verbena is a sedative of mild strength. Its calming effect is useful in reducing nervousness, anxiety, and tension. Moreover, Verbena can be effective in relieving stress headaches with associated neck and upper back tension. It is a good herb for individuals whose digestion is impaired due to work or other related stresses. Through the plant's countering of adrenaline–type stress, digestion and assimilation are enhanced, as are other overshadowed parasympathetic functions.

Verbena is a reliable diaphoretic. If feverish and dry–skinned, Verbena stimulates diaphoresis. In addition, like most other diaphoretic herbs, if there is no fever then the plant is diuretic. It also is stimulating to lactation as are other Vervain family plants, particularly its relative Chaste tree. Verbena may have some modulating effect on the neurotransmitter dopamine and the hormone prolactin. This combined with the plant's sedative qualities will be of help to stressed mothers who cannot produce enough milk for their child.

Some Verbenas have small but inconsistent amounts of cardiac glycosides. Occasionally in sensitive individuals, this can cause the heartbeat to slow and strengthen. The effect is rare but has been observed.

Indications
- » Anxiety/Tension
- » Headache, stress related
- » Indigestion with poor circulation
- » Fevers, dry
- » Lactation, insufficient

Collection
Gather the upper herbaceous portions of Verbena. Snip the individual

stems down to where several sets of leaves remain. Lay out to dry or tincture the herbage fresh.

Preparations/Dosage
»   FPT/DPT (60% alcohol): 30–60 drops 2–3 times daily
»   Herb infusion: 4–6 ounces 2–3 time daily

Cautions
Sensitive individuals may develop contact dermatitis from collecting the plant. Do not use excessive amounts during pregnancy due to Verbena's potential effect on prolactin levels.

Western Black Willow
Salicaceae/Willow Family

Salix gooddingii C.R. Ball *(Salix nigra var. vallicola, S. vallicola)*
Dudley willow, Goodding's willow

Description
Western black willow is very closely related to Black willow of the eastern United States, and can be considered practically identical in terms of botanical morphology. Usually Western black willow starts as a multi–trunked bush. Only later in its growth does it become a tree, and this is largely dependent on available water. The drooping branches give the tree a wide and open crown. Generally the trunks are bowed and leaning, are 2'–3' in diameter at maturity, and are covered by blackish–brown and furrowed bark. The toothed leaves are lanceolate, shiny, and yellowish to light green. Like Cottonwood, Western black willow's male and female flowers develop on separate trees. They form in tubular catkins. The mature fruit have attached cottony fibers, making them easily carried by the wind.

Distribution
From Shasta County, California, the Four Corners area, and the Texas Panhandle, Western black willow ranges southward along most waterways. Look for this tree from 6,000' and lower along streams, washes, springs, and larger bodies of water. Occasionally dense thickets are encountered on flood plains where water is not too far from the surface.

Chemistry
Phenolic glycosides: salicin, fragilin, and salicortin.

Medicinal Uses
Western black willow offers us its main medicinal attribute, that of a chronic/acute pain application, by way of its phenolic glycoside content. Use the bark tea internally for a variety of disturbances: headache, arthritic, and injury pain to name a few. It addresses both the pain of chronic inflammation and acute/recent issues. Western black willow (and relatives) has such a wide ranging application, it should be tried for a majority of conditions that 'hurt'.

Besides being a pain–remedying medicinal plant, Western black willow is a remedy for the urinary tract[26]. Internally the fresh plant tincture made with the buds is quieting to irritative conditions of the genitourinary tract. Like Cottonwood, Western black willow buds soothe urethral and bladder irritation as well as mild prostatitis dependent upon chronic laxity of involved tissues. It particularly excels at diminishing irritation that triggers spermatorrhea, and in both men and women, heightened sexual preoccupation from urogenital irritation/sensitivity. It was once even thought of as an anaphrodisiac for men. For this purpose, it combines well with Chaste tree.

Indications
- » Pain/Inflammation, chronic and acute
- » Irritation, chronic, urinary tract
- » Prostatitis
- » Spermatorrhea
- » Sexual preoccupation from genital irritation

Collection
Gather the young buds in the early spring by stripping them from the branch ends.

Preparations/Dosage
- » FPT: 30–60 drops 3–4 times daily

---

26   I apply here to Western black willow what the Eclectic physicians used Black willow (Salix nigra) for over one hundred years ago.

Cautions

Due to a possible synergistic effect with the tree's glycosides, use caution when mixing Western black willow with blood thinning pharmaceuticals. The chances of Western black willow triggering Reye's syndrome in fever-ish children is remote, but it is best to err on the side of caution and not use it internally in these situations.

Western Mugwort

Asteraceae/Sunflower Family

Artemisia ludoviciana Nutt. *(Artemisia mexicana, Artemisia vulgaris var. mexicana)*
Prairie sagewort, White sagewort, Estafiate

Artemisia douglasiana Besser *(Artemisia ludoviciana var. douglasiana, Artemisia vulgaris var. douglasiana)*
California mugwort, Douglas mugwort, Ajenjo

Artemisia filifolia Torr. *(Artemisia plattensis)*
Sand sagebrush, Sandhill sage, Romerillo

Description

Artemisia ludoviciana's leaves can be entire, occasionally lobed, or even serrated. Always variable in shape, the alternate leaves can be bluish green to silver–gray. The plant is highly successful at reproduction, using both seed and rhizome/stem clones to propagate. Individually, A. ludoviciana's flowers are inconspicuous, but in number, they form noticeable terminal spikes inter–mixed with small leaves. When flowering the plant is upright reaching for the sun, though it is not uncommon for flowering branches to droop in response to stem weakness or weighty flower spikes. Like other Artemisias, this species is fragrant. When the leaves are crushed, they emit a characteristic Sage–like aroma.

Like Artemisia ludoviciana, A. douglasiana roots from stem nodes so it too is found in bunched colonies. This perennial is usually several feet in height, but if conditions are optimal, it can occasion 6'–7'. The leaves are variable but tend to be entire towards the top of the plant. Lower along the stem they are toothed, cleft, or lobed. Above, the leaves are dark green, below, they are silvery due to a dense coating of leaf hair. The small, whitish–cream flowers are clustered in small spikelets, originating from the leaf axils on the upper stem ends.

Artemisia filifolia is a perennial sub–shrub, 3' tall by the same wide. The aromatic leaves are pubescent and are light gray to bluish–green. On upper stems, the leaves are entire and thread–like. Lower leaves are also very thin and narrow, but are usually longer and cleft. They alternate along brownish–grey stems. The small inconspicuous flowers form in clusters on the upper stems. Like most Artemisias of the West, A. filifolia is a late summer to fall bloomer.

Distribution

From Wisconsin and Illinois Artemisia ludoviciana ranges south and west to the east side of the Cascade Range. Truly a ubiquitous western plant, A. ludoviciana is found in many microclimates and bioregions. This highly adaptable plant is encountered anywhere between the Mixed Conifer–Pine Belts to lower desert washes and foothills.

A. douglasiana is found through most of California, Oregon, and eastern Washington. It ranges east to the Rocky Mountains. Look to rocky hillsides, mountain drainages, and streamsides. Artemisia filifolia has a wide distribution throughout the interior West. From Nebraska and Wyoming, the plant is abundant on well–drained sandy soils and rangelands. From these areas, the plant is found south to Colorado, Nevada, western Texas, New Mexico, and Arizona.

Chemistry

For Artemisia ludoviciana: sesquiterpenes: arteannuin b, artemisinin, achillin, anthemidin, artedouglasia oxide, douglanine, ludovicin, tanaparthin–α–peroxide, and tanapartholide b; monoterpenes: borneol, camphor, chrysanthemol, transchrysanthenol, and α–pinene; flavonoids: butein, isoliquiritigenin, isorhamnetin, and quercetin; coumarins: lacarol and scopoletin.

Medicinal Uses

Artemisias of the West are some of the most multi–faceted herbal medicines we employ. Although results can vary somewhat depending on species and climate, these plants share a core group of similarities. Additionally, the plants described here differ from Sagebrush (Artemisia tridentata) mainly in their lack of thujone and related aromatic–dependent harshness.

Firstly, Western mugwort is a medicine for the gastrointestinal tract. All three Artemisias tend to be mild to moderate gastric stimulants with Artemisia ludoviciana being the most energetic. Each plant's gastric stimulation is largely determined by its bitterness. The more bitter, the more stimulation it will provide. Underlying Western mugwort's bitter tonic activity is its seemingly paradoxical cytoprotective effect on gastric and intestinal tissue. Western mugwort, particularly Artemisia filifolia and A. douglasiana, have the ability of stabilizing cellular membranes. These plants also provide cyclooxygenase inhibition, increased glycoprotein (mucus) synthesis, granulocyte degranulation inhibition, as well as transcription factor NF–KB inhibition. These activities protect and heal gastrointestinal tract mucosa from inflammatory responses and conditions. Relatedly most Artemisias have some anti–Helicobacter pylori activity, making them all useful if plagued by stomach–duodenal ulcers. Use Western mugwort as a daily tea for peptic ulcers, gastritis, ulcerative colitis, or other inflammatory conditions affecting the area.

Additionally, Western mugwort is choleretic, increasing bile synthesis and release. If prone to gall stone formation, Western mugwort will thin bile enough to diminish precipitants. Deeper, these plants have a cooling and antioxidant effect on hepatocyte function. These influences tend to reduce elevated liver enzyme levels – all stress markers evident in viral and general hepatitis. In addition, the plant inhibits glutathione depletion within hepatocytes. Western mugwort's hepatoprotective effect can also be of benefit to individuals whom consume excess alcohol, rancid oils, and processed foods with their array of artificial ingredients. Use Western mugwort to buffer these nefarious effects on the liver, although making better dietary choices is paramount in liver health. Several ounces of the cool tea taken before bed is one of the best approaches, if prone to upon waking the next morning, frontal headaches, red–irritated eyes, bad breath, and general liver congestion.

Topically, Western mugwort is mildly antibacterial and antifungal. It is effective against a wide array of microorganisms. It does not provide a strong effect, but it is broad. Artemisia ludoviciana is distinctly inhibiting to HSV (herpes simplex virus), type I and II. For cold sore treatment, the oil or salve in combination with Creosote bush is effective. With clients, I have observed genital herpes outbreaks diminish under internal use of the plant. Added benefit is achieved by topical application. Like its larger cousin, Sagebrush, Western mugwort is effective against a number of intestinal parasites. Drink several cups of tea daily for treatment of traveler's diarrhea (Entamoeba histolytica), giardiasis (Giardia lamblia), pinworm infection, and other infestations affecting intestinal function. Do not underestimate Western mugwort, particularly A. ludoviciana in these situations. The plant contains a number of compounds that are broadly anthelmintic.

The hot tea is a stimulating diaphoretic. Ingested cool with no elevated temperature, Western mugwort is diuretic. The plant tends also to stimulate menses, so is useful in delayed menstruation where the pelvic area feels cold and achy.

Indications
»   Dyspepsia/Gastritis
»   Ulcer, gastric/duodenal
»   Inflammation, intestinal
»   Inflammation, liver, with no hepatic/biliary blockage
»   Infection, bacterial/fungal (external)
»   HSV, type I and II (internal and external)
»   Diarrhea, ameba/giardia
»   Parasites, intestinal
»   Fever, low–moderate temperature
»   Amenorrhea, with pelvic rigidity

Collection
Depending on variety, Western mugwort's foliage is collectable from spring through fall. Gather it without the flowers as the pollen can occasionally trigger hayfever reactions in sensitive individuals. Dry well spaced.

Preparations/Dosage
»   Infusion (cold or standard): 4–6 ounces 2–3 times daily
»   FPT/DPT (50% alcohol): 20–40 drops 2–3 times daily
»   DPT (100% vinegar): 20–40 drops 2–3 times daily
»   Oil/Salve/Wash: as needed

Cautions
Do not use during pregnancy due to Western mugwort's dilating effect on uterine vasculature. Due to the plant's cholagogue properties do not use if there is a biliary blockage.

Other Uses

Artemisia annua, principally used in TCM (Traditional Chinese Medicine) also contains artemisinin, a compound used in conventional medicine as an antimalarial drug. Even whole herb preparations of A. annua have traditional use in intermittent fevers – one hallmark of malaria (Plasmodium falciparum) infection. Even though A. ludoviciana does not contain artemisinin, the plant has related compounds that have potential in resolving Plasmodium infections as well.

Western Peony
Paeoniaceae/Peony Family

Paeonia brownii Douglas ex Hook.
Brown's peony

Paeonia californica Nutt. *(Paeonia brownii subsp. californica)*
California peony

Description

Western peony is a 1'–1½' tall by 2'–3' wide herbaceous perennial. Its leaves, which are vibrantly green and sub–fleshy, are numerous and form from the plant's base. Occasionally they are scarlet tipped when first emerging. Later in the season leaf wilt occurs from lack of rain or intense sun exposure. The solitary large flowers are dark red and occasionally shade to black. The nodding flowers are composed of 5–6 petals, although sometimes they are more numerous. Since the petals still cup the reproductive center when mature, they can be mistaken for not appearing fully developed. As the seed capsules mature the stems droop, and even may touch the ground. The numerous slender tubers on mature plants are vertically oriented. Some botanists place the plant in the Buttercup family.

Distribution

Paeonia californica is found only throughout southern and coastal California. P. brownii has a much larger range: northern California, western Oregon, western Washington, and into Nevada, Utah, Idaho, and Wyoming where extensive stands exists. Sagebrush is a common companion plant throughout its range in the Great Basin Desert.

Chemistry

The specific constituents for Western peony are not known, but they are likely similar to other Paeonias: volatiles, flavonoids, tannins, stilbenoids, triterpenoids, steriodal compounds, and paeonols.

Medicinal Uses

I find Western peony to be a fascinating root medicine. Uniquely aromatic and pigmented, pleasantly peculiar in taste, and easy to dig, it leaves little to be desired as a largely unknown yet potent medicinal plant. I also believe our western species are as effective, if not more so, particularly if recently collected and utilized, than European and Asian species.

Western peony's two primary areas of influence are the uterine and bronchial areas. To these regions the plant is decidedly antispasmodic, lessening to tissue irritation, and generality sedating.

As a medicine that is distinctly sedative to uterine cramps, it should be used as needed on the first or second day of menses. It will reliably ease spasmodic pain, although some women find it more effective started a week or so before the onset of menses. Some women also experience the plant as a mild menstrual stimulant, so it is useful if there is cramping and menses is slow to start, or stop and start. If adrenaline–stress (worry, anxiety, and nervousness) is present then Western peony is doubly indicated – it is a gentle sedative of use in nervous excitability and tension. Unrelated to reproductive issues, many people additionally find Western peony sedating to muscular twitching, mild tremor, and tic activity, especially if these nervous systems manifestations are brought on by stress, worry, etc.

Lastly, regarding reproductive tissue, even if there is no overt spasmodic pain, try it if the area feels irritated, congested, and overly sensitive. It is likely that men too will perceive some relief with the plant if troubled by urogenital and/or prostrate irritation and sensitivity.

Western peony is of value in relieving a spasmodic cough. Its effect on bronchial irritation is of note. It combines well (as a tincture or a cough syrup ingredient) with Ligusticum, Lomatium, and other more powerful expectorants.

Indications

»   Cramps, uterine
»   Dysmenorrhea, with spasm
»   Muscular twitching/Tics/Tremors, from stress

»   Cough, spasmodic

Collection

Select robust plants with corresponding large root masses. Start digging to one side of the plant and work inward towards the roots. Take only peripheral tubers while leaving the inner ones. This will ensure the plant's survival in years to come. After splitting open a tuber, the coloration is normally pale pink–purple; the darker the coloration the stronger the root medicine. The best time to gather is when the new foliage first appears or after flowering.

Preparations

If using Western peony for tea split the tuber length–wise to ensure proper drying. As the root dries, it will darken considerably.

Dosage

»   FPT/DPT (60%): 30–60 drops 1–3 times daily
»   Infusion (cold or standard): 4–6 ounces 1–3 times daily

Cautions

Western peony may interfere with consistent blood coagulation if mixed with blood–thinning pharmaceuticals. Also, do not take it during pregnancy due to the plant's stimulating effect on menses.

Wild Lettuce

Asteraceae/Sunflower Family

Lactuca serriola L. *(Lactuca scariola. L. virosa)*
Prickly lettuce

Description

This annual, or sometimes biannual, grows to be 2′–6′ high. Its leaves are alternately spaced, point upward, and clasp the stem. They are deeply lobed and toothed but occasionally are entire and lanceolate. On the underside of each leaf are spines aligned on the midrib. Flower heads are small, yellow, and Dandelion–like. They are borne on branching flower stalks and close by mid–morning. The seeds, like those of many other composites, are

small and have an attached swirl of whitish fibers making wind dispersal
an effective mode of dispersal. When cut or injured the entire plant exudes
a white milky sap.

Distribution

Introduced from Europe, the plant now exists throughout most of the United States. Like other introduced species, Wild lettuce is found along roadsides, buildings, walkways, and other areas where it is allowed through
neglect and soil–disruption to flourish. Throughout drier areas in the West,
the plant prefers moister soils and semi–shade.

Chemistry

Lactucin, lactucopicrin, lactucic acid, and lactucerin.

Medicinal Uses

Wild lettuce is a sedative best used for mild insomnia and restlessness. Use
it when these problems derive from mental and emotional agitation. It will
be found less effective if insomnia is from physical pain. It curbs agitation
particularly if there is a sensation, either imagined or real, of physical heat,
such as elevated core temperature from fever, dehydration, or exertion. As
a sedative Wild lettuce has some similarities to California poppy. Although
the plant is not in the Poppy family, by effect, it can be considered a 'sub–
opiate', hence the antiquated name, Opium lettuce. Moreover, Wild lettuce
is used in allying a spasmodic cough dependent on bronchial irritation.

Indications

» Insomnia and restlessness from overwork and stress
» Cough, spasmodic, from bronchial irritation

Collection

Lactucarium is the name applied to the concentrated milky juice of several Lactuca species. It can be collected through a number of time consuming methods. The first approach: clip the tops from a good–sized stand of
Wild lettuce. Wait until the milky juice hardens slightly, and then scrape
the milky beads off with a knife or razor blade. Re–snip each plant ¼"–½"
below the original cut and continue on... and on...

The second method is similar to the first. Strip the leaves from the
plant, then with a razor blade make vertical cuts along the plant's stalk.

The exudate can be collected after it hardens or can be sponged up and squeezed out using a small amount of water. Finally, the last method is to collect the whole plant, before flowering, and juice it. Although the resulting juice is not technically lactucarium, the effect of the preparation is practically identical. Whatever method is utilized, dehydrate the milky liquid or juice. This hardened material, typically reddish–brown in color, is lactucarium or close to it.

Preparations
Although the whole plant tincture and leaf infusion are feeble in effect compared to lactucarium, they still have value. When making the tincture of lactucarium the hardened milky material should dissolve completely.

Dosage
» DPT of lactucarium (80% alcohol): 30–60 drops 2–3 times daily
» FPT/DPT (60% alcohol): 60–90 drops 2–3 times daily
» Leaf infusion: 4–8 ounces 2–3 times daily

Cautions
There are no known cautions for Wild lettuce with normal usage.

Wild Licorice
Fabaceae/Pea Family

Glycyrrhiza lepidota Nutt. ex Pursh *(Glycyrrhiza glutinosa)*
American licorice

Description
Wild licorice is a colony–forming perennial bush, spreading either from underground rhizomes or through typical seed reproduction. This deciduous plant stands 1'–3' tall and has erect stems rising from the ground. The leaves are comprised of 11–19 oblong and narrow leaflets. The arrangement is called odd–pinnate because one leaflet always terminates the group. The leaflets are gland dotted at maturity and are slightly sticky when rubbed. The flower spikes originate from the upper part of the plant and arise between leaf and stem joints. The spikes are an arrangement of compact yellowish–white to greenish–white small pea flowers. The burred seedpods

are ½"–¾" long and resemble Cocklebur pods. The beans within are small and reddish–brown.

Distribution

Wild licorice covers a wide range of territory throughout the country. Although the plant is absent from low–elevation arid areas of the Southwest, such as the Sonoran Desert, it can be found throughout most of the West. Look to moist and sandy soils along streams, fields, and roadsides.

Chemistry

Glabidin, glabranin, glepidotin, pinocembrin, and glycyrrhizin.

Medicinal Uses

Use Wild licorice for inflammatory conditions of the stomach dependent upon insufficient gastric secretions, namely mucin and hydrochloric acid. Additionally, the plant is inhibiting to Helicobacter pylori, a bacterium often associated with gastric ulcers[27]. Wild licorice also supports gastric secretion and related membranes by it use as a simple bitter. Many find it allays indigestion, increases appetite, and even reduces feeling of heartburn – a useful combination of effects for a troubled stomach.

Use Wild licorice when there is mild constipation and uncomfortable intestinal movement. The plant shifts fluids to the intestines and hydrates the contents somewhat, normalizing bowel movements. Moreover, the bronchial environment tends to be moistened by the plant. Use it when there is a dry cough and the lungs feel irritated and sore. Wild licorice will be of greatest benefit to individuals whom exhibit the above tendencies and who are under low–grade adrenaline fight or flight stress.

Recent research suggests that Wild licorice as well as European and Chinese species, due to their glabidin contents, are useful in diminishing inflammation, oxidative stress, and the tissue damage of glomerulonephritis. All Licorice's tends to stabilize nephrons and reduce albumin in the

---

27   Gastric ulcers are not solely caused by H. pylori. This is why after a round of conventional antibiotics, designed to eliminate the bacterium, H. pylori does diminish and the corresponding ulcer resolves, but all too often, both reoccur. Typically, there is an underlying stress pattern predisposing the gastric lining to H. pylori colonization. It is only when the surrounding tissues become vulnerable to H. pylori does the bacterium wreak havoc. In fact, H. pylori can be present in the gastric environment and not cause a problem.

urine.

Wild licorice contains insignificant amounts of glycyrrhizin (one of the main bioactive constituents of European and Chinese licorice). It has virtually no effect on mineralocorticoids and the like, making it safe to use in hypertension. The plant can sometimes stimulate menses through its isoflavone content. Its effect in this department is unpredictable so care should be taken if cycles are irregular.

Indications

- » Ulcer, gastric, H. pylori involvement
- » Gastritis/Heartburn
- » Indigestion
- » Constipation
- » Cough, dry
- » Inflammation, chronic, kidney

Collection

Gather Wild licorice's sub–surface rhizomes and taproots. Some stands can develop impressive root networks. In moist and sandy soils, the runners can sometimes be pulled up by hand. Chop the roots into small pieces and dry them normally.

Preparations/Dosage

- » DPT (50% alcohol): 40–60 drops 2–3 times daily
- » Fluidextract: 10–20 drops 2–3 times daily
- » Root decoction: 4–6 ounces 2–3 times daily

Cautions

Due to the plant's unpredictable effect on circulating estrogen levels, do not use it during pregnancy.

Wild Oats

Poaceae/Grass Family

Avena fatua L.
Oatstraw, Oatgrass

Description

Wild oats is a robust annual. It is 2'–4' tall with jointed and hollow stems and corkscrewing leaf blades. Inflorescences form in wide panicles. Individual spikelets droop tassel–like. With rearward stretched awns appearing as spindly legs, they resemble green cockroaches. The small oat seeds mature from late spring to early summer and can remain viable in the ground for nearly 10 years. Cultivated oats (Avena sativa) is another commonly found oat. Often it is difficult to tell the two apart, but upon close study, unlike Wild oats, the bracts of this variety are not hairy.

Distribution

With exceptions pertaining to the Southeast, Wild oats, a European native, is ubiquitous throughout North America. Look for the plant in disturbed and rich soils and around drainage ditches and culverts. Occasionally it can be found along streams and canyon sides.

Chemistry

Vitexin, apigenin, d5–avenasterol, avenacosides a and b, and nuatigenin.

Medicinal Uses

Wild oats primarily exerts its effect on distresses arising from nervous system debility. Think of Wild oats as a nervous system stabilizer. It counteracts agitation from over work and prolonged periods of stress. There is some difficultly in describing what Wild oats actually does. It is not an overt sedative, nor is it particularly stimulating, but this detracts little from the fact that if you are physically and emotionally 'rode hard and put away wet' the plant imparts a sense of stability.

Depressive states arising out of pushing through workloads on the job or at home are lifted. The edginess and frayed–end feeling of quitting nicotine, opiate, or alcohol habits is also lessened. As the late herbalist Michael Moore once stated: 'this is crispy critter medicine'.

Indications

» Depressive states
» Nervous system debility from overwork, stress, or substance withdrawal

Collection

Starting in the spring visit a stand several times a month. It is important not miss the oat in 'milk stage', as there is a window in which this plant is collectable for only about 1–2 weeks. The oat seed matures quickly. When the spikelets are green and just starting to yellow, pick several and squeeze them. While squeezing the spikelet, feel for the 'pop' between thumb and forefinger. This is followed by the milky–preformed seed coming out of the opposite end. At this point, they are prime for tincturing. Strip the spike-lets from the rising stalks. Leave enough seeds on the collective group, so next year they will be equally abundant.

Preparations/Dosage

»   FPT: 30–90 drops 3–4 times daily

Cautions

There are no known cautions for Wild oats.

Other Uses

The whole dried plant, also known as Oatstraw, prepared as a tea is a good source of readily absorbable electrolytes, particularly calcium.

Wild Rhubarb

Polygonaceae/Buckwheat Family

Rumex hymenosepalus Torr. *(Rumex arizonicus, R. salinus, R. saxei)*
Desert rhubarb, Tanner's dock, Cañaigre

Description

Late winter to early spring, Wild rhubarb is one of the first plants to send up small clusters of leaves from beneath the ground. The leaf tips, which are seen first, quickly progress into large, smooth, wavy–margined, and deeply green leaves. At maturity these lower basal leaves are generally 1'–2' long by 2"–4" wide. They progressively become smaller and less abun-dant along the rising flower stalks. The flower clusters are similar to other Docks and are borne on central fleshy stalks. After maturing, the seeds become reddish, waiting in large clusters to be released by the wind. The whole plant is rather succulent and is able to withstand drought through numerous underground tubers. This tactic provides the upper portion with necessary water and nutrients in times of scarcity.

Distribution

Wild rhubarb can be found from western Texas to stretches of the Mohave Desert in California, south from Wyoming, Utah, and Colorado, to Arizona and New Mexico. Look for the plant from 6,000' and lower in sandy and moist soils. Washes, fields, and roadsides are some of its favorite abodes.

Chemistry

Condensed and hydrolyzable tannins; chrysophanol, emodin, and physcion.

Medicinal Uses

Wild rhubarb is used topically for its astringency. External preparations are tightening to surface tissues and will lessen skin irritation and redness from burns, rashes, and scrapes. The plant, being moderately hemostatic is well applied to superficial cuts. Although symptomatic in effect, it can be almost miraculous in limiting the spread of stress or chemical sensitivity rashes. It likely exerts this effect through its inflammatory–prostaglandin mediating properties. In these cases, use the juice liberally as a paint. In addition, the juice as a mouthwash or gargle is soothing and astringing to mouth sores, bleeding gums, and sore throats.

Although Wild rhubarb and closely related Yellowdock (known as Yerba colorado south–of–the–border) do share a number of alterative–type compounds, Wild rhubarb's astringency tends to overshadow all other medicinal possibilities.

Indications

» Cuts/Abrasions/Burns (external)
» Rashes (external)
» Sore throats/Mouth sores (gargle)

Collection

Late winter or early spring when Wild rhubarb's leaves are just starting to show themselves, dig to a depth of about 1', 6"–10" beyond the outer leaves. Slowly work in to the central area underneath the plant. Depending on the softness of the soil, this can sometimes be done with hands alone. Along the way tubers of varying sizes will be found, some will be younger, pale, and flesh–colored, others will be darker, having a rust–brown coloration. Also, some will be dried out, remnant tubers of the year before (these should be discarded). If a healthy tuber[28] is left in the ground it will sprout and growth next year.

Preparations

The following instruction describes how best to make Wild rhubarb root juice, which in many ways is the superior preparation. This method is an adaptation of a technique used by Peter Bigfoot: wash and clean the roots well, as running small pebbles through a juicer is never a good idea. Dice the fresh tubers in ¼″ pieces. Slowly in small handfuls, juice the entire root (periodic cleaning of the metal juicer screen may be necessary as you progress – root fibers tend to collect there). Overall, this is a difficult root to juice and will challenge the best of juicers, but the result is worth the effort.

Pour the juice in a glass container; a mason jar works well. Place the covered Wild rhubarb juice in an area where it is easily observed but will not be disturbed. After several hours, the juice will begin to form two layers. There will be a top layer, deeply rust brown, most likely tannic acid in solution and a bottom layer – mostly remnant pulp and bound tannins. After the two layers have separated fully (24–48 hours), ladle off the top tannin layer and preserve it with 20% grain alcohol (4 parts juice to 1 part undiluted grain alcohol). Discard the remaining yellowish–orange pulp. Once preserved with alcohol, the tannin solution does not need to be refrigerated. The tubers can also be thinly sliced and dried for future use.

Dosage

»   Tannin juice/Root powder/Root decoction: externally as needed

Cautions

Externally there are no known cautions with normal usage.

Other Uses

Some ethnobotanical literature cites Wild rhubarb tubers being used for food. This is strange since they are so high in tannins. Realistically this may be possible only after several changes of water, which itself is a highly

28   It is too bad that more cannot be done with roots. They are some of the easiest to gather.

valued and often scarce substance in most arid places where Wild rhubarb grows. If eaten fresh Wild rhubarb's high concentration of root tannins are so deranging to sensitive mucosal layers, which the mouth and gut are primarily lined with, even if an individual was starving, it would hurt more than help.

The fleshy flower stalks and leaf petioles can be eaten more liberally raw and also are used as a substitute for 'true' Rhubarb in pie recipes. The young and tender leaves can be boiled through a couple of changes of water to remove the bitterness then eaten alone or with other greens.

Wolfberry
Solanaceae/Nightshade Family

Lycium pallidum Miers
Pale wolfberry, Thornbush, Desert thorn, Tomatillo

Description
Wolfberry is a large and dense shrub typically 3′–6′ high. Its branches are thorny, smooth and whitish, and are crowded with clusters of spatula–shaped small leaves, approximately an inch in length. They are pale green and fleshy. The greenish, tubular flowers are often tinged with purple and hang bell–like from leaf clusters. The smooth red fruit are the size of small grapes. They are juicy, contain a number of seeds, are slightly sweet to bitter, and have a subtle nightshade taste. Throughout the West, Lycium is a moderately sized genus. Most Lycium's are similarly formed with the main noticeable differences being berry and leaf size and general stature.

Distribution
From 3,000′–7,000′, Wolfberry can be found throughout the Sonoran, Mojave, and Chihuahuan Deserts. At higher elevations look for Wolfberry among Oak Woodlands and Chaparral Scrub areas. The plant tends to inhabit varying areas such as basins, hillsides, and arroyos. Wolfberry can be found from Texas to Colorado, west to Utah and California, and south to Arizona and New Mexico.

Chemistry
An array of Nightshade family alkaloids; specific constituents are not

known.

Medicinal Uses

The medicinal use of this genus in modern times has only come about in recent years. It is reasonable to speculate that most species can be used alike, however, approach each species with prudence.

In allergic situations use Wolfberry when there is excessive eye and nasal discharge. Combined with Mormon tea its effect on hayfever–type problems often displaces the need for over–the–counter allergy medicines. In addition, when lower respiratory tract tissues are congested and there are accompanying sensations of bronchial tightness Wolfberry can prove opening to the area. The plant's moderate anticholinergic effect shifts nervous system activity away from constricting respiratory tissues. This effect is most useful in mild–moderate humid asthma or other allergic–immune mediated bronchial responses. Wolfberry shrinks tissues and allays hyper–secretion.

Wolfberry's influence is also noticeable in gut– and –intestinal centered distresses. Nausea, intestinal spasm, and over–excitability of these areas respond well to Wolfberry. Moreover, the plant acts well to quell chills, sweating, and nausea (much like drinking the juice of one or two raw potatoes) from over–exposure to chemical herbicides, fertilizers, and other cholinergic toxins.

It is important to note that Wolfberry is a mild drug plant, meaning it suppresses symptoms and does not have much underlying value beyond temporally diminishing distresses. For longer–term use Wolfberry is better used in a formula. Combined with other more supportive herbs, it diminishes surfaces distresses while deeper issues, possibly exaggerated immune responses or stress patterns, can be equally addressed.

Topically the freshly poulticed plant or liniment can be applied to acute stings, swellings, contusions, and other injuries. In this respect, applied externally, Wolfberry acts like other Nightshade family plants. It moderately reduces pain and inflammation similarly to, although weaker than, Datura or Tobacco.

Indications

» Rhinitis
» Breathing, constricted from humid asthma and allergic reaction
» Nausea

» Spasm, intestinal, with or without accompanying diarrhea
» Pain and inflammation from acute injuries (external)

Collection
In the spring or summer when Wolfberry's foliage is hydrated and full, collect the leaves by either stripping them from the young branches or pick individual leaf groupings where they are clustered. Be attentive to the thorns as they can be an inconvenience.

Preparations/Dosage
» FPT/DPT (50% alcohol): 20–30 drops 1–3 times daily
» Leaf infusion: 2–4 ounces 1–3 times daily
» External preparations: as needed

Cautions
Too much Wolfberry is apt to cause dizziness, dry skin and respiratory/gastrointestinal tract membranes, and heat sensations. Do not use Wolfberry during pregnancy, while nursing, or if taking anticholinergic pharmaceuticals.

Other Uses
The fruit can be eaten raw in limited quantities. Beyond a handful or so, the medicinal effect of the plant may become evident. An interesting tasting fruit, they are a combination of bitter and sweet. Try them alone or stewed with other foods.

Yerba Mansa
Saururaceae/Lizard's–Tail Family

Anemopsis californica Hook. & Arn.
Lizard's tail, Swamp root, Yerba manso, Yerba del manso, Bavisa

Description
Yerba mansa[29] is a low–growing herbaceous perennial. Adept at cloning,

29   Popularly known as Yerba mansa, I have always heard the plant referred to locally (southern Arizona/northern Mexico) as Yerba manso/Yerba del manso by both native Hispanics and Indians (Yaqui). The name Yerba mansa, popularized by the

most newer plants develop from creeping stems/lateral roots. Leaves are sub–fleshy and mostly basal. Each blade is oblong to elliptic (sometime cordate) and 2"–6" in length. They develop on long petioles. 5–8 petal–like bracts are white, red–tinged, and arranged disk–like. When flowering the inflorescence is a notable contrast to the green leaf layer beneath. Crush a leaf: it smells part swamp, part minty fragrance.

Distribution

Yerba mansa ranges from California, Nevada, Utah, Colorado, Arizona, New Mexico, western Texas, to Mexico. A desert wetland and ciénega plant, it is found around seeps, alkali springs, and marshes where it tends to be a ground cover – locally abundant, but isolated in distribution[30]. The plant's largest threat is not over–harvesting but habitat loss through development and lowering of the region's water table.

Chemistry

Essential oil (root): α–pinene, cymene, limonene, 1,8–cineole, myrtenol, anethole, piperitone, thymol, methyl eugenol, and elemicin; essential oil (leaf): α–pinene, β–phellandrene, 1,8–cineole, piperitone, methyl eugenol, (e)–caryophyllene, and elemicin.

Medicinal Uses

In a sense Yerba mansa is Ligusticum porteri's (Mountain lovage) lower–country relative. They are related not by botanical association but by a long history of use, medicinal potency, and associated southwestern range: make a trek into the aspen–covered mountains for Ligusticum; the desert ciénegas for Yerba mansa. Like Ligusticum, Yerba santa, and Creosote bush, most people living around the plant and privy to its use, utilized it at

late herbalist Michael Moore, is probably more traditionally in use throughout central–northern New Mexico. Yerba mansa loosely means 'tame herb'. Yerba manso/Yerba del manso means 'tame herb' or 'herb of the tame Indian' or it may be a possible reference to the long–since vanished 'Manso' tribe of southwestern New Mexico.

30   It has been hypothesized by some that these isolated patches were grown from transplanted rhizomes by mobile native Indians living next to springs and seeps. Although fascinating, this seems unlikely: vast expanses, stretching for scores of miles were once reported for the plant. Due to today's much lower water table these great Yerba mansa swaths have been reduced to isolated pockets. This gives the appearance of purposeful planting.

one time or another.

Due mainly to a combination of aromatics and tannins the plant affects a number of regions in a similar manner. Broadly, Yerba mansa is a stimulating astringent – yet, unlike many plants (Oak, Geranium, and Jatropha), its tannin content does not dominate, it accents. The plant will help most chronic/sub–acute respiratory, gastrointestinal, and urogenital complaints that are accompanied by irritation and mucus discharge.

Use Yerba mansa to resolve lingering sore throats and sinus infections. The tincture or tea works well as a gargle or rinse (and/or swallowed). Most find it anaesthetic, soothing, and stimulating to area tissues. In combination with immune stimulants like Echinacea or Myrrh, it will more profoundly affect regional deficiency. The tea can equally be used as a nasal or throat spray. Not particularly expectorant, it makes a useful cough suppressant, especially if the bronchial region feels painful, sore, and chronically irritated. It makes a nice addition to most winter–time cold and flu formulas.

Yerba mansa is well applied to chronic bladder, ureter, and urethra irritations. It is particularly soothing if there is accompanying mucus discharge. The plant is also moderately antimicrobial – certainly this quality assists if the issue is microbial in origin. Men often notice some relief if suffering from prostatitis. Helping to curb infection from bacterial growth/ urine backlog, the plant is also antispasmodic. This assists in better urine passage.

The tea is the choice preparation for any gastrointestinal application. Esophageal, gastric, and intestinal irritations are quieted by Yerba mansa. As long as the situation is accompanied by sensitivity, gas and bloating, and is chronic/sub–acute in nature, Yerba mansa likely be beneficial. It should also be used if there is diarrhea with accompanying intestinal spasms.

2–3 teaspoons of the fresh plant tincture have a pronounced central nervous system influence. It can be used for all types of pain. From that of acute injuries to arthritic flare–ups, it has a soothing analgesic–sedative influence. I've even seen back injury pain significantly diminish with the plant's use.

Externally the herbal oil is one of the best for chronic hemorrhoids. Shrinking to tissue, apply it several times a day, especially before bed. Anal fissures will also heal more quickly with regular application. Cuts, scrapes, and burns will speedily resolve with the poultice, fomentation, or oil/salve. Lastly, in combination with alteratives like Golden smoke or Stillingia, external application will help in diminishing metabolic–centered skin eruptions, boils, and acne.

Indications

» Laryngitis/Pharyngitis, chronic
» Sinusitis, chronic with mucus discharge
» Cough, spasmodic with irritation
» Irritation, urinary tract
» Prostatitis, chronic
» Irritation, gastrointestinal, with gas/bloating,
» Pain, from injury or chronic issue
» Hemorrhoids, chronic (external)
» Fissure, anal, poorly healing (external)
» Cuts/Burns (external)
» Boils/Acne

Collection

Both leaf and root material are gathered for medicine. Leaves are easy enough to collect: grab several by the tops and snip the leaf petioles with pruners. A relatively weighty and large leafed plant, sizable quantities can be collected in relatively short periods of time.

Depending on soil conditions, underground rhizomes can be lateral, vertical, or a combination of the two. Regardless, sandy–loomy soils will make root procurement less difficult. Whatever the soil condition, start on the edge of a stand. Dig a couple of feet down and work around the edge of a group being careful not to split the group in half or remove its center plants. Collect both roots, leaves, and surface runners. Most root material with be sub–surface.

Preparations

Slice the root. It should be pinkish and aromatic, and taste stimulating, astringent, and anesthetic. The leaves will be a little less astringent. The whole plant is medicinal – the fresh plant tincture is the most active internal preparation (I prefer mixing half root material and half herbaceous material when tincturing). The roots are a fair medicine after drying; the leaves, lesser so, but still of service. Use the alcohol intermediate preparation when making the herbal oil.

Dosage
- » FPT/DPT (60%): 30–60 drops 2–3 times daily
- » Standard/Cold infusion of root/herb: 4–6 ounces 2–3 times daily
- » Ointment/Oil/Salve: topically as needed
- » Poultice/Fomentation: topically as needed

Cautions
There are really no cautions for normal usage. Even a cup of tea or a dose of tincture every couple of days should pose no problem during pregnancy.

Other Uses
The plant cultivates easily. The creeping stems simply allowed to root or placed over soil–filled pots is an efficient way of propagation. In a matter of weeks (spring/summer) the stem nodes will root, creating individual plants. Having several potted plants on hand and occasionally collecting leaf material, is a fine method for individual/family use.

Yerba Santa
Boraginaceae/Borage Family

Eriodictyon californicum (Hook. & Arn.) Torr.
California yerba santa, Mountain balm

Eriodictyon angustifolium Nutt.
Narrow–leaved yerba santa

Eriodictyon trichocalyx A.A. Heller
Hairy yerba santa

Description
This erect, 3′–9′ tall shrub has shedding bark and lanceolate to oblong leaves. They are leathery and 2–toned. The upper leaf surface is hairless, or nearly so; the lower surface is densely hairy. The leaves' dual appearance is striking: above they are yellowish–green and often shiny, below they are fuzzy–white. Eriodictyon californicum's and E. trichocalyx's leaves are somewhat wider than E. angustifolium's. When crushed all three species are semi–aromatic and resinous–sticky.

Yerba santa's flower clusters form at branch ends and are open in appearance. All species have funnel shaped corollas. Eriodictyon californicum's inflorescence is white to purple, sparsely hairy, and is the largest of the group. E. angustifolium has the smallest flower. It is white and densely hairy. E. trichocalyx's flower size falls between the other two species. It is white to lavender and also hairy.

Distribution

The epicenter of Eriodictyon californicum's biomass is northern California. With extensive populations of the plant found in various coastal and inland mountain ranges there is no lack of collectable supply. Throughout southern California it is more sporadically found at mid–elevations. Its northern limit stretches to Oregon. Look to disturbed roadside soil, trailsides, and exposed hillsides where other Chaparral–Scrub shrubs are found.

From southeastern California to Utah, Nevada, and Arizona, Eriodictyon angustifolium is found in mid–desert regions. As the most easterly–growing of the genus, the plant seeds well in disturbed soils, especially those that are burnt by fast–moving chaparral fires. I have seen large stands of the plant stop only where the land had not been burnt years before. Sun–exposed hillsides and trail and road sides are other areas to look.

Eriodictyon trichocalyx is a southern California grower. Found in and around the Peninsular and Transverse Ranges, it's successful and common. Like the other species, it's Chaparral–oriented and prefers disturbed soils.

Chemistry

For Eriodictyon californicum: flavonoids: eriodictyol, luteolin, chrysoeriol, apigenin, hispidulin, luteolin, nepetin, jaceosidin, homoeriodictyol, kaempferol, and quercetin.

Medicinal Uses

Yerba santa has a rich history of use in American herbal medicine. Like Creosote bush, everyone in the Southwest privy to plant usage, utilized it for essentially the same thing – an expectorant with decongestant properties. In the past Yerba santa's high esteem was maintained not only because it worked but because of its stability. For herbaceous material, the plant stored and shipped well. It held up through the ravages of time, travel, and elemental exposure leading to a reliable herbal medicine.

Use Yerba santa when suffering from bronchitis or when in need of an expectorant. It not only loosens phlegm, but it also dries the bronchial environment. Unlike other expectorants that tend to increase pulmonary secretions, Yerba santa has a distinct decongesting quality, yet without stimulating cardiovascular functions such as Ephedra. Compounding the plant's useful lung effects, is its antibacterial property. Yerba santa's leaf resins are distinctly bacteriostatic, particularly against gram–positive microbes: Micrococcus spp., Mycobacterium tuberculosis, Sarcina spp., and Streptococcus pyogenes.

Asthmatic congestion, when breathing is accompanied by mucus, responds well to Yerba Santa. Also use the plant in cases of rhinitis or sinusitis caused by allergies and/or infection.

For urinary tract infections the plant is distinctly antimicrobial. Use it in cases of bladder and urethra infection when there is mucus in the urine. For infections that Manzanita does not affect try Yerba Santa as its non–polar compounds tend to eliminate microbes that the latter plant does not. A combination of the two can be used as well.

Indications
» Bronchitis, copious phlegm
» Asthma, humid
» Sinusitis/Rhinitis, copious mucus
» Cystitis/Urethritis, with mucus in the urine

Collection
Gather the leafing tips in the spring or early summer when the new growth is apparent. They should be resinous and somewhat sticky. The leaves can be dried loosely or in wrapped bundles.

Preparations/Dosage
» FPT/DPT (70% alcohol): 30–60 drops 2–3 times daily
» Fluidextract: 10–30 drops 2–3 times daily
» Herb infusion: 2–4 ounces 2–3 times daily

Cautions
There are no known cautions with judicious use.

Other Uses
Due to Yerba santa's ability at masking bitter herbs, it is well–used in

making poor–tasting formulas (especially cough syrups) more palatable. Its composition of 10%–20% of a formula is usually all that is needed, however be sure that its medicinal effects are needed, as part of a combination for respiratory or urinary problems for instance.

For smokers a number of fluffy–leaved Yerba santa species make a good medicated smoke (if there is such a thing). Try the leaves of Felt leaf yerba santa (Eriodictyon crassifolium) or Woolly yerba santa (E. tomentosum) mixed with a good kinnikinnick. Certainly it's best not to smoke anything while suffering from a lung affliction, but if one must, it may be of value.

Yucca
Liliaceae/Lily Family

Yucca elata Engelm.
Soaptree, Spanish bayonet

Yucca schottii Engelm.
Mountain yucca, Hoary yucca

Yucca baccata Torr.
Banana yucca, Blue yucca, Datil

Description
Depending on variety, at maturity Yucca's height can vary anywhere from several to 25'. The leaves of most Yuccas are stiff and pointed. On the tall and slender trunked varieties the old leaves have a tendency to droop making a protective layer over the trunk, much like an un–trimmed palm tree. If enough water and nutrients are available, Yucca produces a flowering stalk, upon which are borne (depending on variety), either fleshy or hard capsule–like fruit. They contain small, black, and circular flattened seeds stacked in several columns. In the West these are long–lived perennials. They are well adapted to their arid environments.

Yucca elata is tall and slender–trunked. It occasionally reaches 15' in height. On mature plants, 2–3 side trunks are not uncommon, although younger plants tend to have 1 small trunk. The bluish–green leaves are 10"–20" long and very narrow with separating margin fibers. The large, showy, and white flowers form from stalks that sprout during the spring. The woody capsule–like fruit contain numerous small black seeds.

Y. schottii in some respects is similar to Y. elata. The plant is stout, thick trunked, and has stiff–leaves. Y. schottii reaches 20'–25' in height and may have 2–3 trunks arising from its base, though 1 trunk is common. The long stiff leaves are stout, pointed, and 1"–2" thick. Fleshy fruit develop after the showy and cream–colored flowers are pollinated.

Y. baccata is a multi–trunked, lower–growing plant. Its lower stems occasionally creep just below the ground's surface. The stiff leaves are pointed and have fibrous margins. The typical cream–colored flowers are followed by fleshy fruit.

Distribution

Yucca elata ranges from west of the Pecos River through southern New Mexico, along the Rio Grande Drainage, southeast–central Arizona, and finally to an isolated grouping in southwestern Utah. As a plant of the Desert Grasslands, it is found from 2,000'–6,000'.

Y. schottii is isolated to southeastern Arizona and southwestern New Mexico. It is a hillside and canyon plant that is commonly found throughout Desert Grasslands and Oak Woodlands. Look for it from 4,000'–7,000'.

Y. baccata has the widest range of the three Yuccas profiled here. From southern Nevada, Utah, Colorado, and southeastern California it ranges south through much of Arizona, New Mexico, and southwestern Texas. Y. baccata enjoys a large array of habitat and elevation ranges. It is a common plant.

Chemistry

Sapogenins: diosgenin, gitogenin, neogitogenin, hecogenin, manogenin, sarsasapogenin, smilagenin, stigmasterol, tigogenin, neotigogenin; steroidal compounds: β–sitosterol, stigmasterol, and campesterol.

Medicinal Uses

Like the many other lesser–known medicinal plants profiled in this book, these species of Yucca are the not commercial varieties. Even though Yucca schidigera is the main commercial source plant, the following Yuccas will be found just as effective.

Yucca produces several therapeutic effects mainly through its influence of intestinal tract membranes and related flora. The plant's saponins form complexes with abnormal colonic flora by–products rendering these toxins, to some degree, inert. Since these saponins are indigestible, the formed complexes are removed with other waste matter from the colon. Therefore, bacterial end–products are unable to exert an inflammatory effect because they literally are stuck to Yucca's saponins, making absorption into systemic circulation less likely.

High protein/high fat/low carbohydrate diet followers will benefit from Yucca's effective binding of ammonia[31] in the colon. This allows it to pass out with the feces and not be reabsorbed through the portal circulation. Thus, liver stress in response to a high protein diet, will diminish.

It is interesting to note that constipation is often a factor in many arthritic/inflammatory conditions. When abnormal microorganisms have more time to interact negatively with intestinal waste matter there is a tendency for our internal environment to become pro–inflammatory. This certainly is one reason why laxative and liver stimulant therapies have a place in treating pain syndromes. Also old vaqueros are known to use the plant to lessen the full body pains of years of hard work and cowboyin'.

Yucca is useful in lowering bile salt and cholesterol re–uptake by the lower duodenum. As above, the binding effect of these saponins can lower blood triglyceride and cholesterol levels.

Indications

»   Arthritis, rheumatoid
»   Pain, chronic, dependent upon constipation
»   LDL/Triglycerides levels, elevated

Collection

Collect the roots and lower trunk in the fall. Yucca's saponin content varies in response to season and species. The highest yields are in the fall when the plant draws back in and again starts the cycle of accumulation for next year's spring growth.

Preparations

Chop the gathered material into ¼"–½" pieces. Lay out on a flat to dry if in

---

31   Ammonia, an end result of protein breakdown, is converted from urea in the colon by colonic flora. If the liver is not able to reconvert ammonia back to urea, because of large protein qualities from diet or impaired renal or liver function, resulting ammonia toxicities can ensue.

an arid place or if in a more humid environment use a dehydrator. Either way the root will dry quickly given its porous nature.

Dosage

It is best to approach Yucca as a short–term plant used concurrently for 3–4 weeks. If longer term use is needed try a rotation of Yucca for 3–4 weeks followed by 1 week of Creosote bush or Turmeric.

» Root decoction: 4–6 ounces 2–3 times daily
» DPT (50% alcohol): 30–60 drops 2–3 times daily
» Fluidextract: 10–30 drops 2–3 times daily
» Capsule (00): 2–3, 2–3 times daily

Cautions

Used in excessive quantities Yucca can cause intestinal distress. Do not use during pregnancy due to the plant's potential altering effect on reproductive hormones.

Other Uses

1–2 ounces of the powdered root can be added to water making a usable soap/shampoo. The fruit from the fleshy varieties are sweet and edible. Collect and eat these when small brown marks of sugar fermentation are just starting to appear on the outer light green surface of the fruit skin. According to Peter Bigfoot, a mountain man herbalist who lives in the Superstition Mountains of Arizona, the seeds will cause gastrointestinal upset.

Therapeutic Index

Cardiovascular

Angina pectoris (Puncturevine)

Cardiac weakness, from age/tobacco heart (Antelope horns, Desert milkweed, Night blooming cereus)

Hypertension, essential (Puncturevine, Spanish needles)

Leg heaviness, fatigue, and fluid retention (Beargrass, Ocotillo)

Tachycardia with hypertension and forceful pulse (Passionflower)

Gastrointestinal

Amebiasis (Crucifixion thorn, Cypress, Desert barberry, Sagebrush, Soapberry, Tree of heaven, Western mugwort)

Constipation (Aloe, Buttonbush, Rayweed, Senna, Velvet ash, Wild licorice)

Cramps, intestinal (Baccharis, Burrobrush, Canyon bursage, Canyon walnut, Datura, Hopbush, Passionflower, Prickly poppy, Sage, Sagebrush, Wolfberry)

Diarrhea (Bird of paradise, Caltrop, Canadian fleabane, Cocklebur, Flat–top buckwheat, Jojoba, Jumping cholla, Limberbush, Ratany, Sumac, Tree of heaven)

Diarrhea with intestinal cramps (Bricklebush, Chinchweed, Marsh fleabane, Yerba mansa)

Dyspepsia (Desert anemone, Bricklebush, Buttonbush, Cottonwood, Desert barberry, Golden smoke, Rayweed, Tarbush, Trumpet creeper, Verbena, Western mugwort, Wild licorice)

Dyspepsia with bloating (Chinchweed, Poreleaf, Beebrush, Dogweed, Juniper, Mountain marigold, Poliomintha, Sagebrush)

Food poisoning (Crucifixion thorn, Cypress, Desert barberry, Sagebrush)

Gastritis (Baccharis, Bird of paradise, Bricklebush, Caltrop, Crownbeard, Dogweed, Jumping cholla, Mallow, Mormon tea, Mountain marigold, Prickly pear, Spanish needles, Trumpet flower, Western Mugwort, Wild licorice, Yerba mansa)

Giardiasis (Cypress, Desert barberry, Tree of heaven)

Hemorrhoids (Crownbeard, Datura, Ocotillo, Ratany, Tobacco, Yerba mansa)

Hemorrhoids, bleeding (Periwinkle, Ratany, Yerba mansa)

Hiccups (Chinchweed)

Inflammation, intestinal (Baccharis, Bird of paradise, Caltrop, Canadian fleabane, Canyon walnut, Scouring rush, Marsh fleabane, Spanish needles, Tree of heaven, Western mugwort, Yerba mansa)

Infection, Candida albicans (Canyon walnut, Desert willow, Trumpet flower)

Malabsorption, nutrient/lipid (Buttonbush, Canyon walnut)

Ulcer, duodenal (Baccharis, Spanish needles)

Ulcer, gastric (Crownbeard, Prickly pear, Spanish needles, Wild licorice)

Ulcer, peptic (Aloe, Desert lavender, Scouring rush, Jumping cholla)

Worms (Crucifixion thorn, Sagebrush, Western mugwort)

Liver–Gallbladder

Congestion, liver and gallbladder (Bricklebush, Buttonbush, Desert barberry, Rayweed, Sagebrush, Tarbush, Velvet ash)

Inflammation, liver (Desert barberry, Western mugwort)

Spasm, gall bladder (Hopbush)

Lymph–Immune

Skin conditions from allergy or autoimmune disturbances, chronic (Golden smoke)

Enlargements, lymph node (Golden smoke, Ocotillo)

Men

Debility, genital (Desert anemone)

Irritation, genital, resulting in excessive sexual activity and preoccupation (Western black willow)

Herpes simplex virus, type II (Creosote bush, Crownbeard, Western mugwort)

Libido, decreased (Desert anemone, Puncturevine)

Prostatitis (Cypress, Cottonwood, Ocotillo, Western black willow, Yerba mansa)

Sperm count, low and poor quality (Puncturevine)

Spermatorrhea (Western black willow)

Trichomoniasis (Crucifixion thorn)

Warts, genital (Creosote bush, Cypress)

Metabolic

Hyperglycemia–NIDDM (Aloe, Bouvardia, Bricklebush, Prickly pear, Trumpet flower)

Gout (Prickly pear)

LDL levels, elevated (Prickly pear, Yucca)

Mouth and Throat

Gingivitis (Cypress, Elephant tree)

Gums, spongy and bleeding (Elephant tree, Limberbush, Ratany, Sumac)

Periodontitis (Elephant tree, Ratany)

Sores, mouth (Wild rhubarb, Limberbush, Mesquite, Mimosa, Ratany, Tamarisk)

Strep throat (Cypress, Desert barberry, Elephant tree, Sage)

Sore throat–general (Cypress, Desert barberry, Wild rhubarb, Elephant tree, Filaree, Jojoba, Mesquite, Sage, Sumac, Tamarisk, Yerba mansa)

Nervous System

Depression (Desert anemone, Syrian rue, Wild oats)

Insomnia/anxiety (Bouvardia, California poppy, Desert lavender, Passionflower, Prickly poppy, Red betony, Verbena, Wild lettuce, Wild oats)

Memory loss/poor cognition/Alzheimer's (Sage)

Seizure activity/tremors/tics (Golden smoke, Passionflower, Tree of heaven, Turpentine bush, Western peony)

Pain

Arthritis, general (Desert anemone, Brittlebush, Clematis, Cottonwood, Elephant tree, Snakeweed, Soapberry, Yerba mansa)

Arthritis, rheumatoid (Beargrass, Clematis, Creosote bush, Soapberry, Yucca)

Injury, acute, with pain (California poppy, Prickly poppy, Camphorweed, Cottonwood, Wolfberry, Yerba mansa)

Injury, acute, with pain and unbroken skin (Datura, Tobacco)

Muscular pain, chronic (Elephant tree, Snakeweed)

Headache, migraine, beginning stages (Clematis, Desert anemone)

Headache, migraine, acute pain (Periwinkle)

Headache, stress (Red betony, Verbena)

Spasm, muscle, from injury (Datura, Passionflower, Yerba mansa)

Renal–Urinary
Debility, general (Desert anemone)

Fluid retention (Elder, Filaree, Scouring rush, Prickly pear)

Incontinence/bed wetting from lack of bladder tone (Cypress)

Inflammation/pain, lower urinary tract (Cocklebur, Filaree, Flat–top buckwheat, Globemallow, Scouring rush, Jumping cholla, Kidneywood, Mallow, Mormon tea)

Inflammation/pain, lower urinary tract, weakened tissues (Cypress, Elephant tree, Juniper, Western black willow, Yerba mansa)

Inflammation with hematuria (Filaree, Scouring rush, Periwinkle, Ratany, Spanish needles)

Infection, alkaline urine (Manzanita)

Infection, general (Cypress, Elephant tree, Juniper, Yerba santa)

Kidney stones, general (Kidneywood)

Kidney stones, preventative (Scouring rush, Jumping cholla, Mallow, Puncturevine)

Kidney stones, uric acid (Jumping cholla, Kidneywood, Prickly pear)

Nephritis, acute (Globemallow, Mallow)

Nephritis, chronic (Cottonwood, Elephant tree, Juniper, Kidneywood, Wild licorice)

Respiratory (Lower)
Asthma, copious phlegm (Wolfberry, Yerba santa)

Asthma, dry, non–spasmodic (Antelope horns, Desert milkweed)

Asthma, general (Creosote bush, Datura)

Bronchitis with copious phlegm and weak cough (Cypress, Elephant tree, Yerba santa)

Bronchitis with difficult expectoration (Antelope horns, Cudweed, Desert milkweed, Ocotillo, Sagebrush)

Bronchitis with dry fever (Cudweed, Sagebrush, Texas ranger)

Cough, dry and painful (Cudweed, Globemallow, Mallow, Wild licorice)

Cough, spasmodic (California poppy, Passionflower, Prickly poppy, Western peony, Wild lettuce, Yerba mansa)

Hemorrhaging, passive (Scouring rush, Ratany)

Pleurisy (Antelope horns, Desert milkweed)

Respiratory (Upper) and Eyes
Conjunctivitis (Desert anemone, Caltrop, Mesquite, Prickly poppy, Spanish needles)

Glaucoma (Desert anemone)

Rhinitis (Brittlebush, Burrobrush, Canyon bursage, Cocklebur, Mormon tea, Wolfberry, Yerba santa)

Sinusitis (Canyon bursage, Burrobrush, Cocklebur, Desert barberry, Elephant tree, Yerba mansa, Yerba santa)

Styes (Desert anemone, Prickly poppy)

Skin
Abscess (Globemallow, Copperleaf, Elephant tree, Leadwort, Mallow)

Actinic keratosis (Creosote bush)

Bedsores (Copperleaf, Cypress, Elephant tree, Leadwort)

Bites, insect, venomous (Creosote bush, Pipevine)

Bites, stings, general (Bird of paradise, Creosote bush, Flat–top buckwheat,

Hopbush, Penstemon, Pipevine, Tobacco)

Bites, snake, venomous (Pipevine)

Boils (Mallow)

Burns form heat and sunburn (Aloe, Crownbeard, Datura, Jumping cholla, Prickly pear, Prickly poppy, Yerba mansa)

Candida infections (Cypress, Desert lavender, Desert willow, Hopbush, Trumpet flower)

Chicken pox (Crownbeard)

Contusions (Aloe, Prickly pear, Sagebrush, Wolfberry)

Dermatitis, dry scabby (Cypress)

Eczema (Creosote bush, Elephant tree, Juniper, Puncturevine, Purple gromwell)

Herpes simplex virus, type I (Creosote bush, Crownbeard, Western mugwort)

Hives, Rashes (Bird of paradise, Burrobrush, Caltrop, Canyon bursage, Wild rhubarb, Filaree, Flat–top buckwheat, Golden smoke, Hopbush, Jojoba, Penstemon, Puncturevine)

Infections, bacterial – Aloe, Creosote bush, California poppy, Cypress, Desert barberry, Desert lavender, Elephant tree, Hopbush, Prickly poppy, Purple gromwell, Sagebrush, Syrian rue, Western mugwort)

Infections, fungal (Aloe, Antelope horns, California poppy, Creosote bush, Cypress, Desert barberry, Desert milkweed, Purple gromwell, Sagebrush, Syrian rue, Tarbush, Western mugwort)

Poison ivy reactions, systemic (Brittlebush)

Poorly healing tissue with tendency towards ulceration (Golden smoke)

Psoriasis (Creosote bush, Desert barberry, Elephant tree, Juniper, Puncturevine, Purple gromwell)

Shingles (Crownbeard)

Scrapes, abrasions, cuts – Acacia, Aloe, Baccharis, Bird of paradise, California poppy, Cocklebur, Cottonwood, Crownbeard, Desert lavender, Wild rhubarb, Elephant tree, Flat–top buckwheat, Hopbush, Limberbush, Marsh fleabane, Mesquite, Mimosa, Mountain marigold, Penstemon, Prickly pear, Prickly poppy, Snakeweed, Spanish needles, Sumac, Tamarisk, Tarbush, Yerba mansa)

Splinters (Globemallow, Copperleaf, Leadwort, Mallow)

Stings, scorpion (Bouvardia)

Ulcers, poorly healing (Copperleaf, Cypress, Elephant tree, Leadwort)

Varicosities/spider veins (Beargrass, Prickly pear)

Vitiligo (Puncturevine)

Warts, common (Antelope horns, Cypress, Creosote bush, Desert milkweed)

Wounds (Aloe, Scouring rush, Marsh fleabane, Penstemon, Purple gromwell, Sagebrush, Spanish needles, Tarbush, Trixis)

Wounds, poorly healing (Copperleaf, Cypress, Elder, Elephant tree, Leadwort, Mountain marigold, Prickly pear, Turpentine bush, Velvet ash)

Women

Anovulatory cycles (Chaste tree)

Cramps, uterine (Desert anemone, Datura, Hopbush, Western peony)

Cramps, uterine with pelvic congestion (Canyon bursage, Burrobrush, Sagebrush, Turpentine bush)

Fibroids, breast and uterine (Desert cotton)

Fibroids, uterine, subserous (Chaste tree)

Herpes simplex virus, type II (Creosote bush, Crownbeard, Western mugwort)

Irritation, genital, resulting in excessive sexual activity and preoccupation (Western black willow)

Inflammation, vaginal and cervical (Filaree, Manzanita)

Lactation, insufficient (Chaste tree, Verbena)

Lactation, to lessen (Sage)

Labor, slowed (Antelope horns, Desert milkweed)

Libido, decreased (Desert anemone)

Menstruation, heavy (Chaste tree, Caltrop, Filaree, Periwinkle, Ratany)

Menstruation, slowed (Desert anemone, Antelope horns, Desert cotton, Desert milkweed, Poliomintha, Sagebrush, Turpentine bush, Western mugwort)

Perimenopause (Chaste tree)

Premenstrual discomfort with breast tenderness, agitation, and anxiety (Chaste tree)

Postpartum tonic (Manzanita)

Trichomoniasis (Crucifixion thorn)

Warts, genital (Creosote bush, Cypress)

Miscellaneous

Connective tissues, hair, nails, skin, and bones, weakened (Scouring rush)

Fever, dry, low–moderate temperature (Desert lavender, Elder, Marsh fleabane, Mountain marigold, Poliomintha, Sage, Verbena, Western mugwort)

Fever with autoimmune inflammation (Desert barberry)

Fever with moderately high temperature, dry skin, strong determination of blood (Cottonwood, Sagebrush, Syrian rue)

Sweating, colliquative (Cocklebur, Sage)

Valley fever (Cypress Desert willow)

Bibliography

Aloe

Chithra, P., G.B. Sajithlal, and Gowri Chandrakasan. "Influence of Aloe Vera on the Glycosaminoglycans in the Matrix of Healing Dermal Wounds in Rats." *Journal of Ethnopharmacology* 59 (1998): 179–186.

D.N. Herndon and J.P. Heggers. "Retardation of Wound Healing by Silver Sulfadiazine is Reversed by Aloe Vera and Nystatin." *Burns* 29 (2003): 834–836.

Seyger, M.M.B., P.C.M. van de Kerkhof, I.M.J.J. van Vlijmen–Willems, E.S.M. de Bakker, F. Zwiers, and E.M.G.J. de Jong. "The Efficacy of a New Topical Treatment for Psoriasis: Mirak." *Journal of the European Academy of Dermatology and Venereology* 11 (1998): 13–18.

Femenia, Antoni, Emma S. Sánchez, Susana Simal, and Carmen Rosselló. "Compositional Features of Polysaccharides from Aloe Vera (Aloe Barbadensis Miller) Plant Tissues." *Carbohydrate Polymers* 39 (1999): 109–117.

Frode, T.S. and Y.S. Medeiros. "Animal Models to Test Drugs with Potential Antidiabetic Activity." *Journal of Ethnopharmacology* 115 (2008): 173–183. Grover, J.K., S. Yadav, and V. Vats. "Medicinal Plants of India with Anti–Diabetic Potential." *Journal of Ethnopharmacology* 81 (2002): 81–100.

Jia, Yimei, Guodong Zhaoa, Jicheng Jia. "Preliminary Evaluation: The Effects of Aloe Ferox Miller and Aloe Arborescens Miller on Wound Healing." *Journal of Ethnopharmacology* 120 (2008): 181–189.

Muller, M.J., M.A. Hollyoak, Z. Moaveni, Tim La H. Brown, T. Reynolds, A.C. Dweck. "Aloe Vera Leaf Gel: A Review Update." *Journal of Ethnopharmacology* 68 (1999): 3–37.

Rodríguez, D. Jasso de, D. Hernández–Castillo, R. Rodríguez–García, and J.L. Angulo–Sánchez. "Antifungal Activity In Vitro of Aloe Vera Pulp and Liquid Fraction Against Plant Pathogenic Fungi." *Industrial Crops and Products* xxx (2004): xxx–xxx.

Sadiq, Yusuf, Agunu Abdulkarim, and Diana Mshelia. "The Effect of Aloe Vera A. Berger (Liliaceae) on Gastric Acid Secretion and Acute Gastric Mucosal Injury in Rats." *Journal of Ethnopharmacology* 93 (2004): 33–37.

Váquez, Beatriz, Guillermo Avila, David Segura, and Bruno Escalante. "Antiinflammatory Activity of Extracts from Aloe Vera Gel." *Journal of Ethnopharmacology* 55 (1996): 69–75.

Verlag, Gustav Fischer. "Antidiabetic Activity of Aloe Vera L. Juice. I. Clinical Trial in New Cases of Diabetes Mellitus." *Phytomedicine* 3, 3 (1996): 241–243.

Antelope Horns

Chiu, F.C. and Watson, T.R. "Conformational Factors in Cardiac Glycoside Activity." *Journal of Medical Chemistry* 28, 4 (1985): 509–515.

Giordani, R., Moulin–Traffort, J., and Regli, P. "Glycosidic Activities of Candida Albicans After Action of Vegetable Latex Saps (Natural Antifungals) and Isoconazole (Synthetic Antifungal)." *Mycoses* 34, 1–2 (1991): 67–73.

Kelley, Bruce D., Glenn D. Appelt, and Jennifer M. Appelt. "Pharmacological Aspects of Selected Herbs Employed in Hispanic Folk Medicine in the San Luis Valley of Colorado, USA: II Asclepias Asperula (Inmortal) and Achillea Lanulosa (Plumajillo)." *Journal of Ethnopharmacology* 22 (1988): 1–9.

Radford, D.J., Gillies, A.D., Hinds, J.A., and Duffy, P. "Naturally Occurring Cardiac Glycosides." *Medical Journal of Australia* 144, 10 (1986): 540–544.

Sady, Michael B. and James N. Seiber. "Chemical Differences Between Species of

Asclepias from the Intermountain Region of North America." *Phytochemistry* 30, 9 (1991): 3001–3003.

Seiber, James N., Carolyn J. Nelson, and S. Mark Lee. "Cardenolides in the Latex and Leaves of Seven Asclepias Species and Calotropis Procrea." *Phytochemistry* 21, 9 (1982): 2343–2348.

Baccharis

Falcao, H.S., I.R. Mariath, M.F.F.M. Diniz, L.M. Batista, and J.M. Barbosa–Filho. "Plants of the American Continent with Antiulcer Activity." *Phytomedicine* 15 (2008): 132–146.

Moreno–Salazar, S.F., R.E. Robles–Zepeda, and D.E. Johnson. "Plant Folk Medicines for Gastrointestinal Disorders Among the Main Tribes of Sonora, Mexico." *Fitoterapia* 79 (2008): 132–141.

Beargrass

Mimaki, Y., Takaashi, Y., Kuroda, M., Sashida, Y., and Nikaido, T. "Steroidal Saponins from Nolina Recurvata Stems and their Inhibitory Activity on Cyclic AMP Phosphodiesterase." *Phytochemisty* 42, 6 (1996): 1609–1615.

Bird of Paradise

Andrade, C.T., E.G. Azero, L. Luciano, and M.P. Goncalves. "Solution Properties of the Galactomannans Extracted from the Seeds of Caesalpinia Pulcherrima and Cassia Javanica: Comparison with Locust Bean Gum." *International Journal of Biological Macromolecules* 26 (1999): 181–185.

Heras, B. de las, K. Slowing, J. Benedí, E. Carretero, T. Ortega, C. Toledo, P. Bermejo, I. Iglesias, M.J. Abad, P. Gómez–Serranillos, P.A. Liso, A. Villar, and X. Chiriboga. "Antiinflammatory and Antioxidant Activity of Plants Used in Traditional Medicine in Ecuador." *Journal of Ethnopharmacology* 61 (1998): 161–166.

Krishna, K.V.S. Rama, K. Hara Kishore, and U.S.N. Murty. "Flavanoids from Caesalpinia Pulcherrima." *Phytochemistry* 63 (2003): 789–793.

Muschietti L., V. Martino, G. Ferraro, J. Coussio, L. Segura, C. Cartana, S. Canigueral, and T. Adzet. "The Anti–Inflammatory Effect of some Species from South America." *Phytotherapy Research* 10, 1 (1996): 84–86.

Patil, Ashok D., Alan J. Freyer, R. Lee Webb, Gary Zuber, Rex Reichwein, Mark F. Bean, Leo Faucette, and Randall K. Johnson. "Pulcherrimins A – D, Novel Diterpene Dibenzoates from Caesalpinia pulcherrima with Selective Activity against DNA Repair–Deficient Yeast Mutants." *Tetrahedron* 53, 5 (1997): 1583–1592.

Pavón, Numa P. and Oscar Briones. "Phenological Patterns of Nine Perennial Plants in an Intertropical Semi–arid Mexican Scrub." *Journal of Arid Environments* 49 (2001): 265–277.

Bouvardia

Jimenez–Ferrer, E. et al. "Antitoxin activity of plants used in Mexican traditional medicine against scorpion poisoning". *Phytomedicine* 12 (2005): 116–122.

Jimenez–Ferrer, E. et al. "The secretagogue effect of the poison from Centruroides limpidus limpidus on the pancreas of mice and the antagonistic action of the Bouvardia ternifolia extract." *Phytomedicine* 12 (2005): 65–71.

Pérez–Gutiérrez, R M et al. "Effect of Triterpenoids of Bouvardia terniflora on blood sugar levels of normal and alloxan diabetic mice." *Phytomedicine* 5 (1998): 475–478.

Pérez–Gutiérrez, R M et al. "Hypoglycemic activity of Bouvardia terniflora, Brickelia veronicaefolia, and Parmentiera edulis". *Salud Publica Mex.* (1998): 40 354–358.

Bricklebush

Beck, John J. and Frank R. Stermitz. "Pyrrolizidine Alkaloids from Brickellia Grandiflora and Cryptantha Jamesii." *Biochemical Systematics and Ecology* 30 (2002): 1079–1081.

Perez–Gutierrez, R.M., Perez–Gonzalez, C., Zavala–Sanchez, M.A., Perez–Gutierrez, S. "Hypoglycemic Activity of Bouvardia Terniflora, Brickellia Veronicaefolia, and Parmentiera Edulis." *Salud Publica Mex* 40, 4 (1998): 354–358.

Brittlebush

Proksch, P., M. Breuer, and H. Budzikiewicz. "Benzofuran Derivatives from Two Encelia Species." *Phytochemistry* 24, 12 (1985): 3069–3071.

Proksch, P., U. Politt, E. Wollenweber, V. Wray, and C. Clark. "Epicuticular Flavonoids from Encelia." *Planta Medica* 54, 6 (1988): 542–546.

Proksch, Peter, Aristotelis Mitsakos, Jutta Bodden, and Eckhard Wollenweber. "Benzofurans and Methylated Flavonoids of Geraea (Asteraceae)." *Phytochemistry* 25, 10 (1986): 2367–2369.

Wisdom, Charles and Eloy Rodriguez. "Seasonal Age–Specific Measurements of the Sesquiterpene Lactones and Chromenes of Encelia Farinosa." *Biochemical Systematics and Ecology* 11, 4 (1978): 345–352.

Wisdom, Charles and Eloy Rodriguez. "Quantitative Variation of the Sesquiterpene Lactones and Chromenes of Encelia Farinosa." *Biochemical Systematics and Ecology* 10, 1 (1978): 43–48.

California Poppy

Beck, Mona–Antonia and Hanns Häberlein. "Flavonol Glycosides from Eschscholtzia Californica." *Phytochemistry* 50 (1999): 329–332.

Chaffee, M.A. and C.W. Gale, III. "The California Poppy (Eschscholtzia Mexicana) as a Copper Indicator—A New Example." *Journal of Geochemical Exploration* 5 (1976): 59–63.

Fabre, Nicolas, Catherine Claparols, Suzanne Richelme, Marie–Laure Angelin, Isabelle Fourasté, and Claude Moulis. "Direct Characterization of Isoquinoline Alkaloids in a Crude Plant Extract by Ion–Pair Liquid Chromatography–Electrospray Ionization Tandem Mass Spectrometry: Example of Eschscholtzia Californica." *Journal of Chromatography A* 904, 1 (2000): 35–46.

Paul, Liane D. and Hans H. Maurer. "Studies on the Metabolism and Toxicological Detection of the Eschscholtzia Californica Alkaloids Californine and Protopine in Urine Using Gas Chromatography–Mass Spectrometry." *Journal of Chromatography B* 789 (2003): 43–57.

Caltrop

Lia, Veronica V., Viviana A. Confalonieri, Cecilia I. Comas, and Juan H. Hunziker. "Molecular Phylogeny of Larrea and Its Allies (Zygophyllaceae): Reticulate Evolution and the Probable Time of Creosote Bush Arrival to North America."

Molecular Phylogenetics and Evolution 21, 2 (2001): 309–320.

Saleh, Nabiel A. M., Mohamed Nabil El–Hadidi, and Ahmed A. Ahmed. "The Chemosystematics of Tribulaceae." *Biochemical Systematics and Ecology* 10, 4 (1982): 313–317.

Camphorweed

Gené, Rosa M., Laura Segura, Tomás Adzet, Esther Marin, and José Iglesias. "Heterotheca Inuloides: Anti–inflammatory and Analgesic Effect." *Journal of Ethnopharmacology* 60 (1998): 157–162.

Lincoln, David E. and Brian M. Lawrence. "The Volatile Constituents of Camphorweed, Heterotheca Subaxillaris." *Phytochemistry* 23, 4 (1984): 933–934.

Morimoto, Masanori, Charles L. Cantrell, Lynn Libous–Bailey, and Stephen O. Duke. "Phytotoxicity of Constituents of Glandular Trichomes and the Leaf Surface of Camphorweed, Heterotheca Subaxillaris." *Phytochemistry* 70 (2009): 69–74.

Canadian Fleabane

Heras, B. de las, K. Slowing, J. Benedía, E. Carretero, T. Ortega, C. Toledo, P. Bermejo, I. Iglesias, M.J. Abad, P. Gómez–Serranillos, P.A. Liso, A. Villar, and X. Chiriboga. "Antiinflammatory and Antioxidant Activity of Plants Used in Traditional Medicine in Ecuador." *Journal of Ethnopharmacology* 61 (1998): 161–166.

Lenfeld, J., O. Motl, and A. Trka. "Antiinflammatory Activity of Extracts from Conyza Canadensis." *Pharmazie* 41, 4 (1986): 268–269.

Todd, Albert M. "Oils of Erigeron and Fireweed." *American Journal of Pharmacy* 59, 6 (1887).

Canyon Bursage

Muschietti, L., V. Martino,G. Ferraro, J. Coussio, L. Segura, C. Cartana, S. Canigueral, and T. Adzet. "The Antiiflammatory Effects of some Species from South America." *Phytotherapy Research* 10, 1 (1996): 84–86.

Wang, P.H., J. XU, and M.Y. WU. "Chemical Constituents of Ragweed (Artemisia Artemisiifolia)." *China Journal of Chinese Materia Medica* 18, 3 (1993): 164–166.

Canyon Walnut

Biancoa, M. A., A. Handajia, and H. Savolainenb. "Quantitative Analysis of Ellagic Acid in Hardwood Samples." *The Science of the Total Environment* 222 (1998): 123–126.

Boelkins, James N., Lloyd K. Everson, and Theodore K. Auyong. "Effects of Intravenous Juglone in the Dog." *Toxicon* 6, 2 (1968): 99–102.

Guarrera, Paolo Maria. "Traditional Antihelmintic, Antiparasitic and Repellent Uses of Plants in Central Italy." *Journal of Ethnopharmacology* 68 (1999): 183–192.

Lopez, A., J.B. Hudson, and G.H.N. Towers. "Antiviral and Antimicrobial Activities of Colombian Medicinal Plants." *Journal of Ethnopharmacology* 77 (2001): 189–196.

Omar, S., B. Lemonnier, N. Jones, C. Ficker, M.L. Smith, C. Neema, Towers, G.H.N., K. Goel, and J.T. Arnason. "Antimicrobial Activity of Extracts of Eastern North American Hardwood Trees and Relation to Traditional Medicine." *Journal of Ethnopharmacology* 73 (2000): 161–170.

Chaste Tree

Böhnert, K. J. "The Use of Vitex Agnus Castus for Hyperprolactinemia." *Quarterly*

Review of Natural Medicine, spring (1997): 19–21.

Brown, Donald J. "Vitex Agnus Castus Clinical Monograph from Quarterly Review of Natural Medicine." *Herbal Research Review,* Summer (1994)

Halaška, M., P. Beles, C. Gorkow, and C. Sieder. "Treatment of Cyclical Mastalgia with a Solution Containing a Vitex Agnus Castus Extract: Results of a Placebo–Controlled Double–Blind Study." *The Breast* 8 (1999): 175–181.

Lauritzen, CH., H.D. Reuter, R. Repges, K.J. Böhnert, and U. Schmidt. "Treatment of Premenstrual Tension Syndrome with Vitex Agnus Castus Controlled, Double–Blind Study Versus Pyridoxine." *Phytomedicine* 4, 3 (1997): 183–189.

Lucks, Barbara Chopin. "Vitex Agnus Castus Essential Oil and Menopausal Balance: A Research Update." *Complementary Therapies in Nursing and Midwifery* 8 (2003): 148–154.

Schellenberg, R. "Treatment for the Premenstrual Syndrome with Agnus Castus Fruit Extract: Prospective, Randomized, Placebo Controlled Study." *British Medical Journal* 322 (2001): 134–137.

Chinchweed

Downum, K. R., D. J. Keil, and E. Rodriguez. "Distribution of Acetylenic Thiophenes in the Pectidinae." *Biochemical Systematics and Ecology* 13, 2 (1985): 109–113.

Clematis

Buzzini, P. and A. Pieroni. "Antimicrobial Activity of Extracts of Vitalba Clematis Towards Pathogenic Yeast and Yeast–Like Microorganisms." *Fitoterapia* (2003).

Kern, John R. and John H. Cardellina II. "Native American Medicinal Plants. Anemonin from the Horse Stimulant Clematis Hirsutissima." *Journal of Ethnopharmocology* 8 (1983): 121–123.

Li, Rachel W., G. David Lin, Stephen P. Myers, and David N. Leach. "Anti–inflammatory Activity of Chinese Medicinal Vine Plants." *Journal of Ethnopharmacology* 85 (2003): 61–67.

Cocklebur

Malik, Mabgel S., Naresh K. Sangwan, and Kuldip Singh Dhindsa. "Xanthanolides from Xanthium Strumarium." *Phytochemistry* 32, 1 (1993): 206–207.

Omar, Abdallah A., Elsayed M. Elrashidy, Nabila A. Ghazy, Ali M. Metwally, Jurgen Ziesche, and Ferdinand Bohlmann. "Xanthanolides from Xanthium Spinosum." *Phtyochemistry* 23, 4 (1984): 915–916.

Copperleaf

Büssing, A., G.M. Stein, I. Herterich–Akinpelu, and U. Pfüller. "Apoptosis–Associated Generation of Reactive Oxygen Intermediates and Release of Pro–Inflammatory Cytokines in Human Lymphocytes and Granulocytes by Extracts from the Seeds of Acalypha Wilkesiana." *Journal of Ethnopharmacology* 66 (1999): 301–309.

Samy, R. Perumal, S. Ignacimuthu, and D. Patric Raja. "Short Communication Preliminary Screening of Ethnomedicinal Plants from India." *Journal of Ethnopharmacology* 66 (1999): 235–240.

Cáceres, Armando, Beatriz López, Sonia González, Ingeborg Berger, Isao Tada, and Jun Maki. "Plants Used in Guatemala for the Treatment of Protozoal Infections. I. Screening of Activity to Bacteria, Fungi and American Trypanosomes of 13

Native Plants." *Journal of Ethnopharmacology* 62 (1998): 195–202.

Reddy, J. Suresh, P. Rajeswara Rao, and Mada S. Reddy. "Wound Healing Effects of Heliotropium Indicum, Plumbago Zeylanicum and Acalypha Indica in Rats." *Journal of Ethnopharmacology* 79 (2002): 249–251.

Irobia, O.N. and A. Bansob. "Effects of Crude Leaf Extracts of Acalypha Torta Against some Anaerobic Bacteria." *Journal of Ethnopharmacology* 43, 1 (1994): 63–65.

Cottonwood

English, S, W. Greenaway, and F.R. Whatley. "Analysis of Phenolics in the Bud Exudates of Populus Deltoides, P. Fremontii, P. Sargentii and P. Wislizenii by GC–MS." *Phytochemistry* 31, 4 (1992): 1255–1260.

Mattes, Benjamin R., Thomas P. Clausen, and Paul B. Reichardt. "Volatile Constituents of Balsam Popular: The Phenol Glycoside Connection." *Phytochemistry* 25, 5 (1987): 1361–1366.

Pearl, Irwin A. and Stephen F. Darling. "Hot Water Phenolic Extractives of the Bark and Leaves of Diploid Populus Tremuloides." *Phytochemistry* 10 (1971): 483–484.

Tiitto, Julkunen Riitta. "A Chemotaxonomic Survey of Phenolic in Leaves of Northern Salicaceae Species." *Phytochemistry* 25, 3 (1986): 663–667.

Creosote Bush

Anesini, Claudia and Cristina Perez. "Screening of Plants Used in Argentine Folk Medicine for Antimicrobial Activity." *Journal of Ethnopharmacology* 39 (1993): 119–128.

Craigo, Jodi, Michelle Callahan, Ru Chih C. Huang, and Angelo L. DeLucia. "Inhibition of Human Papillomavirus Type 16 Gene Expression by Nordihydroguaiaretic Acid Plant Lignan Derivatives." *Antiviral Research* 47 (2000): 19–28.

Grant, Kathryn L., Leslie V. Boyer, and Boyd E. Erdman. "Chaparral Induced Hepatotoxicity." *Intagrative Medicine* 1, 2 (1998): 83–87.

Hyder, Paul W., E.L. Fredrickson, Rick E. Estell, Mario Tellez, and Robert P. Gibbens. "Distribution and Concentration of Total Phenolics, Condensed Tannins, and Nordihydroguaiaretic Acid (NDGA) in Creosotebush (Larrea Tridentata)." *Biochemical Systematics and Ecology* 30 (2002): 905–912.

Quiroga, Emma Nelly, Antonio Rodolfo Sampietro, and Marta Amelia Vattuone. "Screening Antifungal Activities of Selected Medicinal Plants." *Journal of Ethnopharmacology* 74 (2001): 89–96.

Vargas–Arispuro, I., R. Reyes–Baez, G. Rivera–Castaneda, M.A. Martınez–Tellez, and I. Rivero–Espejel. "Antifungal Lignans from the Creosotebush (Larrea Tridentata)." *Industrial Crops and Products* 22 (2005): 101–107.

Verástegui, M. Angeles, César A. Sánchez, Norma L. Heredia, and J. Santos García–Alvarado. "Antimicrobial Activity of Extracts of Three Chihuahuan Desert Major Plants from the Chihuahuan Desert." *Journal of Ethnopharmacology* 52 (1996): 175–177.

Crownbeard

Banerjee, Shanta, Jasmin Jakupovic, Ferdinand Bohlmann, Robert M. King, and Harold Robinson. "A Rearranged Eudesmane and Further Verbesindiol Derivatives from Verbesina Eggersii." *Phytochemistry* 24, 5 (1985): 1106–1108.

Eichholzer, John V., Ivor A. S. Lewis, John K. Macleod, Peter B. Oelrichsa, and Peter

J. Vallelya. "Galegine and a New Dihydroxyalkylacetamide from Verbesina Enceloiodes." *Phytochemistry* 21, 1 (1982): 97–99.

Glennie, C. W. and S. C. Jaint. "Flavonol 3,7–Diglycosides of Verbesina Encelioides." *Phytochemistry* 19, 1 (1980): 157–158.

Crucifixion Thorn

Calzado–Flores, C., E.M. Guajardo–Touche, M. P. Carranza–Rosales, and J.J. Segura–Luna. "In Vitro Anti–Trichomonic Activity of Castela texana." *Proc. West. Pharmacol. Soc.* 41 (1998): 173–174.

Calzado–Flores, C., J. Verde–Star, G. Lozano–Garza, and J.J. Segura–Luna. "Preliminary Acute Toxicological Study of Castela texana." *Proc. West. Pharmacol. Soc.* 41 (1998): 77–78.

Calzado–Flores, C., J. Verde–Star, M. Morales–Vallarta, and J.J. Segura–Luna. "Possible Inhibition of Entamoeba invadens Encystation by Castela texana." *Archives of Medical Research* 31 (2000): S196–S197.

Cudweed

Caceresa, Armando, Alma V. Alvareza, Ana E. Ovandoa, and Blanca E. Samayoa. "Plants Used in Guatemala for the Treatment of Respiratory Diseases. 1. Screening of 68 Plants Against Gram–Positive Bacteria." *Journal of Ethnopharmacology* 31, 2 (1991): 193–208.

Rojas, Gabriela, Juan Lévaro, Jaime Tortoriello, and Victor Navarro. "Antimicrobial Evaluation of Certain Plants Used in Mexican Traditional Medicine For the Treatment of Respiratory Diseases." *Journal of Ethnopharmacology* 74 (2001): 97–101.

Villagómez–Ibarra, J. Roberto, Maricruz Sánchez, Ofelia Espejo, Armida Zúniga–Estrada, J. Martín Torres–Valencia, and Pedro Joseph–Nathan. "Antimicrobial Activity of Three Mexican Gnaphalium Species." *Fitoterapia* 72 (2001): 692–694.

Cypress

Homer, K.A., F. Manji, and D. Beighton. "Inhibition of Peptidase and Glycosidase Activities of Porphyromonas Gingivalis, Bacteroides Intermedius and Treponema Denticola by Plant Extracts." *Journal of Clinical Periodontology* 19, 5 (1992): 305–310.

Lopéz, L., M.A. Villavicencio, A. Albores, M. Martínez, J. de la Garza, J. Meléndez–Zajgla, and V. Maldonado. "Cupressus Lusitanica (Cupressaceae) Leaf Extract Induces Apoptosis in Cancer Cells." *Journal of Ethnopharmacology* 80 (2002): 115–120.

Pauly, Ginette, Abdelhamid Yani, Louis Piovetti, and Colette Bernard–Dagen. "Volatile Constituients of the Leaves of Cupressus Sempervirens." *Phytochemistry* 22, 4 (1983): 957–959.

Piovetti, Louis, Abdelhamid Yani, Georges Combaut, and Anne Diara. "Waxes of Cupressus Dupreziana and Cupressus Sempervirens." *Phytochemistry* 20, 5 (1981): 1135–1136.

Ponce–Macotela, M., I. Navarro–Alegria, M.N. Martinez–Gordillo, R. and Alvarez–Chacon. "In Vitro Effect Against Giardia of 14 Plant Extracts." *Revista De Investigacion Clinica* 46, 5 (1994): 343–347.

Datura

Abena, A.A., L.M. Miguel, A. Mouanga, Th. Hondi Assah, and M. Diatewa. "Evaluation of Analgesic Effect of Datura Fastuosa Leaves and Seed Extracts." *Fitoterapia* 74 (2003): 486–488.

Eftekhar, Fereshteh, Morteza Yousefzadi, and V. Tafakori. "Antimicrobial Activity of Datura Innoxia and Datura Stramonium." *Fitoterapia* 76 (2005): 118– 120.

Evens, William C. and Aim–On Somanabandhl. "Alkoloids of Datura Discolor." *Phytochemistry* 13 (1974): 304–305.

Gnanamani, A., K. Shanmuga Priya, N. Radhakrishnan, and Mary Babu. "Antibacterial Activity of Two Plant Extracts on Eight Burn Pathogens." *Journal of Ethnopharmacology* 86 (2003): 59–61.

Griffin, William J. and G. David Lin. "Chemotaxonomy and Geographical Distribution of Tropane Alkaloids." *Phytochemistry* 53 (2000): 623–637.

Miraldia, Elisabetta, Alessandra Masti, Sara Ferri, and Ida Barni Comparini. "Distribution of Hyoscyamine and Scopolamine in Datura Stramonium." *Fitoterapia* 72 (2001): 644–648

Pate, David W. and John E. Averett. "Flavonoids of Datura." *Biochemical Systematics and Ecology* 14, 6 (1986): 647–649.

Priya, K. Shanmuga, A. Gnanamani, N. Radhakrishnan, and Mary Babu. "Healing Potential of Datura Alba on Burn Wounds in Albino Rats." *Journal of Ethnopharmacology* 83 (2002): 193–199.

Rajesh, G.L. Sharma. "Studies on Antimycotic Properties of Datura Metel." *Journal of Ethnopharmacology* 80 (2002): 193–197.

Desert Barberry

Ivanovska, N. and S. Philipov. "Study on the Anti–Inflammatory Action of Berberis Vulgaris Root Extract, Alkaloid Fractions and Pure Alkaloids." *International Journal Of Immunopharmacology* 18,10 (1996): 553–561.

Janbaz, K.H. and A.H. Gilani. "Studies on Preventive and Curative Effects of Berberine on Chemical–Induced Hepatotoxicity in Rodents." *Fitoterapia* 71 (2000): 25–33.

Ji, Xiuhong, Yi Li, Huwei Liu, Yuning Yan, and Jiashi Li. "Determination of the Alkaloid Content in Different Parts of some Mahonia Plants by HPCE." *Pharmaceutica Acta Helvetiae* 74 (2000): 387–391.

Khin–Maung–U and Nwe–Nwe–Wai. "Effect of Berberine on Enterotoxin–Induced Intestinal Fluid Accumulation in Rats." *J Diarrhoeal Dis Res* 10, 4 (1992): 201–204.

Kostalova, D., A. Kardosova, and V. Hajnicka. "Effect of Mahonia Aquifolium Stem Bark Crude Extract and One of its Polysaccharide Components on Production of IL–8." *Fitoterapia* 72 (2001): 802–806.

Sack, R.B. and J.L. Froehlich. "Berberine Inhibits Intestinal Secretory Response of Vibrio Cholerae and Escherichia Coli Enterotoxins." *Infect Immun* 35, 2 (1982): 471–475.

Shamsa, F., A. Ahmadiani, and R. Khosrokhavar. "Antihistaminic and Anticholinergic Activity of Barberry Fruit (Berberis Vulgaris) in the Guinea–Pig Ileum." *Journal of Ethnopharmacology* 64 (1999): 161–166

Sohni, Y.R., P. Kaimal, and R.M. Bhatt. "The Antiamoebic Effect of a Crude Drug Formulation of Herbal Extracts Against Entamoeba Histolytica In Vitro and in Vivo." *Journal of Ethnopharmacology* 45, 1 (1995): 43–52.

Sohni, Youvraj R. and Ranjan M. Bhatt. "Activity of a Crude Extract Formulation in

Experimental Hepatic Amoebiasis and in Immunomodulation Studies." *Journal of Ethnopharmacology* 54 (1996): 119–124.

Stermitz, F.R., J. Tawara–Matsuda, P. Lorenz, P. Mueller, L. Zenewicz, and K. Lewis. "5'–Methoxyhydnocarpin–D and Pheophorbide A: Berberis Species Components That Potentiate Berberine Growth Inhibition of Resistant Staphylococcusaureus." *Journal of Natural Products* 63, 8 (2000): 1146–1149.

Stermitz, Frank R., Teresa D. Beeson, Paul J. Mueller, Jen–Fang Hsiang, and Kim Lewis. "Staphylococcus Aureus MDR Effux Pump Inhibitors from a Berberis and a Mahonia (Sensu Strictu) Species." *Biochemical Systematics and Ecology* 29 (2001): 793–798.

Yesilada, Erdem and Esra Küpeli. Berberis Crataegina DC. "Root Exhibits Potent Anti–Inflammatory, Analgesic and Febrifuge Effects in Mice and Rats." *Journal of Ethnopharmacology* 79 (2002): 237–248.

Desert Cotton

Bai, Junping and Yuliang Shi. "Inhibition of T–Type Ca2+ Currents in Mouse Spermatogenic Cells by Gossypol, an Antifertility Compound." *European Journal of Pharmacology* 440 (2002): 1–6.

Coutinho, Elsimar Metzker. "Gossypol: A Contraceptive for Men." *Contraception* 65 (2002): 259–263.

Coutinho, Elsimar M., Célia Athayde, Gabriel Atta, Zhi–Ping Gut, Zhen–Wen Chen, Guo–Wei Sang, Edward Emuveyan, Adeyemi O. Adekunle, Japheth Mati, Joseph Otubu, Marcus M. Reidenberg, and Sheldon J. Segal. "Gossypol Blood Levels and Inhibition of Spermatogenesis in Men Taking Gossypol as a Contraceptive." *Contraception* 61 (2000): 61–67.

Fiorini, Céline, Anne Tilloy–Ellul, Stephan Chevalier, Claude Charuel, and Georges Pointis. "Sertoli Cell Junctional Proteins as Early Targets for Different Classes of Reproductive Toxicants." *Reproductive Toxicology* 18 (2004): 413–421.

Hedin, P. A., A.C. Thompson, R.C. Gueldner, and J.P. Minyard. "Constituents of the Cotton Bud." *Phytochemistry* 10 (1971): 3316–3318.

Lane, Harry C. and Michael F. Schuster. "Condensed Tannins of Cotton Leaves." *Phytochemistry* 20 (1981): 425–427.

Waage, Susan K. and Paul A. Hedin. "Biologically Active Flavonoids from Gossypium Arboreum." *Phytochemistry* 23, 2 (1984): 2509–2511.

Desert Lavender

Pandey, V. N. and N. K. Dubey. "Antifungal Potential of Leaves and Essential Oils from Higher Plants Against Soil Phytopathogens." *Soil Biology and Biochemistry* 26, 10 (1994): 1417–1421.

Kuhnt, M., A. Probstle, H. Rimpler, R. Bauer, and M. Heinrich. "Biological and Pharmacological Activities and Further Constituents of Hyptis Verticellata." *Planta Medica* 61, 3 (1995): 227–232.

Bispo, M.D., R.H.V. Mourao, E.M. Franzotti, K.B.R. Bomfim, M. de F. Arrigoni–Blank, M.P.N. Moreno, M. Marchioro, and A.R. Antoniolli. "Antinociceptive and Anti-edematogenic Effects of the Aqueous Extract of Hyptis Pectinata Leaves in Experimental Animals." *Journal of Ethnopharmacology* 76 (2001): 81–86.

Asekun, Olayinka Taiwo, Olusegun Ekundayo, and Bolanle A. Adeniyi. "Antimicrobial Activity of the Essential Oil of Hyptis Suaveolens Leaves." *Fitoterapia* 70 (1999): 440–442.

Rojas, A., Hernandez, L., Pereda–Miranda, R., and Mata, R. "Screening for Antimicrobial Activity of Crude Drug Extracts and Pure Natural Products from Mexican Medicinal Plants." *Journal of Ethnopharmacology* 35, 3 (1992): 275–83.

Desert Milkweed

Chiu, F.C. and T.R. Watson. "Conformational Factors in Cardiac Glycoside Activity." *Journal of Medical Chemistry* 28, 4 (1985): 509–515.

Giordani, R., J. Moulin–Traffort, and P. Regli. "Glycosidic Activities of Candida Albicans After Action of Vegetable Latex Saps (Natural Antifungals) and Isoconazole (Synthetic Antifungal)." *Mycoses* 34, 1–2 (1991): 67–73.

Radford, D.J., A.D. Gillies, J.A. Hinds, and P. Duffy. "Naturally Occurring Cardiac Glycosides." *Medical Journal of Australia* 144, 10 (1986): 540–544.

Sady, Michael B. and James N. Seiber. "Chemical Differences Between Species of Asclepias from the Intermountain Region of North America." *Phytochemistry* 30, 9 (1991): 3001–3003.

Seiber, James N., Carolyn J. Nelson, and S. Mark Lee. "Cardenolides in the Latex and Leaves of Seven Asclepias Species and Calotropis Procrea." *Phytochemistry* 21, 9 (1982): 2343–2348.

Elder

Ahmadiani, A., M. Fereidoni, S. Semnanian, M. Kamalinejad, and S. Saremi. "Antinociceptive and Anti–inflammatory Effects of Sambucus Ebulus Rhizome Extract in Rats." *Journal of Ethnopharmacology* 61 (1998): 229–235.

Bergner, Paul. "Elderberry (Sambucus Nigra, Canadensis)." *Medical Herbalism* 8, 4 (1996–1997).

Buhrmester, Rex A., John E. Ebinger, and David S. Seigler. "Sambunigrin and Cyanogenic Variability in Populations of Sambucus Canadensis L. (Caprifoliaceae)." *Biochemical Systematics and Ecology* 28 (2000): 689–695.

Caceres, Armando, Brenda R. Lopez, Melba A. Giron, and Heidi Logemann. "Plants Used in Guatemala for the Treatment of Dermatophytic Infections. 1. Screening for Antimycotic Activity of 44 Plant Extracts." *Journal of Ethnopharmacology* 31 (1991): 263–276.

Caceres, Armando, Orlando Cano, Blanca Samayoa and Leila Aguilar. "Plants Used in Guatemala for the Treatment of Gastrointestinal Disorders. 1. Screening of 84 Plants Against Enterobacteria." *Journal of Ethnopharmacology* 30 (1990): 55–73.

Hernández, Nancy E., M.L. Tereschuk, and L.R. Abdala. "Antimicrobial Activity of Flavonoids in Medicinal Plants from Tafí del Valle (Tucumán, Argentina)." *Journal of Ethnopharmacology* 73 (2000): 317–322.

Losey, Robert J., Nancy Stenholm, Patty Whereat–Phillips, and Helen Vallianatos. "Exploring the Use of Red Elderberry (Sambucus Racemosa) Fruit on the Southern Northwest Coast of North America." *Journal of Archaeological Science* 30 (2003): 695–707.

McCutcheon, A.R., T.E. Roberts, E. Gibbions, S.M. Ellis, L.A. Babiuk, R.E.W. Hancock, and G.H.N. Towers. "Antiviral Screening of British Columbian Medicinal Plants." *Journal of Ethnopharmacology* 49 (1995): 101–110.

Elephant Tree

Noguera, B., E. Díaz, M.V. García, A. San Feliciano, J.L. López–Perez, and A. Israel. "Anti–Inflammatory Activity of Leaf Extract and Fractions of Bursera Simaruba

(L.) Sarg (Burseraceae)." *Journal of Ethnopharmacology* 92 (2004): 129–133.

Sosa, S., M.J. Balick, R. Arvigo, R.G. Esposito, C. Pizza, G. Altinier, and A. Tubaro. "Screening of the Topical Anti–Inflammatory Activity of some Central American Plants." *Journal of Ethnopharmacology* 81 (2002): 211–215.

Rosas–Arreguín, P., Pablo Arteaga–Nieto, Ramón Reynoso–Orozco, Julio C. Villagómez–Castro a, M. Sabanero–López, Ana M. Puebla–Pérez, Carlos Calvo–Méndez. "Bursera Fagaroides, Effect of an Ethanolic Extract on Ornithine Decarboxylase (ODC) Activity In Vitro and on the Growth of Entamoeba Histolytica." *Experimental Parasitology* 119 (2008): 398–402.

Mormon Tea

Feresin, Gabriela Egly, Alejandro Tapia, Silvia N. López, and Susana A. Zacchino. "Antimicrobial Activity of Plants Used in Traditional Medicine of San Juan Province, Argentine." *Journal of Ethnopharmacology* 78 (2001): 103–107.

Gurni, A. Alberto and Marcelo L. Wagner. "Proanthocyanidins from some Argentine Species of Ephedra." *Biochemical Systematics and Ecology* 12, 3 (1984): 319–320.

Konno, Chohachi, Takashi Taguchi, Misturu Tamada, and Hiroshi Hikino. "Ephedroxane, Anti–Inflammatory Principle of Ephedra Herbs." *Phytochemistry* 18 (1979): 697–698.

Filaree

Saleh, Nabiel A.M., Zeinab A.R. El–Karemy, Ragaa M.A.. Mansour, and Abdel–Aziz A. Fayed. "A Chemosystematic Study of some Geraniaceae." *Phytochemistry* 22, 11 (1983): 2501–2505.

Sroka, Z., H. Rzadkowska–Bodalska, and I. Mazol. "Antioxidative Effect of Extracts from Erodium Cicutarium L." *Z Naturforsch* 49, 11–12 (1994):881–884.

Zielinska–Jenczylik, J., A. Sypula, E. Budko, and H. Rzadkowska–Bodalska. "Interferonogenic and Antiviral Effect of Extracts from Erodium Cicutarium. II. Modulatory Activity of Erodium Cicutarium Extracts." *Arch Immunol Ther Exp (WARSZ)* 36, 5 (1988): 527–36.

Golden Smoke

Abbasoglu, U., B. Sener, Y. Gunay, and H. Temizer. "Antimicrobial Activity of some Isoquinoline Alkaloids." *Archiv Der Pharmazie* 324, 6 (1991): 379–80.

Adams, Michael, Francine Gmunder, and Matthias Hamburger. "Plants Traditionally Used in Age Related Brain Disorders—A Survey of Ethnobotanical Literature." *Journal of Ethnopharmacology* 113 (2007): 363–381.

Chang, Cheng–Kuei and Mao–Tsun Lin. "DL-Tetrahydropalmatine May Act Through Inhibition of Amygdaloid Release of Dopamine to Inhibit an Epileptic Attack in Rats." *Neuroscience Letters* 307 (2001): 163–166.

Chernevskaja, N.I., O.A. Krishtal, and A.Y. Valeyev. "Inhibitions of the GABA–Induced Currents of Rat Neurons by the Alkaloid Isocoryne from the Plant Corydalis Pseudoadunca." *Toxicon* 28 (1990): 727–730.

Ito, Chihiro, Toyoko Mizuno, Tian–Shung Wua, and Hiroshi Furukawa. "Alkaloids from Corydalis." *Phytochemistry* 29 (1990): 2044–2045.

Kleber, E., W. Schneider, H.L. Schafer, and E.F. Elstner. "Modulation of Key Reactions of the Catecholamine Metabolism by Extracts from Eschscholtzia Californica and Corydalis Cava." *Arzneimittelforschung* 45, 2 (1995): 127–31.

Lin, Mao–Tsun, Jhi–Joung Wang, and Ming–Shing Young. "The Protective Effect of DL–tetrahydropalmatine Against the Development of Amygdala Kindling Seizures in Rats." *Neuroscience Letters* 320 (2002): 113–116.

Ma, Wei guang, Yukiharu Fukushi, and Satoshi Tahara. "Fungitoxic Alkaloids from Hokkaido Corydalis species." *Fitoterapia* 70 (1999): 25–265.

Hopbush

Amabeoku, G.J., P. Eagles, G. Scott, I. Mayeng, and E. Springfield. "Analgesic and Antipyretic Effects of Dodonaea Angustifolia and Salvia Africana–Lutea." *Journal of Ethnopharmacology* 75 (2001): 117–124.

Getie, M., T. Gebre–Mariam, R. Rietz, C. Hohne, C. Huschka, M. Schmidtke, A. Abate, and R.H.H. Neubert. "Evaluation of the Anti–Microbial and Anti–Inflammatory Activities of the Medicinal Plants Dodonaea Viscosa, Rumex Nervosus and Rumex Abyssinicus." *Fitoterapia* 74 (2003): 139–143.

Heerden, F.R. van, A.M. Viljoen, and B–E. van Wyk. "The Major Flavonoid of Dodonaea Angustifolia." *Fitoterapia* 71 (2000): 602–604.

Rojas, Alejandra, Lourdes Hernandez, Rogelio Pereda–Miranda, and Rachel Mata. "Screening for Antimicrobial Activity of Crude Drug Extracts and Pure Natural Products from Mexican Medicinal Plants." *Journal of Ethnopharmacology* 35, 3 (1992): 275–283.

Sachdev, Kusum and Dinesh K. Kulshreshtha. "Viscosol, a C–3–Prenylated Flavonoid from Dodonaea Viscosa." *Phytochemistry* 25, 8 (1986): 1967–1969.

Wagner, Hildebert, Christine Ludwig, Lutz Grotjahn, and Mohd S.Y. Khan. "Biologically Active Saponins from Dodonaea Viscosa." *Phytochemistry* 26 (1987): 697–701.

Jojoba

Boven, M. Van, R. Busson, M. Cokelaere, G. Flo, and E. Decuypere. "4–Demethyl Simmondsin from Simmondsia Chinensis." *Industrial Crops and Products* 12 (2000): 203–208.

Cappillino, Patrick, Robert Kleiman, and Claudia Botti. "Composition of Chilean Jojoba Seeds." *Industrial Crops and Products* 17 (2003): 177–182.

Ham, Roeline, Sabien Vermaut, Gerda Flo, Marnix Cokelaere, and Eddy Decuypere. "Digestive Performance of Dogs Fed a Jojoba Meal Supplemented Diet." *Industrial Crops and Products* 12 (2000): 159–163.

York, David A., Lori Singer, Julian Oliver, Thomas P. Abbott, and George A. Bray. "The Detrimental Effect of Simmondsin on Food Intake and Body Weight of Rats." *Industrial Crops and Products* 12 (2000): 183–192.

Juniper

Adams, Robert P. "Systematics of the One Seeded Juniperus of the Eastern Hemisphere Based on Leaf Essential Oils and Random Amplified Polymorphic DNAs (RAPDs)." *Biochemical Systematics and Ecology* 28 (2000): 529–543.

Adams, Robert P., Ernst Von Rudloff, and Lawrence Hogge. "Chemosystematic Studies of the Western North American Junipers Based on their Volatile Oils." *Biochemical Systematics and Ecology* 11, 3 (1983): 189–193.

Adams, Robert P., Thomas A. Zanoni, and Lawrence Hogge. "Analyses of the Volatile Leaf Oils of Juniperus Deppeana and its Infraspecific Taxa: Chemosystematic Implications." *Biochemical Systemics and Ecoclogy* 12, 1 (1984): 23–27.

Adams, Robert P., Thomas A. Zanoni, Ernst Von Rudloff, and Lawrence Hogge. "The South–Western USA and Northern Mexico One–seeded Junipers: their Volatile Oils and Evolution." *Biochemical Systematics and Ecology* 9, 2/3 (1981): 93–96.

Karaman, I., F. Sahin, M. Güllüce, H. Öðütçü, M. Sengül, and A. Adigüzel. "Antimicrobial Activity of Aqueous and Methanol Extracts of Juniperus Oxycedrus L." *Journal of Ethnopharmacology* 85 (2003): 231–235.

San Feliciano, A., M. Gordaliza, J.M. Miguel del Corral, M.A. Castro, M.D. Garcia–Gravalos, and P. Ruiz–Lazaro. "Antineoplastic and Antiviral Activities of some Cyclolignans." *Planta Med* 59, 3 (1993): 246–249.

Tunón, H., C. Olavsdotter, and L. Bohlin. "Evaluation of Anti–Inflammatory Activity of some Swedish Medicinal Plants. Inhibition of Prostaglandin biosynthesis and PAF–Induced Exocytosis." *Journal of Ethnopharmacology* 48 (1995): 61–76.

Kidneywood

Alvarez, Laura and Guillermo Delgado. "C– and O–Glycosyl–á–Hydroxydihydrochalcones from Eysenhardtia Polystachya." *Phytochemistry* 50 (1999): 681–687.

Burns, Duncan T., Barry G. Dalgarno, Paul E. Gargan, and James Grimshaw. "An Isoflavone and a Coumestan from Eysenhardtia Polystachya–Robert Boyle's Fluorescent Acid–base Indicator." *Phytochemistry* 23, 1 (1984): 167–169.

Wächtera, Gerald A., Joseph J. Hoffmann, Todd Furbacher, Mary E. Blake, and Barbara N. Timmermann. "Antibacterial and Antifungal Flavanones from Eysenhardtia Texana." *Phytochemistry* 52 (1999): 1469–1471.

Leadwort

Abdul, Kamal Mohammed and Rao Pinninti Ramchender. "Modulatory Effect of Plumbagin (5–Hydroxy–2–Methyl1–1,4–Naphthoquinone) on Macrophage Functions in BALB/c Mice. 1. Potentiation of Macrophage Bactericidal Activity." *Immunopharmacology* 30 (1995): 231–236.

Ahmad, Iqbal, Zafar Mehmood, and Faiz Mohammad. "Screening of Some Indian Medicinal Plants for their Antimicrobial Properties." *Journal of Ethnopharmacology* 62 (1998): 183–193.

Bhattacharyya, J. and Vicente R. De Carvalho. "Epi–Isoshinanolone from Plumbago Scandens." *Phytochemistry* 25, 3 (1986): 764–765.

Reddy, J. Suresh, P. Rajeswara Rao, and Mada S. Reddy. "Wound Healing Effects of Heliotropium Indicum, Plumbago Zeylanicum and Acalypha Indica in Rats." *Journal of Ethnopharmacology* 79 (2002): 249–251.

Solomon, F. Emerson, A.C. Sharada, and P. Uma Devi. "Toxic Effects of Crude Root Extract of Plumbago Rosea (Rakta chitraka) on Mice and Rats." *Journal of Ethnopharmacology* 38 (1993): 79–84.

Vijayakumar, R., M. Senthilvelan, R. Ravindran, and R. Sheela Devi. "Plumbago Zeylanica Action on Blood Coagulation Profile with and without Blood Volume Reduction." *Vascular Pharmacology* 45 (2006): 86–90.

Wang, Yuan–Chuen and Tung–Liang Huang. "High–Performance Liquid Chromatography for Quantification of Plumbagin, an Anti–Helicobacter Pylori Compound of Plumbago Zeylanica L." *Journal of Chromatography A*, 1094 (2005): 99–104.

Mallow

Billeter, Martin, Beat Meier, and Otto Sticher. "8–Hydroxyflavonoid Glucuronides from Malva Sylvestris." *Phytochemistry* 30, 3 (1991): 987–990.

Classen, B. and W. Blaschek. "High Molecular Weight Acidic Polysaccharides from Malva Sylvestris and Alcea Rosea." *Planta Med* 64, 7 (1998): 640–644.

Giron, Lidia M., Virginia Freire, Aida Alonzo, and Armando Caceres. "Ethnobotanical Survey of the Medicinal Flora Used by the Caribs of Guatemala." *Journal of Ethnopharmacology* 34 (1991): 113–187.

Gonda, R., M. Tomoda, N. Shimizu, and M. Kanari. "Characterization of an Acidic Polysaccharide from the Seeds of Malva Verticillata Stimulating the Phagocytic Activity of Cells of the RES." *Planta Med* 56, 1 (1990): 73–76.

Gonda, Ryoko, Masashi Tomoda, and Noriko Shimizu. "Structure and Anticomplementary Activity of an Acidic Polysaccharide from the Leaves of Malva Sylvestris var. Mauritiana." *Carbohydrate Research* 198 (1990): 323–329.

Grierson, D.S. and A.J. Afolayan. "Antibacterial Activity of some Indigenous Plants Used for the Treatment of Wounds in the Eastern Cape, South Africa." *Journal of Ethnopharmacology* 66 (1999): 103–106.

Schmidgall, J., E. Schnetz, and A. Hensel. "Evidence for Bioadhesive Effects of Polysaccharides and Polysaccharide–Containing Herbs in an ex vivo Bioadhesion Assay on Buccal Membranes." *Planta Med* 66, 1 (2000): 48–53.

Shimizu, N., H. Asahara, M. Tomoda, R. Gonda, and N. Ohara. "Constituents of Seed of Malva Verticillata. VII. Structural Features and Reticuloendothelial System–Potentiating Activity of MVS–I, the Major Neutral Polysaccharide." *Chem Pharm Bull (Tokyo)* 39, 10 (1991): 2630–2632.

Wang, Xing and Greg J. Bunkers. "Potent Heterologous Antifungal Proteins from Cheeseweed (Malva parviflora)." *Biochemical and Biophysical Research Communications* 279 (2000): 669–673.

Manzanita

Dykes, Gary A., Ryszard Amarowicz, and Ronald B. Pegg. "Enhancement of Nisin Antibacterial Activity by a Bearberry (Arctostaphylos Uva–ursi) Leaf Extract." *Food Microbiology* 20 (2003): 211–216.

Grases, F., G. Melero, A. Costa–Bauza, R. Prieto, and J.G. March. "Urolithiasis and Phytotherapy." *International Urology and Nephrology* 26, 5 (1994): 505–511

Marsh Fleabane

Domínguez, Xorge Alejandro and Angeles Zamudio. "b–Amyrin Acetate and Campesterol from Pluchea Odorata." *Phytochemistry* 11 (1972): 1179.

Pérez–García, Francisco, Esther Marín, Salvador Canigueral, and Tomás Adzet. "Anti–Inflammatory Action of Pluchea Sagittalis: Involvemnet of an Antioxidant Mechanism." *Life Sciences* 59, 24 (1996): 2033–2040.

Reyes–Trejo, Benito and Pedro Joseph–Nathan. "Modhephene derivatives from Pluchea Sericea." *Phytochemistry* 51 (1999): 75–78.

Souza, G. Coelho de, A.P.S. Haas, G.L. von Poser, E.E.S. Schapoval, and E. Elisabetsky. "Ethnopharmacological Studies of Antimicrobial Remedies in the South of Brazil." *Journal of Ethnopharmacology* 90 (2004): 135–143.

Mesquite

Adikwu, M.U., O.K. Udeala, and F.C. Ohiri. "Emulsifying Properties of Prosopis African Gum. S.T.P." *Pharma Sciences* 4, 4 (1994): 298–304.

Aqeel, A., Khursheed, A.K., Viqaruddin, A., and Sabiha, Q. "Antimicrobial

Activity of Julifloricine Isolated from Prosopis Juliflora." *Arzneimittel Forschung* 39, 6 (1989): 652–655.

Mimosa

Pavón, Numa P. and Oscar Briones. "Phenological Patterns of Nine Perennial Plants in an Intertropical Semi–Arid Mexican Scrub." *Journal of Arid Environments* 49 (2001): 265–277.

Yusuf, Umi Kalsom, Noriha Abdullah, Baki Bakar, Khairuddin Itam, Faridah Abdullah, and Mohd Aspollah Sukari. "Flavonoid Glycosides in the Leaves of Mimosa Species." *Biochemical Systematics and Ecology* 31 (2003): 443–445.

Mountain Marigold

Abdala, Lidia Rosa. "Chemosystematic Interpretations of the Flavonoids Identified in Tagetes Gracilis (Asteraceae)." *Biochemical Systematics and Ecology* (2003).

Abdala, Lidia Rosa. "Flavonoids of the Aerial Parts from Tagetes Lucida (Asteraceae)." *Biochemical Systematics and Ecology* 27 (1999): 753–754.

Heras, B. de las, K. Slowing, J. Benedí, E. Carretero, T. Ortega, C. Toledo, P. Bermejo, I. Iglesias, M.J. Abad, P. Gómez–Serranillos, P.A. Liso, A. Villar, and X. Chiriboga. "Antiinflammatory and Antioxidant Activity of Plants Used in Traditional Medicine in Ecuador." *Journal of Ethnopharmacology* 61 (1998): 161–166.

Kruger, C.L., M. Murphy, Z. DeFreitas, F. Pfannkuch, and J. Heimbach. "An Innovative Approach to the Determination of Safety for a Dietary Ingredient Derived from a New Source: Case Study Using a Crystalline Lutein Product." *Food and Chemical Toxicology* 40 (2002): 1535–1549.

Piccaglia, Roberta, Mauro Marotti, and Silvia Grandi. "Lutein and Lutein Ester Content in Different Types of Tagetes Patula and T. Erecta." *Industrial Crops and Products* 8 (1998): 45–51.

Night Blooming Cereus

Knight, John C. and George R. Pettit. "Arizona Flora: The Sterols of Peniocereus Greggii." *Phytochemistry* 8 (1969): 477–482.

Ocotillo

Domínguez, X. A., J. O. Velasquez, and D. Guerra. "Extractives from the Flowers of Fouquieria Splendens." *Phytochemistry* 11, 9 (1972): 2888.

Jensen, Søren Rosendal and Bent Juhl Nielsen. "Iridoid Glucosides in Fouquieriaceae." *Phytochemistry* 21, 7 (1982): 1623–1629.

Scogin, Ron. "Leaf Phenolics of the Fouquieriaceae." *Biochemical Systematics and Ecology* 6, 4 (1978): 297–298.

Passionflower

Andersen, Lise, Anne Adsersen and Jerzy W. Jaroszewski. "Cyanogenesis of Passiflora Foetida." *Phytochemistry* 47, 6 (1998): 1049–1050.

Carlini, E.A. "Plants and the Central Nervous System." *Pharmacology, Biochemistry and Behavior* 75 (2003): 501–512.

Dhawan, Kamaldeep and Anupam Sharma. "Antitussive Activity of the Methanol Extract of Passiflora Incarnata Leaves." *Fitoterapia* 73 (2002): 397–399.

Dhawan, Kamaldeep and Anupam Sharma. "Prevention of Chronic Alcohol and Nicotine–Induced Azospermia, Sterility and Decreased Libido, by a Novel

Tri–Substituted Benzoflavone Moiety from Passiflora Incarnata Linneaus In Healthy Male Rats." *Life Sciences* 71 (2002): 3059–3069.

Dhawan, Kamaldeep, Suresh Kumar, and Anupam Sharma. "Anxiolytic Activity of Aerial and Underground Parts of Passiflora Incarnata." *Fitoterapia* 72 (2001): 922–926.

Dhawan, Kamaldeep, Suresh Kumar, and Anupam Sharma. "Comparative Biological Activity Study on Passiflora Incarnata and P. Edulis." *Fitoterapia* 72 (2001): 698–702.

Dhawan, Kamaldeep, Suresh Kumar, and Anupam Sharma. "Suppression of Alcohol–Cessation–Oriented Hyper–Anxiety by the Benzoflavone Moiety of Passiflora Incarnata Linneaus in Mice." *Journal of Ethnopharmacology* 81 (2002): 239–244.

Jaroszewski, Jerzy W., Elin S. Olafsdottir, Petrine Wellendorph, Jette Christensen, Henrik Franzyk, Brinda Somanadhan, Bogdan A. Budnik, Lise Bolt Jørgensen, and Vicki Clausen. "Cyanohydrin Glycosides of Passiflora: Distribution Pattern, a Saturated Cyclopentane Derivative from P. Guatemalensis, and Formation of Pseudocyanogenic a–hydroxyamides as Isolation Artifacts." *Phytochemistry* 59 (2002): 501–511.

Seigler, David S., Guido F. Pauli, Adolf Nahrstedt, and Rosemary Leen. "Cyanogenic Allosides and Glucosides from Passiflora Edulis and Carica Papaya." *Phytochemistry* 60 (2002): 873–882.

Wolfman, Claudia, Hatdee Viola, Alejandro Paladini, Federico Dajas, and Jorge H. Medina. "Possible Anxiolytic Effects of Chrysin, a Central Benzodiazepine Receptor Ligand Isolated from Passiflora Coerulea." *Pharmacology Biochemistry and Behavior* 47 (1994).

Penstemon

Franzyk, Henrik, Soren Rosendal Jensen, and Frank R. Stermitz. "Iridoid Glucosides from Penstemon Secundiflorus and Grandiflorus: Revised Structure of 10–Hydroxy–8–Epihastatoside." *Phytochemistry* 49, 7 (1998): 2025–2030.

Stermitz, Frank R., Andrei Blokhin, Christina S. Poley and Robert E. Krull. "Iridoid Glycosides of Additional Penstemon Species." *Phytochemistry* 37, 5 (1994): 1283–1286.

Wysokinska, H. and Z. Skrzypek. "Studies on Iridoids of Tissue Cultures of Penstemon Serrulatus: Isolation and their Antiproliferative Properties." *J Nat Prod* 55, 1 (1992): 58–63.

Periwinkle

Avijit Banerji and Manas Chakrabarty. "Lochvinerine: a New Indole Alkaloid of Vinca Major." *Phytochemistry* 13 (1974): 2309–2312.

Avijit Banerji and Manas Chakrabarty. "Majvinine: a New Indole Alkaloid of Vinca Major." *Phytochemistry* 16 (1977): 1124–1125.

Rahman, Atta–ur, Abida Sultana, Farzana Nighat, M. Khalid Bhatti, Semra Kurucu, and Murat Kartal. "Alkaloids from Vinca Major." *Phytochemistry* 38, 4 (1995): 1057–1061.

Pipevine

Houghton, Peter J. and Ibironke M. Osibogun. "Flowering Plants Used Against Snakebite." *Journal of Ethnopharmacology* 39 (1993): 1–29.

Moreno, J.J. "Effect of Aristolochic Acid on Arachidonic Acid Cascade and In Vivo Models of Inflammation." *Imrnunopharmacology*, 26 (1993): 1–9.

Mors, Walter B., Maria Celia do Nascimento, Bettina M. Ruppelt Pereira, Nuno Alvares Pereira. "Plant Natural Products Active Against Snake Bite the Molecular Approach." *Phytochemistry* 55 (2000): 627–642.

Shaohua, Zhu, Sunnassee Ananda, Yuan Ruxia, Ren Liang, Chen Xiaorui, and Liu Liang. "Fatal Renal Failure Due to the Chinese Herb "GuanMu Tong" (Aristolochia Manshuriensis): Autopsy Findings and Review of Literature." *Forensic Science International* 199 (2010): e5–e7.

Tian–Shung, W, Amooru G. Damu, Chung–Ren Su, and Ping–Chung–Ko. "Chemical Constituents and Pharmacology of Aristolochia Species." *Studies in Natural Products Chemistry*, 32 (xxxx): 855–1018.

Poreleaf

Guillet, Gabriel, André Bélanger, and John Arnason. "Volitile Monoterpenes in Porophyllum Gracile and P. Ruderale (Asteraceae): Identification, Localization and Insecticidal Synergism with á–Terthienyl." *Phytochemistry* 49, 2 (1998): 423–429.

Prickly Pear

Budinsky, A., R. Wolfram, A. Oguogho, Y. Efthimiou, Y. Stamatopoulos, and H. Sinzinger. "Regular Ingestion of Opuntia Robusta Lowers Oxidation Injury." *Prostaglandins, Leukotrienes and Essential Fatty Acids* 65, 1 (2001): 45–50.

Bwititi, P., C.T. Musabayane, and C.F.B. Nhachi. "Effects of Opuntia Megacantha on Blood Glucose and Kidney Function in Streptozotocin Diabetic Rats." *Journal of Ethnopharmacology* 69 (2000): 247–252.

Frati–Munari, A.C., R. Licona–Quesada, C.R. Araiza–Andraca, R. Lopez–Ledesma, and A. Chavez–Negrete. "Activity of Opuntia Streptacantha in Healthy Individuals With Induced Hyperglycemia." *Archivos de Investigacion Medica* 21, 2 (1990): 99–102.

Fernandez–Lopez, Jose A., Luis Almela. "Application of High–Performance Liquid Chromatography to the Characterization of the Betalain Pigments in Prickly Pear Fruits." *Journal of Chromatography A*, 913 (2001): 415–420.

Galati, E.M., M.M. Tripodo, A. Trovato, N. Miceli, and M.T. Monforte. "Biological Effect of Opuntia Ficus Indica (L.) Mill. (Cactaceae) Waste Matter Note I: Diuretic Activity." *Journal of Ethnopharmacology* 79 (2002): 17–21.

Galati, E.M., S. Pergolizzi, N. Miceli, M.T. Monforte, and M.M. Tripodo. "Study on the Increment of the Production of Gastric Mucus in Rats Treated with Opuntia Ficus Indica (L.) Mill. Cladodes." *Journal of Ethnopharmacology* 83 (2002): 229–233.

Loro, J.F., I. del Rio, L. Pérez–Santana. "Preliminary Studies of Analgesic and Anti–inflammatory Properties of Opuntia Dillenii Aqueous Extract." *Journal of Ethnopharmacology* 67 (1999): 213–218.

Meckes–Lozoya, M. and R. Ibanez–Camacho. "Hypoglycemic Activity of Opuntia Streptacantha Throughout Its Annual Cycle." *American Journal of Chinese Medicine* 17, 3–4 (1989): 221–224.

Medina–Torres, L., E. Brito–De La Fuente, B. Torrestiana–Sanchez, and R. Katthain. "Rheological Properties of the Mucilage Gum (Opuntia Ficus Indica)." *Food Hydrocolloids* 14 (2000): 417–424.

Park, E.–H. and M.–J. Chun. "Wound Healing Activity of Opuntia Ficus–Indica."

Fitoterapia 72 (2001): 165–167.

Park, Eun–Hee, Ja–Hoon Kahng, Sang Hyun Lee, Kuk–Hyun Shin. "An Anti–Inflammatory Principle from Cactus." *Fitoterapia* 72 (2001): 288–290.

Pimienta–Barrios, Eulogio, María Eugenia González del Castillo–Aranda, and Park S. Nobel. "Ecophysiology of a Wild Platyopuntia Exposed to Prolonged Drought." *Environmental and Experimental Botany* 47 (2002): 77–86.

Roman–Ramos, R., J.L. Flores–Saenz, and F.J. Alarcon–Aguilar. "Anti–hyperglycemic Effect of some Edible Plants." *Journal of Ethnopharmacology* 48 (1995): 25–32.

Prickly Poppy

Bandoni, A.L., F.R. Stermitz, R.V.D. Rondina, and J.D. Coussio. "Alkaloidal Content of Argentine Argemone." *Phytochemistry* 14, 8 (1975): 1785–1788.

Stermitz, F.R., R.J. Ito, S.M. Workman and W.M. Klein. "Alkaloids of Argemone Fruticosa and A. Echinata." *Phytochemistry* 12, 2 (1973): 381–382.

Husain, Sajid, R. Narsimha, and R. Nageswara Rao. "Separation, Identification and Determination of Sanguinarine in Argemone and Other Adulterated Edible Oils by Reversed–Phase High–Performance Liquid Chromatography." *Journal of Chromatography* A, 863 (1999): 123–126.

Shenolikar, I.S., C. Rukmini, K.A.V.R. Krisnamachari, and K. Satayanarayana. "Sanguinarine in the Blood and Urine of Cases of Epidemic Dropsy." *Food and Cosmetics Toxicology* 12, 5–6 (1974): 699–702.

Stermitz, Frank R., Don K. Kim and Kenneth A. Lamon. "Alkaloids of Argemone Albiflora, A. Revicornuta, and A. Turnerae." *Phytochemistry* 12, 6 (1973): 1355–1357.

Stermitz, Frank R., Joseph R. Stermitz, Thomas A. Zanoni, and John Gillespie. "Alkaloids of Argemone Subintegrifolia and A. Munita." *Phytochemistry* 13, 7 (1974): 1151–1153.

Verma, S.K., G. Dev, A.K. Tyagi, S. Goomber, and G.V. Jain. "Argemone Mexicana Poisoning: Autopsy Findings of Two Cases." *Forensic Science International* 115 (2001): 135–141.

Puncturevine

Achenbach, Hans, Harald Hübner, Wolfgang Brandta, and Melchior Reitera. "Cardioactive Steroid Saponins and other Constituents from the Aerial Parts of Tribulus Cistoides." *Phytochemistry* 35, 6 (1994): 1527–1543.

Ali, N.A. Awadh, W.–D. Jülich, C. Kusnick, and U. Lindequist. "Screening of Yemeni medicinal plants for antibacterial and Cytotoxic Activities." *Journal of Ethnopharmacology* 74 (2001): 173–179.

Anand, R., G.K. Patnaik, D.K. Kulshreshtha, and B.N. Dhawan. "Activity of Certain Fractions of Tribulus Terrestris Fruits Against Experimentally Induced Urolithiasis in Rats." *Indian Journal of Experimental Biology* 32, 8 (1994): 548–552.

Bhutani, S. P., S. S. Chibber, and T.R. Seshadri. "Flavonoids of the Fruits and Leaves of Tribulus Terrestris: Constitution of Tribuloside." *Phytochemistry* 8, 1 (1969): 299–303.

Gauthaman, K., P.G. Adaikan, and R.N.V. Prasad. "Aphrodisiac Properties of Tribulus Terrestris Extract (Protodioscin) in Normal and Castrated Rats." *Life Sciences* 71 (2002): 1385–1396.

Kirby, Andrew J. and Richard Schmidt. "The Antioxidant Activity of Chinese Herbs for Eczema and of Placebo Herbs." *Journal of Ethnopharmacology* 56 (1997): 103–108.

Lin, Zhi Xiu, J.R.S. Hoult, and Amala Raman. "Sulphorhodamine B Assay for Measuring Proliferation of a Pigmented Melanocyte Cell Line and its Application to the Evaluation of Crude Drugs Used in the Treatment of Vitiligo." *Journal of Ethnopharmacology* 66 (1999): 141–150.

Sangeeta, D., H. Sidhu, S.K. Thind, and R. Nath. "Effect of Tribulus Terrestris on Oxalate Metabolism in Rats." *Journal of Ethnopharmacology* 44, 2 (1994): 61–66.

Wu, Tian–Shung, Li–Shian Shi, and Shang–Chu Kuo. "Alkaloids and Other Constituents from Tribulus Terrestris." *Phytochemistry* 50 (1999): 1411–1415.

Wang, B., L. Ma, and T. Liu. "406 Cases of Angina Pectoris in Coronary Heart Disease Treated with Saponin of Tribulus Terrestris." *Chung His I Chien Ho Tsa Chih Chinese Journal Of Modern Developments* 10, 2 (1990): 68, 85–87.

Wu, G., S. Jiang, F. Jiang, D. Zhu, H. Wu, and S. Jiang. "Steroidal Glycosides from Tribulus terrestris." *Phytochemistry* 42, 6 (1996): 1677–1681.

Purple Gromwell

Grases, F., G. Melero, A. Costa–Bauza, R. Prieto, and J.G. March. "Urolithiasis and Phytotherapy." *International Urology and Nephrology* 26, 5 (1994): 507–511.

Krenn, L., H. Wiedenfeld, and E. Roeder. "Pyrrolizidine Alkaloids from Lithospermum Officinale." *Phytochemistry* 37, 1 (1994): 275–277.

Singh, Fiza, Dayuan Gao, Mark G. Lebwohl, and Huachen Wei. "Shikonin Modulates Cell Proliferation by Inhibiting Epidermal Growth Factor Receptor Signaling in Human Epidermoid Carcinoma Cells." *Cancer Letters* 200 (2003): 115–121.

Weng, X.C., G.Q. Xiang, A.L. Jiang, Y.P Liu, L.L. Wu, X.W. Dong, and S. Duan. "Antioxidant Properties of Components Extracted from Puccoon (Lithospermum Erythrorhizon Sieb. et Zucc.)." *Food Chemistry* 69 (2000): 143–146.

Ratany

Achenbach, Hans, Wolfgang Utz, Humberto Sánchez V., Elsa M. Guajardo Touché, Juia Verde S., and Xorge A. Domínguez. "Neolignans, Nor–neolignans and Other Compounds from Roots of Krameria Grayi." *Phytochemistry* 39, 2 (1995): 413–415.

Guevara, J.M., J. Chumpitaz, and E. Valencia. "The In Vitro Action of Plants on Vibrio Cholerae." *Revista de Gastroenterologia del Peru* 14, 1 (1994): 27–31.

Scholz, E. and H. Rimpler. "Proanthocyanidins from Krameria Triandra Root." *Planta Medica* 55, 4 (1989): 379–384.

Rayweed

Chhabra, B.R., J.C. Kohli, and R.S. Dhillon. "Three Ambrosanolides from Parthenium Hysterophorus." *Phytochemistry* 52 (1999): 1331–1334.

Coates, Wayne, Ricardo Ayerza, and Damian Ravetta. "Guayule Rubber and Latex Content – Seasonal Variations Over Time in Argentina." *Industrial Crops and Products* 14 (2001): 85–91.

Maatooq, Galal T., Ali A. H. El Gamal, Todd R. Furbacher, Tracy L. Cornuelle, and Joseph J. Hoffmann. "Triterpenoids from Parthenium Argentatum x P. Tomentosa." *Phytochemistry* 60 (2002): 755–760.

Proksch, Peter, H. Mohan Behl, and Eloy Rodriguez. "Detection and Quantification of Guayulins A and B in Parthenium Argentatum (Guayule) and F, Hybrids by High–Performance Liquid Chromatography." *Journal of Chromatography* 2, 13 (1981): 345–348.

Rodriguez, Eloy, Hirosuke Yoshioka, and Tom J. Mabry. "The Sesquiterpene Lactone Chemistry of the Genus Parthenium (Compositae)." *Phytochemistry* 10 (1971): 1145–1154

Red Betony

Bilusic' Vundac, Vjera et al. "Content of polyphenolic constituents and antioxidant activity of some Stachys taxa." *Food Chemistry* 104 (2007): 1277–1281.

Háznagy–Radnai, E. et al. "Cytotoxic activities of Stachys species." *Fitoterapia* 79 (2008): 595–597.

Tundis, Rosa et al. "Phytochemical and biological studies of Stachys species in relation to chemotaxonomy: A review". *Phytochemistry* 102 (2014): 7–39.

Sage

Al–Yousuf, M.H., A.K. Bashir, B.H. Ali, M.O.M. Tanira, and G. Blunden. "Some Effects of Salvia Aegyptiaca L. on the Central Nervous System in Mice." *Journal of Ethnopharmacology* 81 (2002): 121–127.

Baricevic, D., S. Sosa, R. Della Loggia, A. Tubaro, B. Simonovska, A. Krasna, and A. Zupancic. "Topical Anti–Inflammatory Activity of Salvia Officinalis L. Leaves: The Relevance of Ursolic Acid." *Journal of Ethnopharmacology* 75 (2001): 125–132.

Gali–Muhtasib, Hala, Christo Hilan, and Carla Khater. "Traditional Uses of Salvia Libanotica (East Mediterranean Sage) and the Effects of its Essential Oils." *Journal of Ethnopharmacology* 71 (2000): 513–520.

Vardar–Unlu, Gülhan, Moschos Polissiou, and Atalay Sokmen. "Antimicrobial and Antioxidative Activities of the Essential Oils and Methanol Extracts of Salvia Cryptantha (Montbret et Aucher ex Benth.) and Salvia Multicaulis (Vahl)." *Food Chemistry* 84 (2004): 519–525.

Lu, Yinrong and L. Yeap Foo. "Polyphenolics of Salvia—A Review." *Phytochemistry* 59 (2002): 117–140.

Miliauskas, G., P.R. Venskutonis, and T.A. van Beek. "Screening of Radical Scavenging Activity of some Medicinal and Aromatic Plant Extracts." *Food Chemistry* 85 (2004) 231–237.

Perry, Nicolette S.L., Chloe Bollen, Elaine K. Perry, and Clive Ballard. "Salvia for Dementia Therapy: Review of Pharmacological Activity and Pilot Tolerability Clinical Trial." *Pharmacology, Biochemistry and Behavior* 75 (2003): 651–659.

Radulescu, Valeria, Silvia Chiliment, and Eliza Oprea. "Capillary Gas Chromatography–Mass Spectrometry of Volatile and Semi–Volatile Compounds of Salvia Officinalis." *Journal of Chromatography A*, 1027 (2004): 121–126.

Savelev, S., E. Okello, N.S.L. Perry, R.M. Wilkins, and E.K. Perry. "Synergistic and Antagonistic Interactions of Anticholinesterase Terpenoids in Salvia Lavandulaefolia Essential Oil." *Pharmacology, Biochemistry and Behavior* 75 (2003): 661–668.

Tepe, Bektas, Dimitra Daferera, Atalay Sokmen, Munevver Sokmen, and Moschos Polissiou. "Antimicrobial and Antioxidant Activities of the Essential Oil and Various Extracts of Salvia Tomentosa Miller (Lamiaceae)." *Food Chemistry* (2003).

Tepe, Bektas, Erol Donmez, Mehmet Unlu, Ferda Candan, Dimitra Daferera, N.T.J. Tildesley, D.O. Kennedy, E.K. Perry, C.G. Ballard, S. Savelev, K.A. Wesnes, and A.B. Scholey. "Salvia Lavandulaefolia (Spanish Sage) Enhances Memory in Healthy Young Volunteers." *Pharmacology, Biochemistry and Behavior* 75 (2003):

669–674.

Wake, George, Jennifer Court, Anne Pickering, Rhiannon Lewis, Richard Wilkins, and Elaine Perry. "CNS Acetylcholine Receptor Activity in European Medicinal Plants Traditionally Used to Improve Failing Memory." *Journal of Ethnopharmacology* 69 (2000): 105–114.

Sagebrush

Gunawardena, K., S.B. Rivera, and W.W. Epstein. "The Monoterpenes of Artemisia Tridentata ssp. Vaseyana, Artemisia Cana ssp. Viscidula and Artemisia Tridentata ssp. Spiciformis." *Phytochemistry* 59 (2002): 197–203.

Kelley, B.D., J.M. Appelt, and G.D. Appelt. "Artemisia Tridentata (Basin Sagebrush) in the Southwestern United States of America: Medicinal Uses and Pharmacologic Implications." *International Journal of the Addictions* 27, 3 (1992): 347–366.

McCutcheon, A.R., S.M. Ellis, R.E.W. Hancock, and G.H.N. Towers. "Antifungal Screening of Medicinal Plants of British Columbian Native Peoples." *Journal of Ethnopharmacology* 44, 3 (1994): 157–169.

Smith, Bruce N., Thomas A. Monaco, Clayton Jones, Robert A. Holmes, Lee D. Hansen, E. Durant McArthur, and D. Carl Freeman. "Stress–Induced Metabolic Differences Between Populations and Subspecies of Artemisia Tridentata (Sagebrush) from a Single Hillside." *Thermochimica Acta* 394 (2002): 205–210.

Scouring Rush

Amarowicz, R., R.B. Pegg, P. Rahimi–Moghaddam, B. Barl, and J.A. Weil. "Free–Radical Scavenging Capacity and Antioxidant Activity of Selected Plant Species from the Canadian Prairies." *Food Chemistry* 84 (2004): 551–562.

Grases, F., G. Melero, A. Costa–Bauza, R. Prieto, and J.G. March. "Urolithiasis and Phytotherapy." *International Urology and Nephrology* 26, 5 (1994): 507–11.

Gurbuz, Iylhan, Osman Ustun, Erdem Yesilada, Ekrem Sezik, and Nalan Akyurek. "In Vivo Gastroprotective Effects of Five Turkish Folk Remedies Against Ethanol–Induced Lesions." *Journal of Ethnopharmacology* 83 (2002): 241–244.

Harrison, C.C. "Evidence for Intramineral Macromolecules Containing Protein from Plant Silicas." *Phytochemistry* 41, 1 (1996): 37–42.

Veit, Markus, Cornelia Beckert, Cornelia Hohne, Katja Bauer, and Hans Geiger. "Interspecific and Intraspecific Variation of Phenolics in the Genus Equisetum Subgenus Equisetum." *Phytochemistry* 38, 4 (1995): 881–891.

Senna

Barbosa, Francisco G., Maria da Conceicao F. de Oliveira, Raimundo Braz–Filho, and Edilberto R. Silveira. "Anthraquinones and Naphthopyrones from Senna Rugosa." *Biochemical Systematics and Ecology* 32 (2004): 363–365.

Djozan, DJ and Y. Assadi. "Determination of Anthraquinones in Rhubarb Roots, Dock Flowers and Senna Leaves by Normal–Phase High Performance Liquid Chromatography." *Talanta* 42, 6 (1995): 861–865.

Fairbairn, J. W. and A.B. Shrestha. "The Distribution of Anthraquinone Glycosides in Cassia Senna L." *Phytochemistry* 6 (1967): 1203–1207.

Snakeweed

Ferdinand Bohlmann, Christa Zdero, Robert M. King, and Harold Robinson. "Gutierrezial and Further Diterpenes from Gutierrezia Sarothrae." *Phytochemistry* 23,

9 (1984): 2007–2012.

Soapberry

Lal, J., S. Chandra, V. Raviprakash, and M. Sabir. "In Vitro Anthelmintic Action of some Indigenous Medicinal Plants on Ascardia Galli Worms." *Indian J Physiol Pharmacol* 20, 2 (1976) 64–68

Albiero, Adriana L. Meyer, Jayme Antonio Aboin Sertié, and Elfriede Marianne Bacchi. "Antiulcer Activity of Sapindus Saponaria L. in the Rat." *Journal of Ethnopharmacology* 82 (2002): 41–44.

Spanish Needles

Alvarez, A., F. Pomar, M.A. Sevilla, and M.J. Montero. "Gastric Antisecretory and Antiulcer Activities of an Ethanolic Extract of Bidens Pilosa L. var. Radiata Schult. Bip." *Journal of Ethnopharmacology* 67 (1999): 333–340.

Alarcon de la Lastra, C., M.J. Martin, C. La Casa, and V. Motilva. "Antiulcerogenicity of the Flavonoid Fraction from Bidens Aurea: Comparison With Ranitidine and Omeprazole." *Journal of Ethnopharmacology* 42, 3 (1994): 161–168.

Brandao, M.G.L., A.U. Krettli, L.S.R. Soares, C.G.C. Nery, and H.C. Marinuzzi. "Antimalarial Activity of Extracts and Fractions from Bidens Pilosa and Other Bidens Species (Asteracea) Correlated With the Presence of Acetylene and Flavonoid Compounds." *Journal of Ethnopharmacology* 57 (1997): 131–138.

Cano, Juan Hernández and Gabriele Volpato. "Herbal Mixtures in the Traditional Medicine of Eastern Cuba." *Journal of Ethnopharmacology* xxx (2004): xxx–xxx.

Dimo, Théophile, Silver Rakotonirina, René Kamgang, Paul V. Tan, Albert Kamanyi, and Marc Bopelet. "Effects of Leaf Aqueous Extract of *Bidens Pilosa* (Asteraceae) on KCl– and Norepinephrine–Induced Contractions of Rat Aorta." *Journal of Ethnopharmacology* 60 (1998): 179–182.

Dimo, Théophile, Silvere V. Rakotonirina, Paul V. Tan, Jacqueline Azay, Etienne Dongo, and Gérard Cros. "Leaf Methanol Extract of Bidens Pilosa Prevents and Attenuates the Hypertension Induced by High–fructose Diet in Wistar Rats." *Journal of Ethnopharmacology* 83 (2002): 183–191.

Geissberger, P. and U. Sequin. "Constituents of Bidens Pilosa L.: Do the Components Found So Far Explain the Use of this Plant in Traditional Medicine?" *Acta Tropica* 48, 4 (1991): 251–261.

Khan, M.R., M. Kihara, and A.D. Omoloso. "Anti–Microbial Activity of Bidens Pilosa, Bischofia Javanica, Elmerillia Papuana and Sigesbekia Orientalis." *Fitoterapia* 72 (2001): 662–665.

Pereira, Rachel L.C., Tereza Ibrahim, Leonardo Lucchetti, Antonio Jorge R. da Silva, and Vera Lucia Goncalves de Moraes. "Immunosuppressive and Anti–Inflammatory Effects of Methanolic Extract and the Polyacetylene Isolated from Bidens pilosa L." *Immunopharmacology* 43 (1999): 31–37.

Rivera, D. and C. Obón. "The Ethnopharmacology of Madeira and Porto Santo Islands, a Review." *Journal of Ethnopharmacology* 46 (1995): 73–93.

Sarg, T.M., A.M. Ateya, N.M. Farrag, and F.A. Abbas. "Constituents and Biological Activity of Bidens Pilosa L. Grown in Egypt." *Acta Pharmaceutica Hungarica* 61, 6 (1991): 317–323.

Tan, Paul V., Théophile Dimo, and Etienne Dongo. "Effects of Methanol, Cyclohexane and Methylene Chloride Extracts of Bidens Pilosa on Various Gastric Ulcer Models in Rats." *Journal of Ethnopharmacology* 73 (2000): 415–421.

Sumac

Homer, K.A., F. Manji, and D. Beighton. "Inhibition of Protease Activities of Perio-dontopathic Bacteria by Extracts of Plants Used in Kenya as Chewing Sticks (Mswaki)." *Archives of Oral Biology* 35, 6 (1990): 421–424.

Saxena, G., A.R. McCutcheon, S. Farmer, G.H.N. Towers, and R.E.W. Hancock. "Antimicrobial Constituents of Rhus Glabra." *Journal of Ethnopharmacology* 42 (1994) 95–99.

Zalacain, A., M. Prodanov, M. Carmona, and G.L. Alonso. "Optimization of Extraction and Identification of Gallotannins from Sumac Leaves." *Biosystems Engineering* 84, 2 (2003): 211–216.

Syrian Rue

Abdel–Fattah, Abdel–Fattah Mohamed, Kinzo Matsumoto, Hatim Abdel–Khalik Gammaz, and Hiroshi Watanabe. "Hypothermic Effect of Harmala Alkaloid in Rats: Involvement of Serotonergic Mechanism." *Pharmacology Biochemistry and Behavior* 52, 2 (1995): 421–426

El–Saad, El–Rifaie. "Peganum Harmala: Its Use in Certain Dermatoses." *International Journal of Dermatology* 19, 4 (1980): 221–222.

Frison, Giampietro, Donata Favretto, Flavio Zancanaro, Giorgio Fazzin, and Santo Davide Ferrar. "A Case of β–Carboline Alkaloid Intoxication Following Ingestion of Peganum Harmala Seed Extract." *Forensic Science International* 179 (2008): e37–e43.

Kartal, M., M.L. Altun, and S. Kurucu. "HPLC Method for the Analysis of Harmol, Harmalol, Harmine and Harmaline in the Seeds of Peganum Harmala L." *Journal of Pharmaceutical and Biomedical Analysis* 31 (2003): 263–269.

Prashanth, D. and S. John. "Antibacterial Activity of Peganum Harmala." *Fitoterapia* 70 (1999): 438–439.

Tamarisk

Nawwar, Mohamed A.M. and Sahar A.M. Hussein. "Gall Polyphenolics of Tamarix Aphylla." *Phytochemistry* 36, 4 (1994): 1035–1037.

Souliman, Ahmed M.A., Heba H. Barakat, Amani M.D El–Mousallamy, Mohamed S.A. Marzouk, and Mohamed A.M. Nawwar. "Phenolics from the Bark of Tamarix Aphyua." *Phytochemistry* 30, 11 (1991): 3763–3766.

Sultanova, N., T. Makhmoor, Z.A. Abilov, Z. Parween, V.B. Omurkamzinova, Atta-ur–Rahman, and M. Iqbal Choudhary. "Antioxidant and Antimicrobial Activities of Tamarix Ramosissima." *Journal of Ethnopharmacology* 78 (2001): 201–205.

Tarbush

M. M. Rao, D.G.I. Kingston and T.D. Spittler. "Flavonoids from Flourensia Cernua." *Phytochemistry* 9 (1970): 227–228.

Mata, Rachel, Robert Bye, Edelmira Linares, Martha Macías, Isabel Rivero–Cruz, Olga Pérez, and Barbara N. Timmermann. "Phytotoxic Compounds from Flourensia Cernua." *Phytochemistry* 64 (2003): 285–291.

Richard E. Estell, Kris M. Havstad, Eddie L. Fredrickson, and Jorge L. Gardea–Torresdey. "Secondary Chemistry of the Leaf Surface of Flourensia cernua." *Biochemical Systematics and Ecology* 22, 1 (1994): 73–77.

Texas Ranger
Blunden, G. et al. "Betaine distribution in the Scrophulariaceae and some previously included families." *Biochemical Systematics and Ecology* 31 (2003): 359–365.

Trotter, Robert T. "Folk remedies as indicators of common illness: examples from the United States–Mexico border." *Journal of Ethnopharmacology* 4 (1981): 207–221.

Tobacco
P.A. Steenkamp, F.R. van Heerden, and B.–E. van Wyk. "Accidental Fatal Poisoning by Nicotiana Glauca: Identification of Anabasine by High Performance Liquid Chromatography/Photodiode Array/Mass Spectrometry." *Forensic Science International* 127 (2002): 208–217.

Tree of Heaven
Dell'Agli, Mario, Germana V. Galli, Silvia Parapini, Nicoletta Basilico, Donatella Taramelli, Ataa Said, Khaled Rashed, and Enrica Bosisio. "Anti–plasmodial Activity of Ailanthus Excelsa." *Fitoterapia* 79 (2008): 112–116.

Hitotsuyanagi, Yukio, Akira Ozeki, Chee Yan Choo, Kit Lam Chan, Hideji Itokawa, and Koichi Takeya. "Malabanones A and B, Novel Nortriterpenoids from Ailanthus Malabarica DC." *Tetrahedron* 57 (2001): 7477–7480.

Stafford, Gary I., Mikael E. Pedersen, Johannes van Staden, Anna K. Jäger. "Review on Plants with CNS–Effects Used in Traditional South African Medicine Against Mental Diseases." *Journal of Ethnopharmacology* 119 (2008): 513–537.

Takeya, Koichi, Hideyuki Kobata, Akira Ozeki, Hiroshi Morita, and Hiden Itokawa. "Quassinoids from Ailanthus Vilmoriniana." *Phytochemistry* 48, 3 (1998): 565–568.

Trumpet Flower
Aguilar–Santamaría, L., G. Ramírez, P. Nicasio, C. Alegría–Reyes, and A. Herrera–Arellano. "Antidiabetic Activities of Tecoma Stans (L.) Juss. ex Kunth." *Journal of Ethnopharmacology* xxx (2009): xxx–xxx. Article in Press.

Binutu, O.A. and B.A. Lajubutu. "Antimicrobial Potentials of some Plant Species of the Bignoniaceae Family." *African Journal of Medicine and Medical Sciences* 23, 3 (1994): 269–273.

Dickinson, E.M. and G. Jones. "Pyrindane Alkaloids from Tecoma Stans." *Tetrahedron* 25, 7 (1969): 1523–1529.

Hammouda, Y. and N. Khalafallah. "Stability of Tecomine, the Major Antidiabetic Factor of Tecoma Stans (Juss.) F. Bignoniaceae." *Journal of Pharmaceutical Sciences* 60, 8 (1971): 1142–1145.

Kunapuli, Satya P. and C.S. Vaidyanathan. "Indole–Metabolizing Enzyme Systems in Tropical Plants." *Phytochemistry* 24, 5 (1985): 973–975.

Lins, Arlete Paulino and Joana D'Arc Felicio. "Monoterpene Alkaloids from Tecoma Stans." *Phytochemistry* 34, 3 (1993): 876–878.

Lozoya–Meckes, M. and V. Mellado–Campos. "Is the Tecoma Stans Infusion an Antidiabetic Remedy?" *Journal of Ethnopharmacology* 14, 1 (1985): 1–9.

Okarter, Temple U., Paul L. Schiff Jr. , Joseph E. Knapp and David J. Slatkin. "Lipid and Phenolic Constituents of Tecoma Radicans." *Phytochemistry* 15, 3 (1976): 436.

Prakash, E.O. and J.T. Rao. "A New Flavone Glycoside from the Seeds of Tecoma Undulata." *Fitoterapia* 70 (1999): 287–289.

Qureshi, S., M.K. Rai, and S.C. Agrawal. "In Vitro Evaluation of Inhibitory Nature of

Extracts of 18–Plant Species of Chhindwara Against 3–keratinophilic Fungi." *Hindustan Antibiotics Bulletin* 39, 1–4 (1997): 56–60.

Roman–Ramos, R., J.L. Flores–Saenz, G. Partida–Hernandez, A. Lara–Lemus, and F. Alarcon–Aguilar. "Experimental Study of the Hypoglycemic Effect of some Antibiabetic Plants." *Archivos de Investigation Medica* 22,1 (1991): 87–93.

Shapiro, Karen and William C. Gong. "Natural Products Used for Diabetes." *Journal of the American Pharmaceutical Association* 42, 2 (2002): 217–226.

Verbena

Hernández, Nancy E., M.L. Tereschuk, and L.R. Abdala. "Antimicrobial Activity of Flavonoids in Medicinal Plants from Tafí del Valle (Tucumán, Argentina)." *Journal of Ethnopharmacology* 73 (2000): 317–322.

Kawashty, S.A. and I.A. El–Garf. "The Favonoid Chemosystematics of Egyptian Verbena Species." *Biochemical Systematics and Ecology* 28 (2000): 919–921.

Western Black Willow

Chrubasik, Sigrun, Elon Eisenberg, Edith Balan, Tuvia Weinberger, Rachel Luzzati, and Christian Conradt. "Treatment of Low Back Pain Exacerbations with Willow Bark Extract: A Randomized Double–Blind Study." *The American Journal of Medicine* 109 (2000): 9–14.

Orians, Colin M., Megan E. Griffiths, Bernadette M. Roche, and Robert S. Fritz. "Phenolic Glycosides and Condensed Tannins in Salix Sericea, S. Eriocephala and their F1 Hybrids: Not All Hybrids are Created Equal." *Biochemical Systematics and Ecology* 28 (2000): 619–632.

Tunón, H., C. Olavsdotter, and L. Bohlin. "Evaluation of Anti–Inflammatory Activity of some Swedish Medicinal Plants. Inhibition of Prostaglandin Biosynthesis and PAF–Induced Exocytosis." *Journal of Ethnopharmacology* 48 (1995): 61–76.

Western Mugwort

Bork, Peter M., M. Lienhard Schmitz, Michaela Kuhnt, Claudia Escher, and Michael Heinrich. "Sesquiterpene Lactone Containing Mexican Indian Medicinal Plants and Pure Sesquiterpene Lactones as Potent Inhibitors of Transcription Factor NF–B." *FEBS Letters* 402, 1 (1997): 85–90.

Fernandez, Salvador Said, Monica Celina Ramos Guerra, Benito David Mata Cardenas, Javier Vargas Villarreal, and Licet Villarreal Trevino. "In Vitro Antiprotozoal Activity of the Leaves of Artemisia Ludoviciana." *Fitoterapia* 76 (2005): 466–468.

Jakupovic, J., R.X. Tan, F. Bohlmann, P.E. Boldt, and Z.J. Jia. "Sesquiterpene Lactones from Artemisia Ludoviciana." *Phytochemistry* 30, 5 (1991): 1573–1577.

Juteau, Fabien, Veronique Masotti, Jean Marie Bessiere, Michel Dherbomez, and Josette Viano. "Antibacterial and Antioxidant Activities of Artemisia Annua Essential Oil." *Fitoterapia* 73 (2002): 532–535.

Lee, K.H. and T.A. Geissman. "Sesquiterpene Lactones of Artemisia Constituents of A. Ludoviciana ssp. Mexicana." *Phytochemistry* 9, 2 (1970): 403–408.

Liu, Yong–Long and T.J. Mabry. "Flavonoids from Artemisia Ludoviciana var. Ludoviciana." *Phytochemistry* 21, 1 (1982): 209–214.

Ruiz–Cancino, Alejandro, Arturo E. Cano, and Guillermo Delgado. "Sesquiterpene Lactones and Flavonoids from Artemisia Ludoviciana ssp. Mexicana." *Phytochemistry* 33, 5 (1993): 1113–1115.

Vega, A.E., G.H.Wendel, A.O.M. and Maria, L. Pelzer. "Antimicrobial Activity of Artemisia Douglasiana and Dehydroleucodine Against Helicobacter Pylori." *Journal of Ethnopharmacology* xxx (2009): xxx–xxx.

Western Peony
Papandreou, Vasiliki, Prokopios Magiatis, Ioanna Chinou, Eleftherios Kalpoutza-
kis, Alexios–Leandros Skaltsounis, and Anthony Tsarbopoulos. "Volatiles with
Antimicrobial Activity from the Roots of Greek Paeonia Taxa." *Journal of Ethnopharmacology* 81 (2002): 101–104
Ikuta, Akira, Kohei Kamiya, Toshiko Satake, and Yasuhisa Saiki. "Triterpenoids
from Callus Tissue Cultures of Paeonia Species." *Phytochemistry* 38, 5 (1995):
1203–1207.

Wild Licorice
Fukai, Toshio, Kazue Satoh, Taro Nomura, and Hiroshi Sakagami. "Antinephri-
tis and Radical Scavenging Activity of Prenylflavonoids." *Fitoterapia* 74 (2003):
720–724.
Fukai, Toshio, Ai Marumo, Kiyoshi Kaitou, Toshihisa Kanda, Sumio Terada, and
Taro Nomura. "Anti–Helicobacter Pylori Flavonoids from Licorice Extract." *Life
Sciences* 71 (2002): 1449–1463.
Fukai, Toshio, Kazue Satoh, Taro Nomura, and Hiroshi Sakagami. "Preliminary
Evaluation of Antinephritis and Radical Scavenging Activities of Glabridin
from Glycyrrhiza Glabra." *Fitoterapia* 74 (2003): 624–629.
Amarowicz, R., R.B. Pegg, P. Rahimi–Moghaddam, B. Barld, and J.A. Weil. "Free–
Radical Scavenging Capacity and Antioxidant Activity of Selected Plant Spe-
cies from the Canadian Prairies." *Food Chemistry* 84 (2004): 551–562.

Wild Rhubarb
Demirezer, L. Omur, Ayse Kuruuzum–Uza, Isabelle Bergere, H.–J. Schiewe, and
Axel Zeeck. "The Structures of Antioxidant and Cytotoxic Agents from Natu-
ral Source: Anthraquinones and Tannins from Roots of Rumex Patientia." *Phy-
tochemistry* 58 (2001): 1213–1217.
Fairbairn, J. W. and F. J. El–Muhtadi. "Chemotaxonomy of Anthraquinones in
Rumex." *Phytochemistry* 11 (1972): 263–268.
Midiwo, J. Ogweno and G. Muriki Rukunga. "Distrubution of Anthraquinone Pig-
ments in Rumex Species." *Phytochemistry* 24, 6 (1985): 1390–1391.
Saleh, Nabiel A.M., Mohamed N. El–Hadidi and Raafat F.M. Arafa. "Flavonoids and
Anthraquinones of some Egyptian Rumex Species (Polygonaceae)." *Biochemical
Systematics and Ecology* 21, 2 (1993): 301–303.
VanderJagt, T.J., R. Ghattas, D.J VanderJagt, M. Crossey, and R.H Glew. "Comparison
of the Total Antioxidant Content of 30 Widely Used Medicinal Plants of New
Mexico." *Life Sciences* 70 (2002): 1035–1040.

Yerba Mansa
Medina, Andrea L., F. Omar Holguin, Sandra Micheletto, Sondra Goehle, Julian A.
Simon, and Mary A. O'Connell. "Chemotypic Variation of Essential Oils in the
Medicinal Plant, Anemopsis Californica." *Phytochemistry* 69 (2008): 919–927.
Medina, Andrea L., Mary E. Lucero, F. Omar Holguin, Rick E. Estell, Jeff J. Posak-
ony, Julian Simon, and Mary A. O'Connell. " Composition and Antimicrobial

Activity of Anemopsis californica Leaf Oil." *J. Agric. Food Chem.* 53, 22 (2005): 8694–8698.

Yerba Santa

Bacon, John D., Gary L. Hannan, Nianbai Fang, and Tom J. Mabry. "Chemosystematics of the Hydrophyllaceae" Flavonoids of Three Species of Eriodictyon." Biochemical Systematics and Ecology 14, 6 (1986): 591–595.

Johnson, Nelson D. "Flavonoid Aglycones from Eriodictyon Californicum Resin and their Implications for Herbivory and UV Screening." Biochemical Systematics and Ecology 11, 3 (1963): 211–215.

Salle, A. J., Gregory J. Jarm, and Lawrence G. Wayne. "Studies on the Antibacterial Properties of Eriodictyon Californicum." From the Department of Bacteriology, University of California, Los Angeles, California (1951).

Yucca

Hussain, I., A.M. Ismail, and P.R. Cheeke. "Effects of Feeding Yucca Schidigera Extract in Diets Varying in Crude Protien and Urea Contents on Growth Performance and Cecum and Blood Urea and Ammonia Concentrations of Rabbits." *Animal Feed Science Technology* 62, (1996): 121–129.

Hussain, I. and P.R. Cheeke. "Effect of Dietary Yucca Schidigera Extract on Rumen and Blood Profiles of Steers Fed Concentrate or Roughage–Based Diets." *Animal Feed Science and Technology* 51 (1995): 231–242.

Wang, Y., T.A. McAllister, C.J. Newbold, L.M. Rode, P.R. Cheeke, and K-J. Cheng. "Effects of Yucca Schidigera Extract on Fermentation and Degradation of Steroidal Saponins in the Rumen Simulation Technique (RUSITEC)1." *Animal Feed Science and Technology* 74 (1998): 143–153.

Glossary

Abscess
An accumulation of pus (defunct leukocytes, damaged tissue cells, and cellular wastes) within tissues or organs either resolving by coming to 'a head' or diminishing internally.

Acetylcholine
Serves as a neurotransmitter throughout the central and peripheral nervous systems, though it is most closely associated with the parasympathetic branch of the autonomic nervous system.

Acetylcholinesterase (AChE)
An enzyme of the central nervous system that breaks down acetylcholine into choline and acetate.

Achene
A term used to describe a seed common to the Sunflower family.

Adaptogen
A somewhat vague term used widely in the herbal medicine field to describe a plant which is capable of increasing an individual's tolerance to stress. Actions of these plants often seem contradictory, at times providing stimulation and at others, sedation. Ginseng is considered a classic adaptogen.

Addison's disease
A life threatening disease caused by tuberculosis or autoimmune involvement. Symptoms of hypotension, abnormal skin pigmentation, weight loss, and weakness are caused by diminished levels of adrenal cortex hormones, cortisol and aldosterone.

Adrenal cortex
The outer layer of the adrenal gland; secretes mineralocorticoids and glucocorticoids.

Adrenal medulla
Inner layer of the adrenal gland; secrets catecholamines epinephrine and norepinephrine.

Adrenaline
(Epinephrine) Both a catecholamine hormone and a neurotransmitter. It is secreted by the adrenal medulla and is used by the sympathetic branch of the central nervous system. It is a prominent physiologic agent in fight or flight reactions and low–grade stress states.

Albumin
A plasma protein crucial in transporting many organic substances – bile acids, hormones, and fatty acids. It is also important in maintaining proper plasma osmotic pressure. Plasma albumin levels diminish in certain renal and hepatic diseases, and if dietary levels of protein are insufficient.

Aldosterone
A mineralocorticoid secreted by the adrenal cortex. It is involved in sodium/potassium dynamics and blood pressure.

Allopathic
Pertaining to present day conventional medicine when solely used to suppress or oppose symptoms, such as steroids for inflammation, analgesics for pain, etc.

Alterative
Pertaining to the quality, or a substance (usually an herbal medicine) that positively alters organs or functions of elimination, detoxification, or immunity.

Alveoli
(Pulmonary alveoli) Small sacs within the lungs where carbon dioxide and oxygen exchange takes place.

Alzheimer's disease
A progressive brain disease with a number of potential causative factors. Senile plaques, neurofibrillary tangles, and loss of acetyltransferase activity are common. Progressed effects are dementia and personality change.

Amebiasis
(Montezuma's revenge or Traveler's diarrhea) An intestinal infection involving Entamoeba histolytica from contaminated food or water. Usually the large intestine is affected but in severe cases infection can migrate to the liver, spleen, brain, lungs, and other areas.

Amenorrhea
The abnormal cessation of menses, often due to extreme weight loss, physical–emotional stress, or the alteration of ovarian hormones.

Amylase
Present in saliva and pancreatic juice, this enzyme breaks down starches into simple sugars.

Anaphrodisiac
That which curbs libido.

Anaphylaxis
A potentially life threatening allergic reaction. Shock and respiratory distress usually accompanies an episode.

Androgen
Any substance, but usually hormonal, that promotes masculinization. Testosterone and androstenedione are examples.

Anesthetic
An agent that causes numbness or reduces/eliminates pain sensations.

Angina pectoris
A particular spasmodic, suffocative pain due to heart tissue ischemia. Radiating left arm pain is a common symptom. An episode may be precipitated by physical exertion and is caused by coronary artery obstruction from plaque buildup.

Annual
Any plant that germinates, then sets seed and dies in one year.

Anorexia
Simply the lack of appetite for food. Anorexia nervosa, more complex than a simple loss of appetite, is considered a mental disorder.

Anovulatory cycle
A menstrual cycle without ovulation.

Antibody
(See Immunoglobulin)

Anticholinergic
Inhibiting to the parasympathetic nervous system. Pertaining to any substance whether pharmaceutical, herbal, or otherwise that lessens gastrointestinal tract, mucosal, and skin secretion and excretion.

Antigen
A substance capable of stimulating a specific acquired immune response. Bacteria and foreign particles are prime examples.

Antiseptic
Inhibiting to the growth and spread of microorganisms.

Antiviral
Inhibiting to virus reproduction or its cellular attachment.

Aphrodisiac
A sexual excitant.

Aphthous stomatitis
(Canker sore) A small white ulcer of the oral mucosa. Stress, immune deficiency, and allergic reaction are common underlying factors.

Apoptosis
The innate process of programed cell death. When operating properly this function is a key cancer inhibitor. Many illnesses are linked to an excess or lack of apoptosis.

Arachidonic acid (AA)
An essential fatty acid intrinsic to prostaglandin, leukotriene, and thromboxane synthesis. It holds a place in both normal cellular process and disease development.

Arrhythmia
Irregular rhythm of the heartbeat.

Asthenic
Weakness; deficiency.

Asthma
A condition of bronchial constriction due to spasm or autoimmune inflammation.

Asthma, humid
Asthma with copious expectoration.

Atherosclerosis
Arterial inflammation in conjunction with plaque deposits. Also known as 'hardening of the arteries'.

Atonic
Lacking normal tone.

Autonomic nervous system
Composed of the sympathetic and parasympathetic nervous systems; mainly involved with visceral function.

Ayurveda
Traditional Indian medicine. Thought to predate Traditional Chinese Medicine, the system describes herbs as having energetic qualities and people being of different constitutional types.

Basophil
A granular leukocyte involved in innate immunity.

Bedsore
Ulcer development from bed confinement. Lack of circulation and continual pressure are factors in development.

Benign prostrate hypertrophy (BPH)
Prostate enlargement associated with age and corresponding DHT levels.

Bifidobacteria
One of a number of gram–positive, anaerobic bacteria belonging to the Bifidobacterium genus. Common species found in the large bowel are B. adolescentis, B. eriksonii, and B. infantis.

Bile
An alkaline liquid secreted by the liver composed of cholesterol, bile salts, phospholipids, bilirubin diglucuronide, and electrolytes. It is essential for fat digestion.

Boil
(Furuncle) A painful, subcutaneous nodule with an enclosed core. Usually caused

by Staphylococci entering through hair follicles, liver and immune deficiencies are common constitutional factors.

Bract
A modified leaf situated at the base of a flower.

Bradycardia
A slowed heart rate, usually slower than 60 beat per minute (although this is considered normal for athletes and young adults).

Bronchitis
Mechanical, bacterial, viral, or allergy induced inflammation of one or more bronchi.

Bronchorrhoea
Excessive lung airway discharge.

Canker sores
(See Aphthous stomatitis)

Cardiac glycoside
Glycosides found in some Cactus, Figwort, Dogbane, and Lily family plants. In therapeutic doses, they are slowing and strengthening to the heart.

Carminative
A term used to describe a medicine that relieves gas pains and bloating.

Catkin
(Ament) A compact male or female, spike–like inflorescence, typically found in Willow or Birch family plants.

Central nervous system
The segment of the nervous system consisting of the brain and spinal cord.

Cervical dysplasia
Cellular changes in the epithelium of the cervix. It is regarded as a precursor to carcinoma. HPV infection is thought to be the main inducer of cervical dysplasia.

Cervicitis
Inflammation of the cervix, either due to infection or injury.

Chicken pox
(Varicella–zoster) A contagious herpes–type virus causing reddened and itching vesicles.

Cholecystokinin (CCK)
Both a hormone secreted by the upper small intestine and by the hypothalamus as a neurotransmitter. It stimulates gallbladder contraction, secretion of pancreatic enzymes, and in response to food it is involved in feelings of satiety and fullness.

Cholesterol
A common sterol produced by the liver and obtained from the diet. It is involved in cell–membrane structure, is a base for steroidal hormones, and is the precursor in bile formation. It is a contributing factor in arterial plaques and in some gallstones.

Choleretic
Either an activity or an agent that stimulates bile production by the liver.

Cholinergic
(Parasympathomimetic) Referring to autonomic nerve fibers that use acetylcholine as a neurotransmitter.

Chologogue
Any substance that stimulates bile release from the gallbladder. Most herbal chologogues are choleretics as well.

Coccidioides immitis
The fungus responsible for Coccidioidomycosis or Valley fever.

Coccidioidomycosis
(Valley fever) The disease caused by Coccidioides immitis. Primary manifestations are cough, fever, and joint pain. The infection is usually self–resolving but can be serious in some racial groups and immune compromised individuals.

Collagenation
The process of collagen formation in cartilage or other tissues.

Colonic flora
Bacterial strains existing in the large intestine, many of which are necessary for gastrointestinal and systemic health.

Condyloma acuminatum
(Venereal or genital warts) caused by Human papillomavirus (HPV). Infectious and sexually transmitted, infection predisposes women to cervical dysplasia.

Conjunctivitis
An inflammation of the conjunctiva, typically involving redness, swelling, and discharge. There can be bacterial, viral, mechanical, or allergic involvement.

Corpus luteum
A temporary glandular mass located in the ovary; secretes progesterone during pregnancy and throughout part of the menstrual cycle.

Corticosteroids
Two groups of hormones secreted by the adrenal cortex: glucocorticoids (cortisol) and mineralocorticoids (aldosterone).

Cortisol
The main glucocorticoid secreted by the adrenal cortex. It is involved in glucose,

protein, and fat metabolism, stress response, and immunity.

Cyclooxygenase
An enzyme or activity involved in prostaglandin synthesis, particularly the inflammatory processes.

Cystitis
Inflammation of the urinary bladder.

Deciduous
Describing a plant that is not evergreen; herbage falling from the plant seasonally.

Dehydroepiandrosterone (DHEA)
An adrenal cortex steroid hormone. It plays a large role as an androgen precursor in premenopausal women and as a major androgen in postmenopausal women. Supplementation in women can be masculinizing.

Dementia
Loss of cognitive ability, memory, and judgement. Alzheimer's disease, stroke, or a variety of neurological diseases are common causes.

Demulcent
A quality or an agent that is soothing and allays irritation of surface tissues. Most in this class are mucilaginous or oily.

Diaphoresis
Perspiration or sweating.

Diaphoretic
A substance that promotes sweating (diaphoresis) or the activity of something that promotes sweating.

5–α–dihydrotestosterone (DHT)
Formed through 5–α–reductase's activity on testosterone, DHT is both an important androgen and one of the main causes of BPH and male pattern baldness.

Dioecious
Imperfect male and female flowers borne on different plants.

Diuretic
A substance that promotes urine excretion or the activity of increasing urine excretion.

Doctrine of Signatures
A philosophy of resemblance applied to herbal medicine popular up until the 17th century. Example: if in some way a plant resembles a heart it is a medicine for that organ.

Dopamine
A catecholamine–type neurotransmitter, widely acting throughout the central nervous system.

Duodenal ulcer
An ulcer of the upper small intestine or duodenum.

Dust cell
(Alveolar macrophage or Alveolar phagocyte) A phagocyte that resides within the lung's alveoli. They ingest inhaled particulate matter and are important in pulmonary immunity.

Dysmenorrhea
Painful menstruation.

Dyspepsia
Faulty digestion, resulting in discomfort, gas, and sometimes, gastrointestinal tract stasis.

Eclectics
A school of medicine existing up until the mid–20th century, devoted to potentiated plant medicines and the treatment of the individual (not just the symptom).

Edema
Increased intercellular fluid buildup from numerous causes, but typically from kidney or heart dysfunction, or venous or lymphatic obstruction.

Emmenagogue
Something that induces menstruation.

Endometriosis
A condition where endometrial tissue develops in other than normal areas (ex. pelvic cavity). Cyclic pain and inflammation are common symptoms.

Endometrium
Inner mucus membrane layer of the uterus.

Entamoeba histolytica
A common ameboid protozoa; the cause of amebiasis. Severe infections may affect the lungs, liver, spleen, and other organs.

Enteric
Of the small intestine.

Enteric coated
A coating applied to a tablet or capsule specially designed to breakdown in the small intestine.

Entire
Referring to the margin of a leaf; not toothed, lobed, or divided, but continuous.

Eosinophil
A granular leukocyte involved in innate immunity; it is specific to parasite defense.

Erythrocyte
(Red blood cell) A main component of blood; responsible for oxygen transport.

Escherichia coli
A gram negative, anaerobic bacterium normally found in the large intestine. The organism typically causes urinary tract infections. Colonization often takes place through poor hygiene and alkaline urine.

Essential oil
The non–polar, volatile oil content of an aromatic plant. Commonly extracted

through distillation. Mint family plants are typical subjects.

Essential hypertension
(Idiopathic or primary hypertension) Elevated blood pressure without organic causes. It is largely a functional problem with sodium intake, weight, and stress as the primary causative agents.

Estrogen
A hormone found in both sexes; necessary for proper female sexual development, reproductive health, and pregnancy.

Eupatory tribe
A division of the Sunflower family. Plants in this division are apt to contain either toxic or non–toxic pyrrolizidine alkaloids. The Brickellia and Eupatorium genera are both in this tribe.

Extracellular fluid
Pertaining to fluid outside of a cell, such as lymphatic fluid.

Fibroid
(Uterine leiomyoma) A benign tumor composed of smooth muscle usually developing in the myometrium of the uterus during a women's 30s or 40s.

Flavonoids
A group of phenolic compounds closely related to tannins; many have therapeutic effects on cell/tissue structure.

Follicle stimulating hormone (FSH)
A pituitary hormone necessary for women's follicle maturation and in men, proper spermatogenesis.

Fusarium
A genus of fungi; a number of species are pathogenic to man.

Gamma–aminobutyric acid (GABA)
A key inhibitory neurotransmitter found throughout the central nervous system.

Gastritis
Inflammation of the stomach often caused from stress, poor diet, mechanical insults, or pharmaceutical side effects.

Gastroenteritis
Inflammation of the stomach and intestinal lining. It can be viral or bacterial initiated, and in some cases, is triggered by intense adrenergic reaction. It is most commonly the result of food poisoning.

Genital warts
(See Condyloma acuminatum)

Giardia
A parasite in humans and in other vertebrates, commonly spread by contaminated food, water, and direct human/animal contact. Giardia lamblia is the most notorious species. The organism attaches itself to the microvilli of the intestinal walls causing diarrhea, nausea, weight loss, and fatigue among other symptoms.

Gingivitis
An acute or chronic inflammation of the gingivae or gums.

Glaucoma
A group of eye diseases caused by increased intraocular pressure. Changes in the optic disk and ultimately blindness occur if left untreated.

Glomerulonephritis
Inflammation of the capillary structures in the glomeruli of the kidney from a residual hemolytic infection or autoimmune involvement.

Glucose–6–phosphate–dehydrogenase deficiency (G6PD)
A genetic deficiency causing, to varying degrees, hemolytic anemia.

Glutathione
An important naturally occurring tripeptide involved in detoxification and antioxidant functions.

Glycogen
The primary storage carbohydrate found in liver and muscle tissue. It is broken down to glucose.

Gout, primary
Affecting 30–50 year old men and post–menopausal women, symptoms are due to improper purine metabolism resulting in urate crystals forming around the joints

and as urinary deposits. If left unchecked it can be painful and debilitating.

Granulocyte
Typically a neutrophil, basophil, or eosinophil that contains immunologic granules that when released heighten inflammatory–defense processes.

Helicobacter pylori
(Campylobacter pylori) A gram–negative bacterium involved in gastric ulcer formation and gastritis.

Hematuria
Blood in the urine.

Hemolysis
The collapse of red blood cell membranes resulting in the liberation of hemoglobin. This can be caused from a myriad of factors but most predominantly, it is triggered by autoimmune reaction, snake venom, microorganisms, and some plant saponins.

Hemolysis, intravascular
Severe red blood cell breakdown within blood vessels.

Hemorrhoids
A varicosity affecting the anal region.

Hemostatic
An activity or something that slows or stops blood flow; typically astringents or other substances that have a localized or systemic vasoconstrictive effect.

Hepatitis C
Inflammation of the liver caused by the hepatitis C virus. This chronic infection is typically the result of contaminated blood transfusions or intravenous drug use.

Hepatocyte
A liver cell.

Herbaceous
Herb–like. Describing a plant or a portion of a plant that is non–woody.

Herpes zoster
(See Shingles)

Homeopathy
A system of medicine founded by Samuel Hahnemann. 'Like treats like' and infinitesimal doses are hallmarks of this system.

Human papillomavirus (HPV)
A significant group of viruses responsible for common and genital warts, cervical dysplasia, and most cases of cervical cancer.

Hyaluronidase
A class of enzymes that breakdown hyaluronic acid. They occur naturally in various tissues and in bee and snake venoms. It is surmised one reason Echinacea is useful in limiting some of the deleterious effects of snakebite is through its antihyaluronidase activity.

Hydrochloric acid (HCL)
Solutions of hydrogen chloride secreted by gastric parietal cells in response to hormonal, local, or nervous system stimulation; necessary for initial protein breakdown in the stomach.

Hydrophilic
(See hygroscopic)

Hydrophobic
Insoluble in water; lacking polar constituents.

Hygroscopic
Absorbing water or having water–interacting polar groups.

Hyperglycemia
Elevated blood glucose levels.

Hyperglycemia, post–prandial
Elevated blood glucose levels after meals.

Hypertension
(See Essential hypertension)

Hypoglycemia
Lowered blood glucose levels.

Immunoglobulin
A specific immune system molecule (IgM, IgG, IgA, IgD, and IgE) that interacts only with a particular antigen. They are classed by individual function.

Immunoglobulin E (IgE)
An antibody that has a significant role in the allergic process.

Influenza
(Flu) A highly variable group of RNA viruses belonging to a single sub–type. They affect both people (usually the young and old) and animals.

Insomnia
Inability to sleep.

Insulin dependent diabetes mellitus (IDDM)
(Juvenile onset or Type I) Onset usually occurs in late childhood or in the early teens and is characterized by the destruction of the pancreatic beta cells by viral

infection or autoimmune reaction. There is some genetic predisposition as well. Lack of endogenous insulin is the hallmark of IDDM. Reliance upon exogenous insulin is necessary, otherwise hyperglycemia and corresponding problems result. IDDM is difficult to treat solely with natural therapies.

Interleukin
A broad group of immunologic compounds (cytokines). Many are produced by T–lymphocytes and macrophages. They are involved in an array of immunologic activities, including inflammatory responses.

Intermittent claudication
Usually dependent upon atherosclerosis and/or smoking, this lack of circulation to the extremities causes pain, cramping, and numbness.

Interstitial cystitis
Chronic inflammation of urinary/bladder tissue. Research points to bladder wall dysfunction/damage.

Interstitial fluid
Fluid between cells or tissue, as opposed to intracellular fluid.

Intraocular pressure
Pressure within the eye. When elevated it is associated with glaucoma.

Involucre
A whorl of bracts at the base of a flower.

Ischemia
Lack of blood in an area. Often due to blood vessel constriction or damage (atherosclerosis).

Isotonic
A solution that has the same tonicity as the tissues that are exposed to the solution. Most notable are eyewash solutions that have roughly the same tonicity/salinity as ocular membranes or tears.

Keratin
The main protein group that forms the skin, hair, and nails.

Keratinocyte
(Malpighian cell) A keratin producing epidermal cell.

Kupffer cell
A line of phagocytic cells residing in the liver.

Lactobacillus
A genus of naturally occurring bacteria found in the mouth, intestine, and vagina. In proper concentrations the bacteria plays a role in surrounding tissue health.

Lanceolate
Widest below the middle; narrow and tapering to the tip.

Latex
A milky sap from a plant.

Leukocyte
(White blood cell) A granular or non–granular type cell, largely involved in immunologic processes.

Leukotriene
A group of immunologically active compounds responsible for leucocyte movement and inflammatory responses.

Lipolysis
The breakdown of fat.

Lithiasis
The formation of urinary tract deposits/concretions.

Litholysis
The breakdown of urinary tract deposits.

Low density lipoprotein (LDL)
A group of lipoproteins involved in the transport of cholesterol from the liver to peripheral tissues. Elevated levels usually reflect poorly on cardiovascular health.

Luteinizing hormone (LH)
A pituitary hormone that promotes ovulation and progesterone secretion. In men, it is important in the formation of the teste's Leydig cells.

Lymphocyte
Divided into T–lymphocytes and B–lymphocytes they are responsible for humoral and cellular immunity. Closely associated with acquired immunity.

Macrophage
A mononuclear phagocyte widely distributed throughout varying tissues. It comprises one of the first lines of defense in response to pathogens; part of the body's innate cellular immunity.

Malaria
An infectious disease caused by the protozoa genus Plasmodium. It is transmitted through mosquito bites.

Mast cell
Intrinsic to the inflammatory–allergic response, these cells release histamine and heparin containing granules.

Melanocyte
Surface skin cells that synthesize the pigment melanin.

Menopause
The cessation of menstruation due to insufficient reproductive hormones. Naturally occurring in the 4th or 5th decade.

Menorrhagia
Excessive menstruation.

Menorrhalgia
(See Dysmenorrhea)

Menorrhea
Normal menstruation.

Micrococcus
A genus of gram–positive bacterial; found in soil, water, and dairy products.

Microsporum
A genus of ringworm–type fungi causing skin and hair infections.

Microvasculature
The finer circulatory vessels of the body.

Mineralocorticoids
Mainly aldosterone secreted by the adrenal cortex necessary in proper water and electrolyte balance. This group of adrenal hormones causes water and sodium retention and potassium loss.

Monoamine oxidase
Enzymes responsible for the breakdown of an array neurotransmitters or similar agents, i.e. serotonin, norepinephrine.

Monocyte
These phagocytic leukocytes are formed within bone marrow and eventually migrate to tissues where they develop into macrophages.

Monoecious
Separate male and female flowers borne on the same plant.

Montezuma's revenge
(See Amebiasis)

Mucin
The main component of mucus; composed of glycoproteins, glycolipids, and polysaccharides.

Mucor
A genus of fungi. Many species form on decaying bread; some are pathogenic to humans.

Mucus
Composed of mucin, inorganic salts, and leukocytes. Secreted by mucus membranes and is necessary for proper functioning of many organs and tissue groups.

Multiple sclerosis
A disease where demyelination of white (sometimes gray as well) matter in the central nervous system causes weakness, incoordination, and other CNS disturbances. There is a significant autoimmune component.

Mutagenic
Causing genetic change. A description applied especially to cancer–causing agents.

Myasthenia gravis
An autoimmune disorder affecting acetylcholine receptor sites. Symptoms of fatigue and muscular weakness, especially affecting the eyes, face, and throat are common.

Mycobacterium
A large family of gram–positive bacteria. A number of species are pathogenic, causing diseases such as tuberculosis and leprosy.

Natural killer cells (NK cells)
Large, granular lymphocytes which play a significant part in innate immunity.

Nephritis
Inflammation of the kidneys.

Nephron
A functional unit of the kidney. The majority of renal activities are carried out by nephrons.

Nightshade alkaloids
Alkaloids found in the Nightshade family. Many of these compounds have profound anticholinergic effects. Atropine and scopolamine are two of these compounds that are still used in conventional medicine.

Nocturnal emission
(See Spermatorrhea)

Non–insulin dependent diabetes mellitus (NIDDM)
(Adult onset or Type II) Chronic hyperglycemia as a result of a sedentary lifestyle and poor dietary choices (although there is some genetic predisposition). Typically, insulin levels are normal or even elevated. The situation is closely related to the notorious 'Syndrome X'. If insulin sensitivity is left impaired, cardiovascular and peripheral nervous system disturbances can ensue.

Norepinephrine
(Noradrenaline) A catecholamine acting as a hormone and neurotransmitter. Secreted by the adrenal medulla and the sympathetic nervous system, it is largely involved in stress (fight or flight) reactions.

Oblanceolate
Lance shaped, but slightly rounded towards the end of the leaf and narrower towards the leaf stem.

Obovate
Egg–shaped.

Oncotic pressure
The force that counterbalances capillary blood pressure.

Orthostatic hypotension
A fall in blood pressure and associated sensations when quickly standing or moving from a static position.

Panicles
Flowers maturing in branched groupings from the bottom of the cluster, up.

Parasympathetic
The cholinergic branch of the autonomic nervous system involved in rest, repair, and nutritive functions of the body.

Parenchymal cells
Functional cells of an organ or group of tissues, as opposed to structural cells.

Pelvic inflammatory disease (PID)
A description of general inflammation of the reproductive area in women. STDs are the most common cause. Associated with endometriosis and infertility.

Pepsin
A proteolytic enzyme derived from pepsinogen by hydrochloric acid. It is responsible for the bulk of gastric protein breakdown.

Perennial
A plant that lives three years or more.

Perimenopause
The period before menopause when reproductive hormones and their effects within the body become irregular.

Periodontitis
Inflammation of the tissues surrounding the teeth. Often a progression of chronic gingivitis, it can ultimately cause tooth and bone loss.

Peripheral
Away from the center.

Peripheral vascular disease
Vascular disturbance of the larger non–truck circulatory vessels. Usually associated with atherosclerosis, ischemia, and thrombosis

Peristalsis
The wave–like contraction of the alimentary canal and other tubular organs/ducts which serve to move contents.

Petiole
A leaf stalk.

Phagocytosis
A process by which white blood cells – macrophages and neutrophils – engulf and eliminate particulate material or microorganisms deemed harmful to the internal environment.

Pharyngitis
Inflammation of the pharynx.

Pimple
A pustule usually on the upper parts of the body, commonly a result of Acne vulgaris.

Pinnae
(Pinna) a leaflet of a pinnate leaf.

Pinnate
A compound leaf with leaflets arranged on both sides of the axis.

Pinnatifid
Pinnately cleft, narrow lobes of a leaf not reaching the mid–vein.

Pinworms
(Enterobius vermicularis, formally called Ascaris vermicularis or Oxyuris vermicularis) Nematode type worms that can colonize the upper large intestine. Common in children and causes anal itching. Infection can occasionally spread to female genitals and bladder.

Pistillate
Used to describe a female flower. A flower lacking stamens.

Placenta
A temporary organ that forms between the mother and fetus. It provides blood borne nutrients, hormones, and other necessary substances for the fetus's development.

Plasmodium falciparum
The main protozoa that causes malaria.

Platelet activating factor (PAF)
A compound produced by an array of immunologic and tissue cells designed to stimulate certain immune functions, platelet aggregation, inflammation, and allergic response.

Platelet aggregation
The clumping together of platelets often triggered by injury or a number of metabolic syndromes.

Pleurisy
An acute or chronic inflammation of the lung and thoracic cavity's serous membrane or pleura. Fever, dry cough, and stitch in the side are common symptoms.

Portal vein
The vein that carries enriched blood from the digestive organs to the liver.

Postpartum
(Postnatal) The period following birth. During this time (4–6 weeks) the mother's body is returning to pre–pregnancy conditions while the newborn adapts to external life.

Progesterone
A reproductive hormone secreted by the corpus luteum, placenta, and in small quantities, by the adrenal cortex. Aside from uterine preparatory and pregnancy sustaining effects, altered circulating levels of the hormone is a factor in premenstrual discomforts and menstrual cycle irregularities.

Prolactin
Traditionally defined as a hormone secreted by the anterior pituitary responsible for lactation. Research suggests the hormone has a broader role in chronic stress states.

Prostaglandin
A diverse group of naturally occurring compounds involved in a wide array of physiological responses. Many are pro–inflammatory, cellular excitants.

Prostatitis
Inflammation of the prostate.

Proteolytic enzyme
An enzyme that breaks down protein into smaller polypeptides by splitting peptide bonds. In supplement form they are used as digestive aids and as antiinflammatories.

Protozoa
Simple, single celled organisms; many are parasitic.

ation.ation ation-ation ation -ation ation

Psoriasis
A syndrome of inflammation and excessive cellular production affecting the skin, joints, and even nails. Red and scaly patches of skin called psoriatic plaques are common. Cause of the disease is an issue of debate. Both autoimmune reaction and excessive growth of skin cells have been implicated as possible factors.

Psychosomatic
Having physical symptoms that originate from the mind or emotions.

Pubescent
Hair–like quality.

Pyorrhea
(See Periodontitis)

Pyrrolizidine alkaloids
A group of compounds common in the Sunflower and Borage families responsible for liver inflammation and subsequent hepatocyte breakdown.

Raceme
An unbranched, elongated group of flowers with pedicels.

Raynaud's syndrome and disease
Severity seems to be the main dividing line between the two types. Vasoconstriction of the smaller vessels in the extremities, resulting in discolored, painful, and cold fingers and/or toes. In severe cases ulceration and infection can develop. Smoking and stress are the main aggravators.

5–α–reductase
The enzyme responsible for the conversion of testosterone to DHT.

Reye's syndrome
Usually occurring as a result of an acute viral infection (often respiratory centered or associated with chicken pox). Fever, vomiting, elevated liver enzyme levels, and brain swelling are common. This childhood syndrome is rare, but can result in seizures and death. Aspirin use in febrile conditions has been linked as a possible factor.

Rheumatoid arthritis
Chronic joint inflammation usually affecting the hands and feet. It is autoimmune mediated and if left untreated leads to lack of mobility and joint deformation.

Rhinitis
Inflammation of nasal mucus membranes; a typical hayfever response.

Ringworm
A non–specific term for a fungal infection affecting the skin. Often developing in a ring–like pattern, numerous fungal strains are causative agents.

Roundworm
(Nematode) An organism from the nematode class; many are intestinal parasites.

Rubefacient
Something that reddens the skin, usually through vasodilation.

Salmonella
A genus of gram–negative bacteria. Many species cause food poisoning.

Samara
A winged fruit, common in the Fraxinus and the Ailanthus genera.

Scrofula (Scrofuloderma)
A tuberculous or similar infection affecting the skin and underlying lymph nodes particularly of the neck area.

Scrofulous
A somewhat antiquated term; afflicted with scrofula or having a scrofula–like appearance.

Seborrheic dermatitis
(Cradle cap, seborrheic eczema, or seborrhea) A chronic skin condition characterized by redness and yellow scaly patches on the trunk, groin, face, and/or scalp. Allergic and constitutional factors are involved.

Seminal vesicle
A pair of glands situated next to the urinary bladder; their secretions comprise approximately 60% of semen.

Sequela
A complication or condition arising from an initial disease or injury.

Serrate
Designating a toothed margin; saw–like.

Shigella
A gram–negative bacteria in the Enterobacteria family. Many cause severe diarrhea/dysentery.

Shingles
(Herpes zoster) More common in the elderly and in immune compromised individuals, shingles manifests as nerve pain and corresponding vesicles over affected dermatomes. Occurrence is normally on one side of the body and is thought to involve expression of latent varicella–zoster virus – called Herpes ophthalmicus when the virus affects the trigeminal nerve.

Simple
An undivided leaf that is not separated into leaflets. Describing an herb used singly, not in formula.

Sinusitis
Inflammation of the sinuses. Typical causes are allergic reaction or bacterial, viral, or fungal infections. Poor tissue health and local immunity are predisposing factors.

Spasmolytic
Antispasmodic.

Spermatorrhea
Involuntary and excessive discharge of semen without copulation; excessive wet dreams or nocturnal emission.

Spikelet
The flower cluster of grasses and sedges, or a secondary spike.

Staminate
Used to describe a male flower bearing only stamens, not pistils.

Staphylococcus
A genus of gram–positive, anaerobic bacteria; many are pathogenic.

Strep throat
Streptococcus infection affecting the throat.

Streptococcus
A gram–positive genus of bacteria. Most species are pathogenic, notably S. pyogenes.

Streptomycetes
A genus of fungus–like aerobic bacteria. Many conventional antibiotics are derived from this group. A number of species are pathogenic.

Succus entericus
Secretions of the small intestine containing enzymes, hormones, and mucus.

Sudorific
Diaphoretic; an agent that causes sweating.

Sympathetic nervous system
A branch of the autonomic nervous system closely associated with fight or flight/ stress responses.

Sympathomimetic
(Adrenergic) Having sympathetic nervous system–like effects (postganglionic fibers).

Tachycardia
Accelerated heartbeat; usually greater than 100 beat per minute.

Taiga
Meaning forest in Russian. A circumboreal forest zone existing below the tundra.

Tepal
A specialized sepal or petal; common in the Passionflower family.

Testosterone
A major male sex hormone produced in the testes. It is crucial for bone and muscle growth and sperm formation in the male.

Thyroid stimulating hormone (TSH)
(Thyrotropin) a pituitary hormone that is necessary in the thyroid's normal functioning. Low levels can be an indicator of hyperthyroidism.

Thyroxine (T$_4$)
A pro–hormone secreted by the thyroid gland. It is transformed into T$_3$ at tissue sites.

Thromboxane
An eicosanoid responsible for platelet aggregation and vasoconstriction.

Thrush
(Candidiasis or yeast infection) Called oral thrush when limited to the mouth region.

Tinnitus
Ringing in the ear. Causes range from local injury to cardiovascular disease.

Tobacco heart
Cardiovascular weakness caused from years of smoking.

Tomentose
Covered by soft, matted hair.

Tonsillitis
Inflammation of the small rounded masses of lymph tissue (palatine tonsils) located near the back of the tongue. This normally occurs through heightened leukocyte activity.

Traveler's diarrhea
(See Amebiasis)

Trichophyton
A genus of fungi known to cause skin, nail, and hair infections.

Trifoliate
Three–leaved.

Triiodothyronine (T_3)
A thyroid hormone responsible for the majority of that gland's cellular effects.

Ulcerative colitis
(Crone's disease) Chronic inflammation affecting the mucosa and submucosa of the colon wall. Symptoms are abdominal pain, diarrhea, and ulceration. Autoimmune involvement is typical.

Ureter
The urinary tube arising from the kidney leading to the bladder.

Ureteritis
Inflammation of the ureter.

Urethra
The urinary tube leading from the bladder to the body's exterior.

Urethritis
Inflammation of the urethra.

Uric acid
The end result of purine (RNA–DNA) catabolism in primates. Gout is a disorder of excess uric acid.

Vaginitis
Inflammation of the vagina. There is usually a bacterial/fungal/viral component.

Vagus nerve
A key parasympathetic cranial nerve involved in viscera innervation. It affects the digestive tract, lungs, heart, liver, and other areas. Certain herbs (Asclepias) stimulate vagus nerve function, particularly when digestive function is depressed by stress.

Vasoconstriction
Blood vessel constriction.

Vasodilation
Blood vessel dilation.

Vermifuge
An agent that kills or expels parasites.

Verruca vulgaris
Common wart. A member of the larger HPV group.

Vertigo
The illusionary sensation of (the body or surroundings) revolving. Often associated with inner ear or CNS disorders.

Very low density lipoprotein (VLDL)
Transports triglycerides from the intestine and liver to adipose and muscle tissues. High levels of VLDLs are associated with atherosclerosis.

Vitiligo
A chronic pigmentary disorder resulting in depigmented skin. A hyperpigmented border may surround these white patches. It is possibly autoimmune mediated with some genetic predisposition.

Volatile oil
Non–polar aromatics that disperse easily through sun exposure or through other forms of heat such as boiling.

Vulnerary
An agent that encourages wound healing.

White blood cell
(See leukocyte)

Index

A

abortifacient 23
abrasion 44, 97, 170, 202, 237, 269
abscess 107, 109, 144, 161, 166, 249, 287, 319
Abutilon spp. 142
Acacia 43, 44, 45, 191, 288
  angustissima 43
  constricta 43
  durandiana 43
  greggii 43
Acaciella angustissima 43
Acaciopsis constricta 43
Acalypha indica 92
  lindheimeri 91
  neomexicana 91
Acerates asperula 49
acetylcholine 61, 319
acetylcholinesterase 146, 215, 319
AChE. See acetylcholinesterase
acne 80, 119, 276, 336
actinic keratosis 97, 287
adaptogen 319
addison's disease 319
adrenal cortex 319
  medulla 319
adrenaline 50, 64, 265, 319
Africa 46, 82, 92, 161, 190
Agave 54, 55
Ailanthus altissima 107, 118, 243
Ailanto 243
Ajenjo 256
Alamo 93
Alberta 143, 156
albumin 319
aldosterone 319, 320, 333
Alfilaria 138
Alfilerillo 138
Algarroba 171
Algerita 116
allergy 66, 78, 79, 99, 118, 119, 226, 272, 320, 321, 323, 339, 340
Alligator juniper 155
Allthorn 100
Aloe 45, 46, 47, 48, 112, 199, 223, 285, 286, 288
  barbadensis 45
  ferox 45

perfoliata var. vera 45
  vulgaris 45
Aloysia triphylla 57
  wrightii 56
Altamisa 56
alterative 72, 146, 320
alveoli 108, 143, 320, 326
alzheimer's disease 146, 215, 216, 320, 325
Ambrosia ambrosioides 77
  artemisiifolia 78
  deltoidea 78
  monogyra 78
  salsola 78
  trifida 78
amebiasis 118, 120, 285, 320, 333, 341
amenorrhea 50, 115, 219, 250, 259, 320
American black elderberry 131
  elder 131
American Indian 133, 149
Amsinckia 207
amylase 320
Anacardiaceae 231
analgesic 70, 112, 179, 218, 242
Anaphalis 104
anaphrodisiac 83, 255, 320
anaphylaxis 320
androgen 320
Anemone patens 114
  tuberosa 113
Anemopsis californica 273
angina pectoris 204, 205, 285, 321
Anil de muerto 98
Animas Mountains 60
anorexia 119, 321
anovulatory cycle 83, 288, 321
Antelope horns 49, 50, 51, 126, 127, 163, 285, 287, 288, 289
Antennaria 104
antibody 78, 330
anticholinergic 54, 112, 272, 273, 321, 334
antifungal 50, 80, 97, 127, 133, 218, 237, 238, 258
antioxidant 30, 96, 97, 215, 328
antispasmodic 80, 261
anxiety 70, 83, 124, 187, 253
Anza–Borrego State Park 134
aphthous stomatitis 321
Apocynaceae 189
apoptosis 321

arachidonic acid 321
Arctostaphylos spp. 166
Argemone mexicana 203
   spp. 201
Argentina 59, 241
Aristolochiaceae 191
Aristolochia fangchi 192
   manshuriensis 192
   porphyrophylla 191
   watsonii 61, 191
Arizona 44, 53, 54, 56, 59, 63, 66, 69, 71,
      72, 73, 77, 79, 80, 84, 87, 91, 92, 93,
      103, 105, 111, 114, 117, 121, 123,
      125, 129, 131, 141, 143, 147, 149,
      151, 153, 156, 159, 160, 163, 169,
      172, 175, 179, 181, 186, 191, 194,
      196, 198, 206, 208, 210, 212, 214,
      217, 223, 225, 227, 229, 232, 234,
      236, 238, 239, 242, 244, 246, 247,
      251, 252, 253, 257, 269, 271, 274,
      278, 281, 283
   butternut 79
   cypress 105
   poppy 71
   snakeroot 191
   walnut 79
Arkansas 44, 49
Arnica 73, 74
arrhythmia 182, 322
Arrowweed 169
Artemisia annua 260
   douglasiana 256
   filifolia 256
   ludoviciana 256
   ludoviciana var. douglasiana 256
   mexicana 256
   plattensis 256
   tridentata 217, 257
   vulgaris var. douglasiana 256
   vulgaris var. mexicana 256
arthritis 47, 66, 88, 94, 96, 97, 115, 218, 226,
      228, 282, 286, 338
   rheumatoid 55, 88, 96, 218, 226, 338
Asclepiadaceae 49, 125
Asclepias albicans 126
   asperula 49
   erosa 126
   linaria 126
   subulata 125

   tuberosa 126
Asclepiodora asperula 49
Ashy limberbush 162
Asia 82
Aspen 93, 94, 188
Asteraceae 52, 62, 65, 73, 74, 77, 84, 89,
      98, 103, 129, 147, 169, 178, 196, 210,
      217, 225, 229, 237, 245, 248, 256, 262
asthma 50, 97, 135, 272, 279, 287, 322
astringent 106, 167
Athel 236
atherosclerosis 322, 331, 336, 343
Atlantic Ocean 75
Australia 149
autonomic nervous system 322
Avena fatua 266
   sativa 267
Ayurveda 161, 322

B

Baboquivari Mountains 196
Baboquivaris 60
Baccharis 52, 53, 285, 288
   glutinosa 52
   pteronioides 52
   ramulosa 52
   salicifolia 52
   sarothroides 52
   viminea 52
Balsam poplar 94
Banana yucca 280
Barberry 80
Barberry family. See Berberidaceae
Bark scorpion 61
Barometer bush 239
basophil 322, 329
Batamote 52
Bavisa 273
Bayberry 118, 135
Beardtongue 188
Beargrass 54, 55, 285, 286, 288
bedsore 107, 109, 249, 287, 322
Beebrush 56, 57, 285
Bee sage 123
Beggar's ticks 229
benign prostrate hypertrophy 322
Berberidaceae 116
Berberis fremontii 116

C

H

Hackberry 160
Hairy yerba santa 277
Hamula 62
Haplopappus laricifolius 248
Harmal 234
hayfever 66, 177, 178, 259, 272, 338. See
   also rhinitis
HCL. See Hydrochloric acid
heart 50, 51, 126, 127, 181, 186, 204, 243,
       321, 323, 325, 326, 341, 342
  enlargement 50, 181
  palpitations 181
  stimulant 50
  tobacco 285
Heartleaf limberbush 162
Heath family 106, 167. See also Ericaceae
Hedeoma incana 194
  spp. 194
Hediondilla 95
Helianthus cernuus 237
Helicobacter pylori 161, 258, 265, 329
hematuria 72, 139, 230, 329
hemolysis 93, 120, 329
hemorrhage 72, 76, 139, 190, 209, 221, 231,
   287
hemorrhoids 99, 100, 112, 183, 184, 190,
   209, 242, 243, 276, 285, 329
hemostatic 75, 139, 221, 269, 329
Hemp 30
hepatitis 329
hepatocyte 329, 338
herpes simplex virus 97, 258, 286, 288,
   289
Heterotheca grandiflora
  subaxillaris 73
Hibiscus coulteri 142
  denudatus 142
  spp. 142
hiccups 85
Hidalgo County 159
Hierba de alacran 160
Hippochaete hyemalis 220
histamine 96, 332
hives 72, 78, 163, 288
Hoary yucca 280
Hojansen 237
Hojase 237

Holacantha emoryi 100
Holly–grape 116
Hollyhock 165
Honey mesquite 171
Honeysuckle family. See Caprifoliaceae
Hopbush 121, 148, 149, 150, 285, 288
Hopi 85, 147, 148
  tea 147
Horsetail 222
Horsetail family. See Equisetaceae
Horseweed 74
hot flashes 83
HPV. See human papillomavirus
HSV. See herpes simplex virus
human papillomavirus 97, 107, 324, 329
Humulus 149
hydrochloric acid 57, 63, 68, 124, 130, 218,
   230, 265, 330, 335
hydrophobia 61
hyperglycemia 47, 61, 200, 248, 286, 330,
   331, 334
hypertension 186, 187, 205, 230, 231, 243,
   266, 285, 327, 330
hypoglycemia 330
hypotension 319, 335
hypothyroidism 119
Hyptis emoryi 123

I

Idaho 63, 260
IDDM. See diabetes mellitus, insulin
   dependent
Illinois 129, 257
immunity 108, 144
immunoglobulin 321, 330
Imperial Valley 101
Incienso 65
incontinence 106, 109
India 46, 92, 161, 203
Indian–fig 200
Indian mallow 142
  spice 82
indigestion 19, 57, 64, 68, 85, 94, 114, 115,
   120, 130, 211, 219, 238, 248, 251,
   253, 266
infection
  bacterial 47, 97, 119, 150, 202, 207, 235,
   238, 259, 288

T–cell 108
TCM. See Traditional Chinese Medicine
Tecoma stans 247
Telegraph plant 73
tendinitis 136
Tepopote 176
Tessaria sericea 169
testosterone 320, 341
Texas 44, 46, 53, 54, 56, 59, 63, 69, 72, 80,
        86, 87, 91, 93, 105, 111, 117, 127,
        129, 131, 143, 147, 156, 163, 167,
        169, 172, 175, 181, 186, 191, 194,
        198, 208, 210, 212, 225, 227, 232,
        236, 238, 239, 242, 246, 247, 251,
        252, 253, 254, 257, 269, 271, 274, 281
    betony 211
    ranger 239, 240
    virgin's bower 86
Texas ranger 287
Thelesperma gracile 147
    longipes 147
    megapotamicum 147
    scabiosoides 147
    subnudum 147
Thornbush 271
Thread–leaf snakeweed 225
Three seeded mercury 91
    fans 208
thromboxane 47
thrush 107, 118, 120, 341
Thuja 167
Thurberia thespesioides 121
    thurberi 121
Thymophylla acerosa 129
    pentachaeta 129
thyroid 119, 181, 207, 341, 342
thyroxin 119
thyroxine 119
Tobacco 73, 99, 241, 242, 243, 272, 285,
        286, 341
tobacco heart 50, 285
Tobaco loco 241
Toloache 110
Tomatillo 271
tonsillitis 183, 215, 216, 341
Tornillo 171
Torote 134
Toxicodendron diversilobum 232
    rydbergii 232

Traditional Chinese Medicine 161, 204,
        260, 322
Trans–Pecos Texas 44, 93, 117
traveler's diarrhea 109, 118, 320, 341
Tree of heaven 53, 102, 243, 244, 245, 285,
        286
    tobacco 241
Tribulus brachystylis 71
    californicus 71
    fisheri 71
    grandiflorus 71
    terrestris 203
Trichomonas vaginalis 102
trichomoniasis 102
Trichophyton 118, 341
Triiodothyronine 119, 342
Trixis 245, 246, 288
    californica 245
Trompetilla 60
Tronadora 247
Tropical America 59, 111, 161, 186
True aloe 45
Trumpet creeper 248, 285
    flower 127, 247, 248, 285, 286, 288
Tunas 198
Turkish red 235
Turmeric 283
Turpentine bush 226, 248, 249, 286, 288,
        289
Tylenol 132

U

ulcer
    duodenal 53, 68, 285
    external 92
    gastric 47, 100, 161, 199, 221, 259, 266,
        285
    peptic 285
    stomach 99
ulcerative colitis 75, 231, 342
urethritis 136, 279, 342
uric acid 153, 199, 204, 205, 287, 342
urinary tract 106, 108, 117, 139, 157, 167,
        220, 279
urination
    painful 90, 157, 220
Utah 69, 84, 93, 114, 117, 169, 172, 194,
        242, 251, 253, 260, 269, 271, 274,

Xerocassia armata 222
Ximenesia encelioides 98
  microptera 98

Y

Yaqui 273
Yellow bird of paradise 58
Yellowdock 269
Yerba colorado 269
  de la negrita 142
  de la víbora 225
  del indio 191
  del manso 273
  del pasmo 52, 248
  del sapo 77
  del vaso 65
  del venado 196
  mansa 118, 135, 209, 273, 274, 275, 285,
      286, 287, 288
  manso 273
  santa 240, 278, 279, 280
Yucca 54, 96, 227, 280, 281, 282, 283, 286
  baccata 280
  schidigera 280
  schottii 280
Yuma 163

Z

Zuni 85
Zygophyllaceae 71, 95, 203, 234

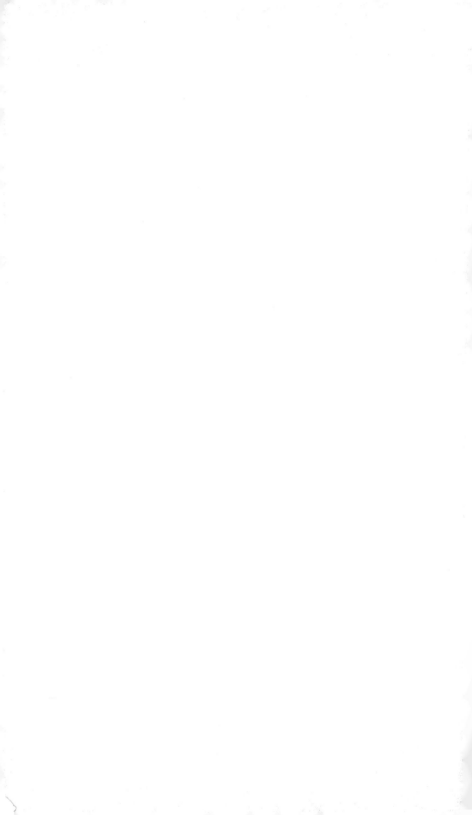